PRAISE FOR *REIMAGINING GLOBAL HEALTH*

"It is a challenging task to provide a novel and comprehensive view of global health—a dynamic arena for action and an increasingly attractive academic field. *Reimagining Global Health* does this with scholarly rigor and political courage. This book will become essential reading for all those working in clinical, public health, and policy roles to address the daunting health disparities of our times."

—**JULIO FRENK**, Dean of the Harvard School of Public Health, Former Minister of Health of Mexico (2000–2006)

"The past decade has seen an unprecedented explosion of interest in the health and welfare of marginalized communities around the world. *Reimagining Global Health* offers a critical approach to the contemporary global health landscape while also tracing its historical antecedents and suggesting a way forward. This seminal work by leading figures in the field is a crucial next step for those interested in grappling with the modern reality of global health inequity. Without question, *Reimagining Global Health* is a salient volume that will shape global health research, practice, and knowledge for many years to come."

—**AMBASSADOR MARK DYBUL**, Executive Director of the Global Fund to Fight AIDS

"Inspired by practicing physicians like two of the authors of this book—Paul Farmer and Jim Kim, who won't take no for an answer when it comes to the universal right to health—many undergraduates, medical students, and professionals have turned to global health as their specialty and their calling. Before now, this nascent field did not have a unifying conceptual approach, let alone a text. This book, based on the authors' decades of practice and years of successfully teaching global health at Harvard, masterfully fills this gap. It presents a strong vision of health as a biological and social phenomenon, and it illustrates how academics from different disciplines, as well as practitioners, must work together to understand not only what works but also how it can be sustainably delivered. Avoiding both cynicism and blind optimism, this book, like the authors in their work, is hopeful, practical, and demanding. It will become an unavoidable reference in the field."

—**ESTHER DUFLO**, Department of Economics, MIT, and author of *Poor Economics*

Rich case studies and incisive biosocial analysis throw the central importance of humility, constancy, and imagination into bold relief."

—**DR. AGNES BINAGWAHO**, Minister of Health of Rwanda; Senior Lecturer, Harvard Medical School; Clinical Professor of Pediatrics, Geisel School of Medicine at Dartmouth

"This inspiring book transforms the field of global health into a revolutionary global movement for human rights to combat the needless suffering imposed by North/South social inequality. The authors' historical, practice-based, and theoretical arguments wrench the field out of its colonial-missionary roots and attack the contemporary greedy behemoths of Bio-Tech, Big Pharma, for-profit healthcare, and cost-benefit neoliberal triage logics to make 'Health for All' a real possibility, as well as a universal human right to be enforced by political will, funding, and democratic access to technology."

—**PHILIPPE BOURGOIS**, author of *Righteous Dopefiend* and of *In Search of Respect: Selling Crack in El Barrio*

"*Reimagining Global Health* is a well-written text based on extensive research, teaching, and practical experience. The fact that it is based on three years of teaching a course implies that it has been finely honed by responses from students. It is superbly researched and written and provides many new angles and fresh perspectives."

—**SOLLY BENATAR**, Professor, Dalla School of Public Health and Joint Centre for Bioethics, University of Toronto

The publisher gratefully acknowledges the generous support
of the Chairman's Circle of the University of California
Press Foundation, whose members are:

Stephen A. and Melva Arditti
Elizabeth and David Birka-White
Ajay Shah and Lata Krishnan
James and Carlin Naify
William and Sheila Nolan
Barbara Z. Otto
Loren and Frances Rothschild
Patricia and David Schwartz
Sidney Stern Memorial Trust
Howard Welinsky and Karren Ganstwig
Lynne Withey

Reimagining Global Health

CALIFORNIA SERIES IN PUBLIC ANTHROPOLOGY

The California Series in Public Anthropology emphasizes the anthropologist's role as an engaged intellectual. It continues anthropology's commitment to being an ethnographic witness, to describing, in human terms, how life is lived beyond the borders of many readers' experiences. But it also adds a commitment, through ethnography, to reframing the terms of public debate—transforming received, accepted understandings of social issues with new insights, new framings.

Series Editor: Robert Borofsky (Hawaii Pacific University)

Contributing Editors: Philippe Bourgois (University of Pennsylvania), Paul Farmer (Partners In Health), Alex Hinton (Rutgers University), Carolyn Nordstrom (University of Notre Dame), and Nancy Scheper-Hughes (UC Berkeley)

University of California Press Editor: Naomi Schneider

Reimagining Global Health

An Introduction

Paul Farmer
Jim Yong Kim
Arthur Kleinman
Matthew Basilico

UNIVERSITY OF CALIFORNIA PRESS
Berkeley · Los Angeles · London

University of California Press, one of the most
distinguished university presses in the United States,
enriches lives around the world by advancing scholarship
in the humanities, social sciences, and natural sciences.
Its activities are supported by the UC Press Foundation
and by philanthropic contributions from individuals and
institutions. For more information, visit www.ucpress.edu.

University of California Press
Berkeley and Los Angeles, California

University of California Press, Ltd.
London, England

Library of Congress Cataloging-in-Publication Data

Reimagining global health : an introduction / [edited by]
Paul Farmer . . . [et al.].
    p.   cm. (California series in public anthropology ;
v. 26)
   Includes bibliographical references and index.
   ISBN 978-0-520-27197-5 (cloth : alk. paper)
   ISBN 978-0-520-27199-9 (pbk. : alk. paper)
   ISBN 978-0-520-95463-2 (ebook)
   I. Farmer, Paul, 1959–   II. Series: California series in
public anthropology ; 26.
   [DNLM: 1. World Health.   2. Health Services
Accessibility.   WA 530.1]
   RA418
   362.1   dc23   2013010762

Manufactured in the United States of America

21
10   9   8

The paper used in this publication meets the minimum
requirements of ANSI/NISO Z39.48–1992 (R 2002)
(*Permanence of Paper*).

Contents

List of Illustrations and Tables   *vii*

Preface by Paul Farmer   *xiii*

1 Introduction: A Biosocial Approach to Global Health   *1*
*Paul Farmer, Jim Yong Kim, Arthur Kleinman,
Matthew Basilico*

2 Unpacking Global Health: Theory and Critique   *15*
Bridget Hanna, Arthur Kleinman

3 Colonial Medicine and Its Legacies   *33*
*Jeremy Greene, Marguerite Thorp Basilico, Heidi Kim,
Paul Farmer*

4 Health for All? Competing Theories and Geopolitics   *74*
*Matthew Basilico, Jonathan Weigel, Anjali Motgi, Jacob Bor,
Salmaan Keshavjee*

5 Redefining the Possible: The Global AIDS Response   *111*
Luke Messac, Krishna Prabhu

6 Building an Effective Rural Health Delivery Model in Haiti
and Rwanda   *133*
*Peter Drobac, Matthew Basilico, Luke Messac, David Walton,
Paul Farmer*

7 Scaling Up Effective Delivery Models Worldwide   *184*

Jim Yong Kim, Michael Porter, Joseph Rhatigan, Rebecca Weintraub, Matthew Basilico, Cassia van der Hoof Holstein, Paul Farmer

8 The Unique Challenges of Mental Health and MDRTB: Critical Perspectives on Metrics of Disease   *212*

Anne Becker, Anjali Motgi, Jonathan Weigel, Giuseppe Raviola, Salmaan Keshavjee, Arthur Kleinman

9 Values and Global Health   *245*

Arjun Suri, Jonathan Weigel, Luke Messac, Marguerite Thorp Basilico, Matthew Basilico, Bridget Hanna, Salmaan Keshavjee, Arthur Kleinman

10 Taking Stock of Foreign Aid   *287*

Jonathan Weigel, Matthew Basilico, Paul Farmer

11 Global Health Priorities for the Early Twenty-First Century   *302*

Paul Farmer, Matthew Basilico, Vanessa Kerry, Madeleine Ballard, Anne Becker, Gene Bukhman, Ophelia Dahl, Andy Ellner, Louise Ivers, David Jones, John Meara, Joia Mukherjee, Amy Sievers, Alyssa Yamamoto

12 A Movement for Global Health Equity? A Closing Reflection   *340*

Matthew Basilico, Vanessa Kerry, Luke Messac, Arjun Suri, Jonathan Weigel, Marguerite Thorp Basilico, Joia Mukherjee, Paul Farmer

Appendix: Declaration of Alma-Ata   *355*

Notes   *359*

List of Contributors   *453*

Acknowledgments   *459*

Index   *463*

Illustrations and Tables

FIGURES

1.1 Mortality rates for children under the age of five, by level of household wealth / 8

1.2 Inequity in infant mortality rates between countries and within countries, by mother's education / 8

2.1 Refugees from the Rwandan genocide at a camp in Kibumba, Democratic Republic of the Congo / 21

2.2 Max Weber, influential social theorist / 23

2.3 Biopower, a concept developed by Michel Foucault / 29

3.1 A colonial medical officer takes a blood sample from an individual suffering from sleeping sickness / 39

3.2 Pears' Soap advertisement: the moral language of health and the "civilizing process" / 45

3.3 "A Congo Child's Appeal," requesting donations for a missionary hospital / 48

3.4 The dangers of the Broad Street pump / 52

3.5 A yellow fever cage in Ancón Hospital, Panama / 54

3.6 Cuban physician and scientist Dr. Carlos Finlay / 55

3.7 Sanitary engineers laying tile drains, construction of the Panama Canal / 56

3.8 A Rockefeller Foundation microscopist working in Panama / 57

3.9 The McKeown Hypothesis: bronchitis, pneumonia, and influenza / 65

3.10 The McKeown Hypothesis: tuberculosis / 65

3.11 Decline in AIDS mortality in the United States following the development of HAART / 66

4.1 A "barefoot doctor" in the People's Republic of China / 76

4.2 Halfdan Mahler, director-general of the World Health Organization, 1973–1988 / 78

4.3 Alma-Ata International Conference on Primary Health Care, 1978 / 79

4.4 Rockefeller Foundation's conference center in Bellagio, site of the 1979 Conference on Selective Primary Health Care / 82

4.5 Prime Minister Margaret Thatcher and President Ronald Reagan / 85

4.6 Economists Friedrich von Hayek and Milton Friedman / 86

4.7 Woman administering oral rehydration therapy to a child / 95

4.8 Jim Grant, executive director of UNICEF, 1980–1995 / 97

4.9 Annual lending by the World Bank's Health, Nutrition, and Population Division, 1970–2011 / 108

5.1 Development assistance for health, 1990–2007, by disease / 112

5.2 Deaths from HIV/AIDS in the United States, 1987–2008 / 117

5.3 Demonstration organized by the Treatment Action Campaign, South Africa, 2000 / 121

5.4 Activists interrupt one of Al Gore's presidential campaign events / 123

5.5 Prices of first-line HIV/AIDS drug regimens, branded versus generic, 2002 / 125

5.6 Dr. Peter Mugyenyi attends President Bush's State of the Union address, 2003 / 128

6.1 François and Jean-Claude Duvalier / 138

6.2 A view of Cange / 143

6.3 The Péligre Dam / 143

6.4 Voluntary HIV testing in Cange and Lascahobas, 2002–2003 / 162

6.5 HIV case detection in Lascahobas, 2002–2003 / 162

6.6 Ambulatory patient clinic visits in Lascahobas, 2002–2003 / 163

6.7 Tuberculosis case detection in Lascahobas, 2002–2003 / 163

6.8 Prenatal care clinic visits in Lascahobas, 2002–2003 / 164

6.9   Vaccinations administered in Lascahobas, 2003 / *164*

6.10 The new Lascahobas clinic in 2010 / *165*

6.11 Rwinkwavu District Hospital, Rwanda, before and after the IMB scale-up / *174*

6.12 Butaro Hospital, Rwanda / *177*

6.13 Loss of life and economic damages in major disasters / *179*

7.1   The care delivery value chain / *190*

7.2   AMPATH HIV program scale-up / *192*

7.3   Olyset manufacturing process at A to Z Textile Mills, Tanzania / *196*

7.4   Health system framework outlined by the WHO / *197*

8.1   Suicide rates in selected countries, by gender / *222*

8.2   An age-weighting mechanism that can be used in calculating the global burden of disease / *227*

8.3   Estimated disease burden and health expenditures, Morogoro, Tanzania / *229*

8.4   A "TB family" in Lima, Peru, whose plight starkly portrayed the limits of DOTS treatment / *236*

8.5   Outcomes for seventy-five "incurable" MDRTB patients in Peru / *238*

8.6   MDRTB patients receiving treatment versus those in need, 2004–2008 / *240*

9.1   Economist Amartya Sen and philosopher Martha Nussbaum / *256*

9.2   The Nuremberg War Crimes Trials, 1945–1946 / *265*

9.3   Eleanor Roosevelt, a champion of the Universal Declaration of Human Rights / *266*

9.4   Treatment Action Campaign's Zackie Achmat and President Nelson Mandela / *276*

9.5   Home built by PIH's Program on Social and Economic Rights / *278*

9.6   Pablo Picasso's *Head of the Medical Student* / *284*

10.1 Development assistance for health, 1990–2007, by channel of assistance / *288*

10.2 Development assistance from developed countries, 2000–2010 / *289*

10.3 Growth and governance / *290*

10.4   Aid and growth in Africa, 1970–1999 / *291*

10.5   Perception versus reality regarding U.S. foreign assistance / *300*

11.1   Millennium Development Goals / *304*

11.2   The drug development pipeline / *315*

11.3   The long tail of endemic noncommunicable diseases in Rwanda, 2004 / *322*

12.1   ACT UP protest in New York City, June 1993 / *343*

12.2   Student Global AIDS Campaign, 2005 march in Washington, D.C. / *346*

MAPS

1.1   Average life expectancy in countries grouped by WHO region and income, 2004 / *7*

3.1   Mortality rates among troops of European descent in areas of colonial expansion, 1817–1838 / *40*

3.2   John Snow's map of the 1854 cholera outbreak in London / *51*

3.3   The progress of smallpox eradication, 1955–1977 / *70*

6.1   Haiti's Central Plateau / *142*

7.1   Distribution of polio cases in India, 1998–2002 / *188*

8.1   Suicide rates per 100,000 population, 2007 / *217*

8.2   Human resources for mental health, 2005 / *218*

TABLES

1.1   Leading causes of death, countries grouped by income, 2004 / *4*

1.2   Leading causes of burden of disease (disability-adjusted life years), countries grouped by income, 2004 / *6*

2.1   Max Weber: Modes of authority / *24*

3.1   Factors affecting the success of eradication efforts: malaria versus smallpox / *69*

6.1   Characteristics of tuberculosis in Sector 1 versus Sector 2 patients / *153*

6.2   Health and development indicators in Rwanda and Haiti, 2008 / *166*

7.1 Advantages of public-sector health systems in democracies / 201

8.1 Disease burden of mental disorders compared to resource allocation / 214

8.2 DALY disability classes and severity weighting / 226

9.1 The relationship of civil and political rights to social and economic rights / 269

11.1 Major characteristics of the most prevalent neglected tropical diseases / 317

11.2 Cancers amenable to prevention, early detection, and treatment in low- and middle-income countries / 325

Preface

PAUL FARMER

This book, several years in the making, derives from a class titled Case Studies in Global Health: Biosocial Perspectives, first taught at Harvard College in 2008. That same year, several articles appeared in the U.S. popular press noting that global health was a hot topic among students.[1] New class offerings and even undergraduate degrees in global health were being offered in over a dozen American universities. Such programs, sometimes hastily concocted, presented what was termed a new discipline.

But global health, while a marked improvement on its forebear "international health," remains a collection of problems rather than a discipline. The collection of problems explored in this book and in complementary teaching materials—problems ranging from epidemics (from AIDS to polio to noncommunicable diseases) and the development of new technologies (preventatives, diagnostics, treatments) to the effective delivery of these technologies to those most in need—all turn on the quest for *equity*.

The just and equitable distribution of the risk of suffering and of tools to lessen or prevent it is too often the unaddressed problem in global health. No one sets out to ignore equity, but the way we frame issues of causality and response typically fails to give it due consideration. Equity is less the proverbial elephant in the room than the elephant lumbering around a maze of screens dividing that room into a series of confined spaces.

This myopia is changing. We are starting to lift our heads to see the entire room and the elephant in it. The roots of global health are to be found, we argue in chapter 3, in colonial medicine, a series of practices in which the concept of equity played a small role, and in international health, which gained prominence through nineteenth-century efforts to control the spread of epidemics between countries and became a precursor of this past decade's efflorescence of interest in global health. During the latter decades of the twentieth century, discussions of equity and justice occurred but in a peculiarly parochial manner, with certain givens: the world was divided into three worlds (first, second, third) or, more typically, into nation-states separated by borders across which pathogens readily moved, even as resources were stuck in customs.

Combining anthropology, sociology, history, political economy, and other "resocializing disciplines" with fields like epidemiology, demography, clinical practice, molecular biology, and economics allows us to build a coherent new field that might better be termed "global health equity."[2] It is this multidisciplinary approach, which leads us from the large-scale to the local and from the social to the molecular, that permits us to take a properly *biosocial* approach to what are, without exception, biosocial problems. Such is the central thesis of this book, and also the approach adopted in each chapter.

. . .

If global health is now merely a collection of problems, what might it take to forge a new discipline? Historians of science know what investments were required to build modern chemistry, physics, genetics, or molecular biology: basic principles had to be demonstrated, labs had to be funded, and institutions had to be reorganized, often over several decades. What might it take to build a science of health care delivery that is properly biosocial? Since the biological and the social have traditionally been handled by different disciplines, building the field will certainly demand a multidisciplinary approach. More than theoretical understanding, articulating the biological and the social aspects of health care delivery will require significant new investments in research and training, which are, happily, the principal concerns of a university.[3]

For both ethical and pedagogic reasons, research and training cannot occur without engaging in the *delivery* of health care to the sick (or to those likely to become sick). This reality is what drives doctors and nurses to spend most of their time training in teaching hospitals and clinics rather than in labs, classrooms, or libraries. It also drives our conviction that building a science of health care delivery will be a more complex challenge than that encompassed by most of the current mottoes and proclamations of our research universities.

How might we integrate research and training and service to build the field already known (if prematurely) as "global health," whether in settings of poverty or of plenty? This question is largely ignored by nongovernmental organizations (NGOs) and other service providers, public and private. It's also too rarely posed within the university, in part because it's clear that honest answers will invoke the need for substantial new investments and that these investments should be especially—commensurately—large in settings of great poverty. It's hard enough to conduct research on health disparities in rich countries and harder still to explore them in the poorest ones, unless there is a clear commitment to addressing them. Most study-abroad experiences in global health take place in affluent or middle-income settings as opposed to the poorest places: in South Africa rather than Burundi; in Brazil rather than Haiti; in France rather than Moldova, to name a few cases. But this habit falls short of the mission implied in the words "global health."

It's not that there aren't important questions to be answered in South Africa, Brazil, China, Russia, France, or the United States; there are many questions, and investigating them in such countries will help to inform a genuinely *global* health, as we've argued many times.[4] Disparities of wealth, like epidemics, transcend national and other administrative borders and remind us of links, rather than disjunctures, between settings of affluence and privation. But many of our students want to follow the economic gradient down to some of the poorest and most disrupted places on the face of the earth. They want to learn how to work in the places that are in greatest need of modern medicine and public health. A new generation of students and trainees has been explicit about the importance of equity, as Richard Horton, editor of *The Lancet,* noted recently: "Global health is an attitude. It is a way of looking at the world. It is about the universal nature of our human predicament. It is a statement about our commitment to health as a fundamental quality of liberty and equity."[5]

It is for this new generation of students and trainees, who draw on precisely this commitment, that we wrote this book. These students are to be found at Harvard and other research universities in the United States, just as they are to be found in Europe and India and China and Brazil and in the places we work as service providers (Haiti, Burundi, Rwanda, Lesotho, the Navajo Nation, and elsewhere). They are found everywhere, regardless of nationality, region, religion, clinical specialty, or social status, since they do indeed constitute a global generation and have embraced, as Horton observes, a commitment to equity.

But global health needs to move well beyond an attitude. To substantiate that attitude, we need to build a new discipline. This book's authors and contributors believe that global health must be "more than just a hobby." This was the title of an editorial I wrote in the *Harvard Crimson,* in an effort to convince the members of our own university that resources dedicated to global health were investments in the university's core mission; similar arguments apply to other research universities as well.[6]

. . .

In writing this preface, I have mentioned at least a half-dozen relevant scholarly disciplines as institutions ranging from public health providers and NGOs to teaching hospitals and research universities. Is it really necessary to take such a complex approach to what some would consider straightforward problems? The issues with which global health is concerned are many and various, and a book like this one addresses a varied public, including undergraduates, medical and nursing students, students of public health, members and supporters of NGOs, and others seeking to understand global health equity. We believe that what we have to say should matter as well to managers, policymakers, and all those seeking to improve health care delivery in the community, the clinic, and the hospital. Taken together with its supplementary materials available online, this book is meant to be a "toolkit" (a term imposed on us by our students) offered to practitioners, including experienced ones, of global hope.

Undergraduates who hope to address health disparities have a long road ahead of them. For future physicians, there is a traditional path outlined by our institutions of training: first the BA, then medical school, followed by internship, residency, and sometimes fellowship. After clinical training, if an academic path is pursued, comes the transition to practitioner-teacher: from trainee to faculty member. Each teacher of this undergraduate course at Harvard has been through precisely this course of training, the sort of training that for generations has produced cardiologists, infectious-disease practitioners, oncologists, psychiatrists, and every other kind of medical specialist.

But what path lies before the student planning a career in global health? Less than ten years ago, almost no such training opportunities existed; they are only now being created. The authors of this book and other materials would be proud to be thought of as midwives to a long-overdue delivery. As the collection of problems turns into a discipline, there will be more and more demand for training and credentialing at every level.

Doctors are, as noted, only a small part of what is needed. Nurses, laboratory technicians, and managers are equally necessary, as are those born in resource-poor settings who have great talent but almost no chance to start up the same professional ladder. For example, there is plenty of cancer in the rural reaches of Haiti and Rwanda, but there are no oncologists, nor are there any oncology training programs. There is plenty of trauma in the hills and mountains of rural Nepal, but orthopedists are rare or absent. If global health is to be "more than just a hobby," it must embrace the training challenges on both sides of the rich-poor divide. For every Harvard student trained, there must be at least a dozen more in the developing world who would benefit from training. No sustainable model of global health ignores the challenge of training in radically different settings (Cambridge, Massachusetts, and Mirebalais, Haiti, say). Yet most resource-rich universities seek to avoid this unpleasant reality. While they recognize the relevance of global health and acknowledge the need for bilateral training programs, generously funded tracks are absent.[7]

A comprehensive view would see and acknowledge the truly global pool of talent out there. Our students and trainees, at every level and in every setting, want us to build this new field; faculty and administrators agree, as do colleagues and patients around the globe. Linking service to training and research will help elevate global health to the level of academic prestige afforded genetics, say, or systems biology.

So why haven't we caught up with the aspirations of our constituents? When historians look back at the current era, I believe that they will see twenty-first-century medicine in the broad biosocial perspective outlined in this book. They might note the worldwide eradication of smallpox in 1977; the promise and failure of universal primary care ("health for all by the year 2000"); the decline of public and private funding of public health systems ("structural adjustment"); the advent of new or "emerging" epidemics, most notably AIDS and drug-resistant infections, whether bacterial or viral or parasitic; the socialization for scarcity evident in late twentieth-century debates over new epidemics (usually taking the form of pitting prevention and care); the sudden injection of new funds to fight these epidemics in the first years of the twenty-first century; the success of these efforts (which showed that sometimes treatment *is* prevention); and the positive synergies that emerged from these investments, which led, when used wisely, to what was termed "health systems strengthening."

Finally, I hope that historians will note the role of universities and NGO partners who sought to contribute to the burgeoning discipline of global health, which came to include, however tardily, training and research programs focused on global health equity. Building such programs for college students, medical students, interns, residents, and junior faculty at Harvard and its teaching hospitals has not been easy. The training of medical professionals is heavily subsidized by the U.S. government, and this funding remains unavailable for those who see health equity in truly global terms. In other words, the training and research agenda of our country hasn't yet caught up with programs like the President's Emergency Plan for AIDS Relief and the Global Fund to Fight AIDS, Tuberculosis and Malaria, which are among the most ambitious global health programs in history.

The need to catch up is real. When I started my medical training at Harvard in 1984, there were three other students (of the one hundred fifty in our class) who reliably expressed interest in global health. A quarter-century later, that number has swelled to fifty. A third of the students plan careers addressing health disparities in resource-poor settings; more than half are interested in global health equity as defined in this book. Indeed, training programs do not keep pace with demand.

. . .

Yet building training and research programs is just one part of reimagining global health. An even bigger part lies in addressing health disparities directly, by delivering high-quality services to those who have never before enjoyed them. That said, a division of labor (between service and research and training) is important and indeed necessary. We believe that conceptual work can inform service, research, and training—and it is this dimension of global health need that a textbook can seek to address.

The training materials developed for this undergraduate course, for "Introduction to Social Medicine" (required at Harvard Medical School), and for the Global Health Delivery courses offered with the Harvard School of Public Health all draw on key theoretical constructs we deemed important to the practice of global health work, whether at the level of policymakers or practitioners.[8] Useful concepts—from Foucault's "biopower" to Berger and Luckmann's "social construction of knowledge" to Merton's exploration of the "unintended consequences of purposive social action," which we consider in the second chapter of this volume—are largely absent from the global public health literature. Someone might justifiably ask whether such notions are necessary to achieve global health equity, or whether they are simply too abstract, philosophical, and speculative. We contend that such concepts inform the biosocial analysis requisite for meaningful action based on understanding of complex problems in complex settings. These concepts can also inform frameworks justifying efforts to address health disparities—health as a human right, public health as a public good, and health services as investments in economic development, for example.

It is good to have the desire and the capacity to practice medicine and an orientation that supports the public good. But when issues of implementation lead to pragmatic quandaries, it is essential to have deep and broad analyses of the problems. One case in point: the interaction of NGOs and what are considered "failing" public health care systems. A medical provider working with a global health NGO might be led to think that the most efficient path to ensuring the best care for the many is to replace public systems with private charitable care, the kind of care the contributors to this volume are, perhaps, most familiar with. But no private entity can meet the whole range of interlocking needs of a system to support healthy human lives, and no NGO is capable of conferring *rights* to those in need of them. NGOs can at most establish a provider-client relation within a framework of legal rights that only a state can confer. This textbook seeks to make evident the links between what are here called neoliberal policies and the witting or unwitting weakening of public-sector health systems.

The course on which *Reimagining Global Health* is based was designed by anthropologists who are also practicing physicians. The original course description read:

> This new undergraduate course will examine a collection of global health problems deeply rooted in rapidly changing social structures that transcend national and other administrative boundaries. The faculty will draw on field experience in Asia, Africa, and the Americas to explore several case studies (addressing AIDS, tuberculosis, malaria, mental illness, and other topics) and a diverse literature (including epidemiology, anthropology, history, and clinical medicine). This course seeks to introduce students to selected topics in a rapidly emerging and poorly defined field, with a focus on how broad biosocial analysis might be used to improve the delivery of

services designed to lessen the burden of disease, especially among those living in poverty.

The undergraduate course has been taught yearly since 2008. As we developed it, we worked with an overlapping group of colleagues at Harvard Medical School and its teaching hospitals to reconfigure a course called Introduction to Social Medicine, which was taken by all first-year medical students.[9] That reconfiguration benefitted from being the product of a group of like-minded practitioners; like all such collective efforts, it relies heavily on the limited experience of people accustomed to working together in certain times and places. We also worked with colleagues at Harvard Business School, the Brigham and Women's Hospital, and the Harvard School of Public Health to develop a series of "cases" (which means something quite different than it would in, say, an anthropology course) for students seeking to focus their careers on improving the delivery of health services broadly defined. One result, the Global Health Effectiveness Program, was one of the first joint teaching efforts ever between Harvard's schools of medicine and public health, entities that are physically separated by no more than a hundred yards. We developed new pedagogic materials that critically explore efforts to address some of the ranking problems of global health, from specific epidemics to the development of new technologies to the effective delivery of these tools.[10]

. . .

In January of 2010, a large earthquake destroyed much of Port-au-Prince, the capital city of a country in which we (working with thousands of colleagues, most of them Haitian) were trying to advance the cause of global health equity by addressing disparities directly. The quake leveled Haiti's only large city and claimed, by some counts, a quarter of a million souls.[11] Less than a month after completing the second iteration of our courses for undergraduates and medical students, we found ourselves contemplating Haiti's ruined medical and training infrastructure. Here was an emergent global health crisis, occurring quite literally before our eyes. How might we marshal the resources of the university, and other partners, to assuage the suffering of the injured and of those who, while not injured directly, were unable to access the services they needed?

In the immediate short term, all our focus was on saving lives. In looking back over those first weeks after the quake—itself a daunting exercise[12]—it's possible to conclude that academic medical centers made a pretty decent showing. One of the greatest problems in an earthquake, inevitably, is crush injuries. From across the world, teams of surgeons and anesthesiologists and skilled surgical nurses traveled to Haiti to preserve life and, when possible, limb. Academic medical centers and NGOs joined Haitian authorities and able-bodied citizens seeking to provide relief. Support was widespread: by some estimates, more than half of all American households donated to earthquake relief.

In those first weeks, surgical teams saved thousands of lives—when they could build field capacity or invest in decent and undamaged infrastructure. But many first-time visitors found it difficult to function. Haiti's health care system, public and private, had been weak, disorganized, and overtaxed well before January 12, 2010. The zoo of NGOs working in Haiti prior to the quake was poorly coordinated and little supervised by Haitian authorities, local or national, and even less coordinated with each other. In other words, the chaos of those first weeks was by no means the result of the disaster alone.

The collapse of schools and clinical facilities in Port-au-Prince led some to speak of "building back better." In this view, the quake offered a chance to reimagine the city and its commons—from parks to schools to medical centers. The revelatory shock of the quake served to interrogate, and sometimes undermine, views of public health that had dominated timid efforts in the latter part of the twentieth century. If a reimagined view of global health offers, to paraphrase Richard Horton, a new way of looking at the world, what might a commitment to health equity look like in post-quake Haiti?

Like some of our students, those of us who were experienced Haiti hands found ourselves torn between pessimism and hope, between inaction and bold initiatives. Whenever ambitious efforts to reimagine health care delivery won out, plans for new and improved hospitals and a proper health system were drawn up, and efforts to build new training programs proliferated. But plans and charrettes and reimagined medical centers were one thing; funding and implementation were quite another. As this book goes to press, more than three years after the quake, only a handful of hospitals have been rebuilt, and none of the downed university structures have been restored. The former Ministry of Health is a vacant lot, raked smooth. But one care delivery institution "reimagined" in the days after the earthquake has been designed and built and opened. The Hôpital Universitare de Mirebalais seeks to link service delivery for the poor to training and research, precisely as outlined in so many chapters of this book. It links the dynamism of NGOs and other parts of the private sector to the mandate and need in the public sector. It is beautiful and modern and done.

Sadly, the forces of globalization and decline were not finished with Haiti. The most water-insecure country in the Western Hemisphere, Haiti was primed for a major cholera epidemic even before the quake, as sober reviews noted.[13] Imagining a robust response to cholera was easy. But a more anemic response prevailed behind closed doors and in conference rooms.

With more than a million displaced people living in camps and enduring repeated calls for an end to the distribution of free potable water (on the grounds that it was neither sustainable nor cost-effective, or that it was cutting into the business of water purveyors), some public health experts nonetheless, and of course incorrectly, predicted that cholera was "unlikely to occur" in Haiti.[14] It is hard, as we show in this book, to make claims of causality regarding epidemic disease. But one plausible scenario involved this political economy of proximity.[15] Sewage from one of the United Nations peacekeeper camps leaked directly into a tributary of Haiti's largest river—an unintended consequence, surely, but not an altogether unpredictable one. Regardless of its origin, the cholera pathogen spread rapidly throughout the region drained by the river system and then, more slowly during the dry season, across the country and into the Dominican Republic and beyond.

Building or rebuilding a proper water and sanitation system in Haiti would take, in the best case, many years. Clearly, tens of thousands of lives were in peril in any scenario that involved only slow forms of prevention; faster (if shorter-acting) modes of prevention, from handwashing to vaccination, were necessary and complementary, as were efforts to identify and treat every cholera case.[16] The same quarrels over prevention versus care registered in this book's accounting of twentieth-century epidemics occurred in the midst of the twenty-first century's largest cholera epidemic. The quarrels were generated by the same socialization for scarcity that has marked all health investments in settings of poverty or for the poor who live in affluent countries.[17]

This is a very personal preface, for a number of reasons. One is because this book, and the large quantity of teaching material we've developed over the past few years, represent a significant personal investment for many of us. Another, of course, is that the faculty (and many of the teaching fellows) have dedicated their careers to this effort.

Finally, this preface is personal because the quake and its aftershocks permeated my experience of teaching more than I could say comfortably in a classroom.

Despite the quake and its aftermath, my faith in the importance of the effort required to reimagine global health remains unshaken. If anything, the experience of the Haitian quake, which was mostly wretched, redoubled my own commitment to linking direct experience in settings such as Haiti to tools from social theory that might allow us to understand the consequences, intended and unintended, of social action and of inaction.

If anthropology, history, and the other resocializing disciplines share a common analytic purpose, it is to render whole what is hard to see as such. It is also to acknowledge that human experience of suffering in pain or injury—and of the individuals and institutions that seek to redress suffering—are difficult to render as abstractions of models or theories. Every account is partial, and none could hope to capture the complexity of human experience.[18] This book's chief shortcoming is that every report or case or chapter or review is thus necessarily and avowedly partial. Acknowledging partiality sometimes helps us to interrogate facile claims of causality. Many of these claims will be revealed, in time, to be immodest or flat-out wrong. The history of medicine and public health has repeatedly taught us that humility should infuse our practice and our teaching and all claims of causality. But humility need not lead to paralysis, and we hope that the reader is not caught between unreflective activism and an informed but ultimately paralytic skepticism.

We counsel neither, for long experience has shown us that this too is a false dichotomy, and more dangerous than most. Inaction is not a real option but rather an illusion, one maintained with difficulty in even the tallest ivory towers or most gated retreats. We live in one world, not three, and "reimagining global health" requires resocializing our understanding of it. We've tried to do as much in this book, and we invite you to join us.

Introduction

A Biosocial Approach to Global Health

PAUL FARMER, JIM YONG KIM, ARTHUR KLEINMAN, MATTHEW BASILICO

A VIEW FROM THE FIELD

Mpatso has been coughing for months. Coughing consumes his energy and his appetite, and he loses weight with every passing week. When his skin begins to sag, he takes the advice of his relatives and makes the two-hour journey to a health center. There Mpatso learns that he has AIDS and tuberculosis. In his village in rural Malawi—an agrarian, landlocked nation in Southern Africa, hard hit by both diseases—Mpatso's diagnosis carries a very poor prognosis. Malawi, like most of the countries in sub-Saharan Africa, faces the combined challenges of poverty, high burden of disease, and limited health services in the public sector. But Mpatso's case is an exception: shortly after he arrives at the Neno District Hospital—a public hospital built with the help of NGOs in a small town in the rural reaches of southern Malawi—he is seen by a team of clinicians. That same afternoon, Mpatso is diagnosed and begins treatment for both diseases. The treatment involves a dizzying number of pills, but his are delivered daily by a community health worker who also helps him follow his therapeutic regimen. His life will likely be prolonged by decades.

Down the hall from Mpatso's exam room, a neighbor gives birth with the support of a nurse-midwife. In an adjacent room, six women are in labor under the watchful eye of the clinical staff and within a few yards of a clean, modern operating room. In this and in many other respects, Neno District Hospital differs from most health facilities in the region (and throughout rural sub-Saharan Africa). The hospital is a comprehensive primary care facility, providing ambulatory care for hundreds of patients each day. It has one hundred and twenty beds, a tuberculosis ward, a well-stocked pharmacy, and an electronic medical records system. The facility is staffed by doctors and nurses from the Ministry of Health and from Partners In Health. In one of the poorest and most isolated areas in Malawi, a robust local health system is delivering high-quality care, free of charge to the patients, as a public good for public health.

How was this system put in place in a country where effective health services are typically unavailable, and how can comprehensive health systems be built across the "developing world" (perhaps better labeled the "majority world")? How is the double burden of poverty and disease experienced by individuals like Mpatso or his neighbors across the border in Mozambique? How can history and political economy help us understand the skewed distributions of wealth and illness around the globe? These are a few of the questions that motivate our investigation of global health equity.

BIOSOCIAL ANALYSIS

As the preface notes, global health is not yet a discipline but rather a collection of problems. The authors of this volume believe that the process of rigorously analyzing these problems, of working to solve them, and of transforming the field of global health into a coherent discipline demands an interdisciplinary approach. Describing the forces that led Mpatso to fall ill with tuberculosis—a treatable infectious disease that has been banished to history books in most of the rich world yet continues to claim some 1.4 million lives per year worldwide—requires an intrinsically *biosocial* analytic endeavor. The roots of the limited health care infrastructure in rural Neno District, a former British colony long on the periphery of the global economy, are historically deep and geographically broad.

Most textbooks of public health have been written by epidemiologists, and we of course draw heavily from this field, relying as well on insights from clinical medicine and from public health disciplines such as health economics. But the course we teach at Harvard College (like the courses we have long taught at Harvard Medical School and the hospitals with which we're affiliated) is not the same as those taught by public health specialists. We who have developed this course and edited this book are jointly trained in clinical medicine and in anthropology or political economy. Thus we also seek to critique prevailing global health discourse with what we have termed the resocializing disciplines—anthropology, sociology, history, political economy.[1] Our approach hinges on social theory, explored in the second chapter, and aims to interrogate claims of causality widely stated in the literature on global health.

Our experience as medical practitioners has also shaped our approach to this volume. As we demonstrate in chapter 6, adapting a fully interdisciplinary investigation to basic questions—how did Mpatso become ill, and why?—has directly informed our practice. We see this close coupling of inquiry and implementation—the "vitality of praxis"—as central to our work: traversing the space between reflection and pragmatic engagement is necessary in any attempt to distill a core body of information about global health. Limitations exist in any team's knowledge of a particular field, and this book is of course based on material with which we are especially familiar, including the work of Partners In Health, the focus of chapter 6.

AN OVERVIEW OF HEALTH DISPARITIES: THE BURDEN OF DISEASE

We begin by taking a look at the global distribution of poor health and the factors that structure it. Globally, heart disease was the leading killer worldwide in 2004 (see table 1.1); cerebrovascular disease and chronic obstructive pulmonary disease ranked in the top five. This picture looks different, however, when we compare high- and low-income countries. Five of the leading causes of death in low-income countries—diarrheal diseases, HIV/AIDS, tuberculosis, neonatal infections, and malaria—are treatable infectious illnesses that are not found on the leading list of killers in high-income countries. Tuberculosis, malaria, and cholera continue to claim millions of lives each year because effective therapeutics and preventatives remain unavailable in most of the developing world. Although effective therapy for HIV has existed since 1996, and treatment now costs less than $100 per year in the developing world, AIDS is still the leading infectious killer of young adults in most low-income countries. In fact, 72 percent of AIDS-related deaths occur in a single region, sub-Saharan Africa, which is also the world's

TABLE 1.1 LEADING CAUSES OF DEATH, COUNTRIES GROUPED BY INCOME, 2004

Disease or Injury	Deaths (millions)	Percent of Total Deaths	Disease or Injury	Deaths (millions)	Percent of Total Deaths
World			*Low-Income Countries*		
1. Ischemic heart disease	7.2	12.2	1. Lower respiratory infections	2.9	11.2
2. Cerebrovascular disease	5.7	9.7	2. Ischemic heart disease	2.5	9.4
3. Lower respiratory infections	4.2	7.1	3. Diarrheal diseases	1.8	6.9
4. COPD^a	3.0	5.1	4. HIV/AIDS	1.5	5.7
5. Diarrheal diseases	2.2	3.7	5. Cerebrovascular disease	1.5	5.6
6. HIV/AIDS	2.0	3.5	6. COPD^a	0.9	3.6
7. Tuberculosis	1.5	2.5	7. Tuberculosis	0.9	3.5
8. Trachea, bronchus, lung cancers	1.3	2.2	8. Neonatal infections^b	0.9	3.4
9. Road traffic accidents	1.3	2.2	9. Malaria	0.9	3.3
10. Prematurity and low birth weight	1.2	2.0	10. Prematurity and low birth weight	0.8	3.2
Middle-Income Countries			*High-Income Countries*		
1. Cerebrovascular disease	3.5	14.2	1. Ischemic heart disease	1.3	16.3
2. Ischemic heart disease	3.4	13.9	2. Cerebrovascular disease	0.8	9.3
3. COPD^a	1.8	7.4	3. Trachea, bronchus, lung cancers	0.5	5.9
4. Lower respiratory infections	0.9	3.8	4. Lower respiratory infections	0.3	3.8
5. Trachea, bronchus, lung cancers	0.7	2.9	5. COPD^a	0.3	3.5
6. Road traffic accidents	0.7	2.8	6. Alzheimer and other dementias	0.3	3.4
7. Hypertensive heart disease	0.6	2.5	7. Colon and rectum cancers	0.3	3.3
8. Stomach cancer	0.5	2.2	8. Diabetes mellitus	0.2	2.8
9. Tuberculosis	0.5	2.2	9. Breast cancer	0.2	2.0
10. Diabetes mellitus	0.5	2.1	10. Stomach cancer	0.1	1.8

SOURCE: World Health Organization, *The Global Burden of Disease, 2004 Update* (Geneva: World Health Organization, 2008), 12, table 2.

NOTE: Countries are grouped by 2004 gross national income per capita: low income ($825 or less), high income ($10,066 or more). For a list of countries grouped by income, see World Health Organization, *The Global Burden of Disease, 2004 Update*, annex C, table C2.

^{a} COPD = chronic obstructive pulmonary disease.

^{b} This category also includes other noninfectious causes arising in the perinatal period, which are responsible for about 20 percent of deaths shown in this category.

poorest. Diarrheal diseases are often treatable by simple rehydration interventions that cost pennies, yet diarrheal diseases rank third among killers in low-income countries.

Table 1.2 presents similar data, this time using a measure that takes into account both disability and death. This measure, the disability-adjusted life year (DALY), which is a way of quantifying years lost to poor health, disability, and early death, is not without its flaws; we will explore them in chapter 8. DALYs show a similar picture of health disparities between high- and low-income countries. It is also apparent that noninfectious conditions—such as birth asphyxia and birth trauma—are disproportionately distributed in low-income countries. Like the treatable infectious diseases just described, these forms of morbidity and mortality are often preventable with modern medical interventions and are thus much rarer in the wealthier parts of industrialized countries. Another stark picture of this disparity can be seen in map 1.1: despite some improvements over the last two decades, average life expectancy in low- and middle-income countries in sub-Saharan Africa stands at 49.2 years—fully 30.2 years less than life expectancy in high-income countries.

The relationship between gross domestic product (GDP) and health is one starting point for an examination of global health inequities. But national measures of wealth such as GDP and GNP (gross national product) are well worth pulling apart. "Domestic" and "national" data often (perhaps always) obscure local inequities, such as those seen within a nation, state, district, city, or other local polity. Figure 1.1, compiled by the World Health Organization's Commission on Social Determinants of Health, illustrates one example of the substantial differences in health outcomes between rich and poor households within single countries. Figure 1.2, from the same report, highlights another measure of social status across countries—in this case, mother's education level—that correlates with health outcomes such as infant mortality. The impact of social class, among other social, political, and economic factors, on health is taken as a given in this book, as it is in others. We will grapple with the many layers of these inequities throughout the text, beginning with a theory of structural violence in chapter 2. We will delve into the complexities of causation and the structures that pattern both the risk of ill health and access to modern health services, even as we explore effective and ineffective interventions in global health. Why is Mpatso able to attain good health care

TABLE 1.2 LEADING CAUSES OF BURDEN OF DISEASE (DISABILITY-ADJUSTED LIFE YEARS), COUNTRIES GROUPED BY INCOME, 2004

Disease or Injury	DALYs (millions)	Percent of Total DALYs	Disease or Injury	DALYs (millions)	Percent of Total DALYs
World			*Low-Income Countries*		
1. Lower respiratory infections	94.5	6.2	1. Lower respiratory infections	76.9	9.3
2. Diarrheal diseases	72.8	4.8	2. Diarrheal diseases	59.2	7.2
3. Unipolar depressive disorders	65.5	4.3	3. HIV/AIDS	42.9	5.2
4. Ischemic heart disease	62.6	4.1	4. Malaria	32.8	4.0
5. HIV/AIDS	58.5	3.8	5. Prematurity and low birth weight	32.1	3.9
6. Cerebrovascular disease	46.6	3.1	6. Neonatal infections and other[a]	31.4	3.8
7. Prematurity and low birth weight	44.3	2.9	7. Birth asphyxia and birth trauma	29.8	3.6
8. Birth asphyxia and birth trauma	41.7	2.7	8. Unipolar depressive disorders	26.5	3.2
9. Road traffic accidents	41.2	2.7	9. Ischemic heart disease	26.0	3.1
10. Neonatal infections and other[a]	40.4	2.7	10. Tuberculosis	22.4	2.7
Middle-Income Countries			*High-Income Countries*		
1. Unipolar depressive disorders	29.0	5.1	1. Unipolar depressive disorders	10.0	8.2
2. Ischemic heart disease	28.9	5.0	2. Ischemic heart disease	7.7	6.3
3. Cerebrovascular disease	27.5	4.8	3. Cerebrovascular disease	4.8	3.9
4. Road traffic accidents	21.4	3.7	4. Alzheimer and other dementias	4.4	3.6
5. Lower respiratory infections	16.3	2.8	5. Alcohol use disorders	4.2	3.4
6. COPD[b]	16.1	2.8	6. Hearing loss, adult onset	4.2	3.4
7. HIV/AIDS	15.0	2.6	7. COPD[b]	3.7	3.0
8. Alcohol use disorders	14.9	2.6	8. Diabetes mellitus	3.6	3.0
9. Refractive errors	13.7	2.4	9. Trachea, bronchus, lung cancers	3.6	3.0
10. Diabetes mellitus	13.1	2.3	10. Road traffic accidents	3.1	2.6

SOURCE: World Health Organization, *The Global Burden of Disease, 2004 Update* (Geneva: World Health Organization, 2008), 44, table 12.

NOTE: Countries are grouped by 2004 gross national income per capita: low income ($825 or less), high income ($10, 066 or more). For a list of countries grouped by income, see WHO, *The Global Burden of Disease, 2004 Update*, annex C, table C2.

[a] This category also includes other noninfectious causes arising in the perinatal period apart from prematurity, low birth weight, birth trauma, and asphyxia. These noninfectious causes are responsible for about 20 percent of DALYs shown in this category.

[b] COPD = chronic obstructive pulmonary disease.

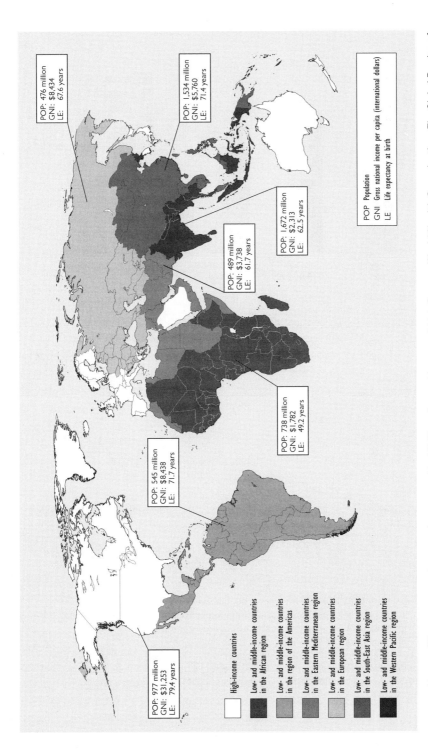

MAP 1.1. Average life expectancy in countries grouped by WHO region and income, 2004. Source: World Health Organization, *The Global Burden of Disease, 2004 Update* (Geneva: World Health Organization, 2008), 5, map 1.

POP: 476 million
GNI: $8,434
LE: 67.6 years

POP: 1,534 million
GNI: $5,760
LE: 71.4 years

POP: 489 million
GNI: $3,738
LE: 61.7 years

POP: 1,672 million
GNI: $2,313
LE: 62.5 years

POP: 738 million
GNI: $1,782
LE: 49.2 years

POP: 545 million
GNI: $8,438
LE: 71.7 years

POP: 977 million
GNI: $31,253
LE: 79.4 years

POP   Population
GNI   Gross national income per capita (international dollars)
LE   Life expectancy at birth

High-income countries

Low- and middle-income countries in the African region

Low- and middle-income countries in the region of the Americas

Low- and middle-income countries in the Eastern Mediterranean region

Low- and middle-income countries in the European region

Low- and middle-income countries in the South-East Asia region

Low- and middle-income countries in the Western Pacific region

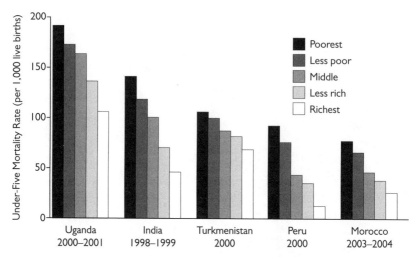

FIGURE 1.1. Mortality rates for children under the age of five, by level of household wealth. Source: *Closing the Gap in a Generation: Health Equity through Action on the Social Determinants of Health,* Final Report of the Commission on Social Determinants of Health (Geneva: World Health Organization, 2008), 30, fig. 2-2.

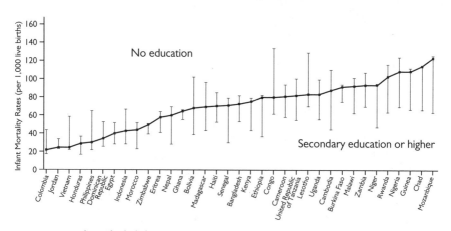

FIGURE 1.2. Inequity in infant mortality rates between countries and within countries, by mother's education. The continuous dark line represents average infant mortality rates for countries; the endpoints of the vertical bars indicate the infant mortality rates for mothers with no education and for mothers with secondary or higher education within each country. Source: *Closing the Gap in a Generation: Health Equity through Action on the Social Determinants of Health,* Final Report of the Commission on Social Determinants of Health (Geneva: World Health Organization, 2008), 29, fig. 2-1.

despite living in rural Malawi, while so many others in similar circumstances cannot?

DEFINING TERMS

Questions quickly arise in any study of this field: what do we mean when we use key terms such as "public health," "international health," and "global health"? What do we mean by "global health delivery"? More fundamentally, how should we define "health" itself? The World Health Organization (WHO) defines health as a state of physical, mental, and social well-being. But is this how Mpatso understands health? Can any definition of health capture the subjective illness experiences of individuals in different settings around the globe?[2] Beyond the direct experiences of individuals are social, political, and economic forces that drive up the risk of ill health for some while sparing others. Some have called this *structural violence*.[3] Such social forces become embodied as health and disease among individuals.

Though they share the goal of improving human health, "public health" and "medicine" are in many ways distinct. Public health focuses on the health of populations, while medicine focuses on the health of individuals. But in reifying the distinctions between them, we risk perpetuating unhelpful visual field defects in both professions. Clinical insights inform public health practice, and public health analysis guides the distribution of medical resources. But we believe both clinical medicine and public health must utilize the resocializing disciplines to address the fundamentally biosocial nature of global health problems. Microbes such as HIV and *Mycobacterium tuberculosis* cannot be understood properly at the molecular, clinical, experiential, or population level without analysis spanning the molecular to the social. Jonathan Mann, a physician and public health expert, put it this way: "Lacking a coherent conceptual framework, a consistent vocabulary, and consensus about societal change, public health assembles and then tries valiantly to assimilate a wide variety of disciplinary perspectives, from economists, political scientists, social and behavioral scientists, health systems analysts, and a range of medical practitioners."[4] All fields have myopias. The restricted gaze of each discipline can illuminate certain global health problems; but only when they are taken together with a fully biosocial approach can we build, properly, the field of global health.

A word on the term "global health": An antecedent term, "international health," emphasized the nation-state as the base unit of comparison and implied a focus on relationships among states. Global health should more accurately encapsulate the role of nonstate institutions, including international NGOs, private philanthropists, and community-based organizations. Pathogens do not recognize international borders. But much churn—social and microbial—is introduced at borders.[5] Further, we seek to examine health disparities not only among countries but also within them, including our own. Boston (like Cape Town and São Paolo and Bangkok) has some of the world's finest hospitals but also great disparities in burden of disease and access to care; it is on the globe, too.

A final note on definitions: "global health delivery" refers to the provision of health interventions, a process distinct from discovering or developing such interventions through laboratory research or clinical trials. Global health delivery begins with the question "how can a health system efficiently provide health services to all who need them?" More efficient and equitable delivery of existing health interventions could save tens of millions of lives each year. But even the best models of global health delivery cannot alone raise the standard of health care available to people worldwide. The health of individuals and populations is influenced by complex social and structural forces; addressing the roots of ill health—including poverty, inequality, and environmental degradation—requires a broad-based agenda of social change.

ORGANIZATION OF THIS BOOK

The chapters in this volume have been drafted by course faculty, guest lecturers, teaching fellows, and—in many instances—former students from our Harvard undergraduate courses, including "Case Studies in Global Health: Biosocial Perspectives." In developing the syllabus and course content, we observed that despite the wealth of scholarship in global health equity, there were few introductory texts addressing it; almost none adopted biosocial perspectives. In reviews of the first year of the course, students encouraged us to find ways to make the course material accessible beyond our Harvard classrooms. We decided that this book could achieve two aims: make our course material available to a broader audience, and help to fill the gap of introductory materials on global health.

An exhaustive treatment of global health would be impossible in a single volume; our goal here is to introduce some of the principal challenges and complexities that confront those pursuing global health equity. We also outline some of the accomplishments of this endeavor, very often drawing on our own experiences as physicians, teachers, and activists. This experience occurs in the clinic and the classroom and the field; it is rooted in time and place. For this reason, *Reimagining Global Health* does not seek to offer a comprehensive review of a vast literature but rather to use our field experience in Haiti, Rwanda, Malawi, China, Peru, the United States, and elsewhere to raise important issues and to link these examples to some of the key readings in a number of disciplines and from an even wider array of settings. We also seek to think hard about future challenges by taking stock of what has happened in the past and by drawing on concepts familiar to us.

The book is divided into twelve chapters. Chapter 2 lays out a framework of social theories relevant to the most important questions in global health. We have found these theories helpful in understanding both the material covered in this volume and our own experience within the field of global health. Though we assume no background knowledge in social theory, we draw on work by some of the great theorists of the past century, including Max Weber and Michel Foucault, as well as more recent health-focused work, such as the notion of social suffering offered by Arthur Kleinman, Veena Das, and Margaret Lock. For readers with some background in social theory, we hope that our focus on health will elicit new insights and spur consideration of the relevance of other theoretical frameworks.

Chapters 3, 4, and 5 continue to build an analytic framework by examining three key historical periods critical to an understanding of global health today. Chapter 3 offers an account of colonial medicine and its legacies. One such legacy is the development of major global health institutions, including the World Health Organization; another is the notion of setting priorities for health interventions in the developing world. We trace the ways in which the economic and political priorities of wealthy nations informed assumptions about other populations and corresponding modalities of intervention. These trends have often continued to structure academic inquiry and the design of health interventions well beyond the colonial era. We also study global fascination with the power of biomedical intervention, such as the development of the first antibiotics and the pesticide DDT, in the context of two of the most important global health campaigns of the Cold War era: the smallpox and malaria eradication campaigns, which achieved markedly different results.

Chapter 4 analyzes two pivotal and tumultuous decades for international public health, the mid-1970s to the mid-1990s. They profoundly influenced health systems in developing countries and shaped contemporary discourse among global health policymakers. The chapter begins with the antecedents of the 1978 International Conference on Primary Health Care, in Alma Ata, Kazakhstan, where delegates from around the world adopted the goal "health for all by the year 2000." We then trace the rising influence of neoliberalism and the shift toward a *selective* primary health care approach in the 1980s. Chapter 4 details how these geopolitical shifts led to the rise of the World Bank as perhaps the most influential institution in global health during the 1990s and considers the effects of its approach on the health of the global poor.

In Chapter 5, we examine one of the most astonishing events in the history of global health: the AIDS movement. Why, after a decade of austerity and fatalism in the face of yawning health inequities around the world, did rich countries begin to devote billions of dollars in new resources to global AIDS treatment efforts? Describing the rise of the U.S. President's Emergency Plan for AIDS Relief (PEPFAR) and the Global Fund to Fight AIDS, Tuberculosis and Malaria, we suggest that a broad coalition of practitioners, patients, policymakers, advocates, and researchers helped to expand the notion of "possible" in global health. Global policy and resource flows shifted dramatically, demonstrating the elasticity of assumptions such as "limited resources" and "appropriate technology" and underscoring the force of vibrant social movements in global health.

Chapters 6, 7, and 8 build on the historical and theoretical frameworks set out in earlier chapters and confront many of the key questions in global health, beginning with those posed by Mpatso's experience. Chapter 6 contextualizes these historical trends at the point of care by exploring the resuscitation of public-sector health systems in Haiti and Rwanda, focusing on the experiences of Partners In Health. It offers a chance to see the biosocial approach in practice in the principles behind the organization's strategy and in the delivery of context-specific health interventions.

Chapter 7 outlines a generalizable framework for effective global health delivery. We begin by defining several principles of global health delivery and then analyze contemporary efforts to strengthen health systems in resource-poor settings. The chapter calls for a true "science of global health delivery" capable of improving health system performance around the globe—in areas poor and rich.[6]

Chapter 8 investigates the social construction of disease categories and health metrics in the context of mental illness and multidrug-resistant tuberculosis—two pathologies that pose unique challenges to global health practitioners. The history and political economy of these illnesses illustrate many of the themes treated in this text and highlight the role of biosocial analysis in unpacking some of the complexities of global health. We hope the chapter will offer lessons for other global health challenges that, unlike AIDS, rarely see media attention and are widely misunderstood—often at the expense of those who encounter them as illness experience.

Chapter 9 examines moral aspects of global health work, including the human rights tradition. It traces the genealogy of several ethical frameworks invoked by practitioners, examining their core premises and also the practical implications of their application in global health. Many people are led to global health work by an intuitive sense that it is the right thing to do; we believe that a critical investigation of several moral frameworks can both facilitate productive introspection and expand the sphere of discourse for public engagement in global health.

The last three chapters (10, 11, and 12) sketch the landscape of global health today. Chapter 10 critically examines the rise in foreign assistance for health and development. The chapter goes beyond the question "does foreign aid work?" to ask "*how* does aid work?" What lessons have been learned during the past decades that might improve foreign aid and global health in the decades to come?

Chapter 11 outlines a number of key global health priorities for the next decade. It suggests that scaling up the model of health care delivery and health system strengthening introduced in chapter 7 offers great promise in addressing these priorities. Such an effort offers a platform to reduce the burden of disease, address social determinants of health, and build long-term care delivery capacity that will allow us to adapt to new demands as they arise. But such scale-up and the ability to advance global health equity will not be possible without broad-based social change—which is the subject of chapter 12, the concluding chapter of *Reimagining Global Health*. Those who have written it have studied and worked together for many years and hope our shared experience will be useful to readers, just as we hope to continue learning from others seeking to pursue the elusive goal of health for all.

2

Unpacking Global Health

Theory and Critique

BRIDGET HANNA, ARTHUR KLEINMAN

This chapter introduces a "toolkit" of social theories relevant to global health work. We believe that social theory can help students and practitioners understand and interpret the nature, effects, and limitations of medical and public health interventions. As examples in this book illustrate, well-intentioned global health and development projects can have unintended—and at times undesirable—consequences. Careful evaluation of the conditions that enable such consequences can help practitioners design better programs and cultivate a habit of critical self-reflection, which would surely be an asset to global health scholarship and delivery.

Most global health practitioners are focused primarily on *action:* providing services and seeking to improve the health of individuals and populations. Like the many leaders of public health and sanitation initiatives who preceded them, practitioners of global health have rarely had much exposure to, or patience for, the application of social theory to the problems they face. Evaluation of global health work usually focuses on measuring program effectiveness. Social theory has often been relegated to the domain of post-hoc analysis by scholars writing in academic journals, sometimes years or decades after their insights might have been used to improve the delivery of care.

The divide between theory and practice has many roots. Some scholars point to the troubled legacy of political Marxism, in which various interpretations of Karl Marx's writings were used as the basis for radical, and sometimes violent, reconstruction of the social order. In addition, the involvement of social scientists, particularly anthropologists, in enabling and justifying the violence of colonialism, and the scientific racism that provided its ideological cover (traced in chapter 3), has led to serious reflection regarding the role of social science in global health and humanitarian work. This history has provided ample cause for the inward turns of deconstructionism and self-criticism that have preoccupied much of anthropology for the past thirty years.

This period also coincided, however, with the rise of medical anthropology as a discipline and the emergence of a new perspective: that of the physician-anthropologist. The physician-anthropologist authors of this volume are examples of those who have used tools from medical anthropology to hone a vision of health equity and social justice. For example, the nongovernmental organization Partners In Health drew on social theory to critique and improve its approach to health care delivery, as chapter 6 explores. It is in this new but vibrant tradition of medical anthropology that we ground our approach to social theory for global health. Effective global health leaders must consider problems from multiple perspectives. They must measure the effects of interventions and explain the meanings of those effects to diverse actors, in diverse places, and at different moments.

Max Weber, an early twentieth-century German sociologist and one of the architects of modern social science, defined sociology as "the science whose object it is *to interpret the meaning of social action* and thereby give a causal explanation of *the way in which this action proceeds and the effect which it produces.*"[1] Weber saw sociology as a science in the sense that it could identify certain causal relationships between social forms. But, as an anti-positivist, he believed that these relationships were not as "ahistorical, invariant, or generalizable"[2] as those studied by natural scientists. Rather, Weber sought to interpret the meanings of cultural norms, symbols, and values that connect people to structures such as bureaucratic institutions of the state.

Today, anthropology and other modes of social analysis still seek to "interpret the meaning of social action." The social theories outlined in this chapter can be used to help explain why certain global health initiatives succeed while others fail. These theories elucidate the social determinants of health: the nature and causes of poverty and inequity. The specific social theories discussed here are by no means the only pertinent ones, but they are particularly relevant to navigating the complexities of global health delivery.

BIOSOCIAL ANALYSIS AND THE SOCIOLOGY OF KNOWLEDGE

Most medical research focuses exclusively on the biologic causes of disease. A biosocial approach posits that such biologic and clinical processes are inflected by society, political economy, history, and culture and are thus best understood as interactions of biological and social processes. Biosocial analysis of global health challenges reaches across disciplines and breaks down the boundaries that separate them; for example, understanding questions of resource optimization, which are usually reserved for economists, also requires insights from anthropologists and health practitioners. One central illustration of the biosocial nature of disease is the correlation between disease risk and poverty. We will revisit this relationship often in this volume under various names (such as structural violence and social suffering) and in the context of different diseases (such as malaria, AIDS, and multidrug-resistant tuberculosis).

Other concrete examples include the link between psychological and economic depression and the rise in rates of disability associated with increased unemployment. Likewise, economic status, education level, cultural traditions, and access to infrastructure all influence dietary habits, a crucial determinant of heart disease and obesity. The global epidemic of type 2 diabetes mellitus is attributable in part to greater sugar intake. To add complexity to the issue of culture and diet, one must also consider mental health. For example, Anne Becker and colleagues conducted dietary studies in Fiji and found that as tourism grew and infrastructure was developed, the diets of the native people shifted toward Western eating habits. Rates of anorexia and bulimia rose as television watching became popular and displaced other cultural events and large family meals.[3] None of these phenomena can be examined properly in the absence of biosocial analysis.

A biosocial approach demands the reconciliation and occasional disruption of multiple frames of knowledge. A medical student will learn, for instance, that the cause of cerebral malaria is the protozoa *Plasmodium falciparum* and that the treatments of choice include quinine or artemisinin-based combination therapy, whereas an epidemiologist or a public health planner might view the cause as undrained breeding grounds for the mosquito vector and recommend draining standing water, providing mosquito nets, and spraying DDT. All the while, residents of an endemic area and ethnographers who speak with them might assert that the cause of malaria is the unequal distribution of land under the local system of tenancy and might protest that DDT's environmental effects make its use unacceptable.

How should global health practitioners navigate these multiple ontological claims? Differential values assigned to diverse categories of evidence—in this case, whether the problem is deemed biological, environmental, or economic—will shape the proposed solution and its ultimate effect. This is particularly clear in the case of malaria. Although the biological view of malaria causality largely won out over the geographic and sociological views in the 1970s, some historical analyses of malaria burden suggest that land development and distribution are as important as technological interventions in eliminating malaria.[4] To help clarify these multiple explanatory frameworks, we introduce biosocial perspectives and the sociology of knowledge.

In 1966, sociologists Peter Berger and Thomas Luckmann published *The Social Construction of Reality,* which defines the sociology of knowledge as "whatever passes for knowledge in a society, regardless of the ultimate validity or invalidity (by whatever criteria) of such 'knowledge.'"[5] Berger and Luckmann begin by explaining how people form shared mental conceptions about the world: when any group of people—whether they are sailors marooned on a desert island, first-year medical students, or commodities traders on Wall Street—find themselves together, they construct norms to govern their relations. As jokes, habits, and practices are passed on to subsequent generations, they become freighted with meaning and assume the status of immanent rules. If these individuals have children or initiate others into their community, the newcomers will over time experience these historicized habits as natural rules. Berger and Luckmann call this process *institutionalization,* in which "reciprocal typification of habitualized action by types of actors" leads to the eventual objectification of that habitualized action as an institution.[6] Assumptions and accidents become historicized into truths, and knowledge is created.

"To understand the state of the socially constructed universe at any given time, or its change over time," Berger and Luckmann write, "one must understand the social organization that permits the definers to do their defining. Put a little crudely, it is essential to keep pushing questions about the historically available conceptualizations of reality from the abstract 'What?' to the socially concrete 'Says who?'"[7] It is through this process that people's knowledge and beliefs about the world—all human knowledge, including science, "regardless of its ultimate validity or invalidity"—become legitimized in society, and the world can be said to be "socially constructed."

The mechanisms of legitimation are useful to keep in mind in any field; for global health analysis, legitimation helps explain how practices become institutionalized. When transformed into policies backed by organizations with claims of authority, legitimized knowledge comes to exert social control over individuals. People feel pressure to obey rules and conventions that have become dissociated from human agents and are instead imbued with coercive power because they have been legitimated and institutionalized. For example, individuals may choose to exercise and follow a "healthy" diet because public health norms recommend these behaviors; doctors may be unable to give patients an already-proven vaccine because it hasn't yet received World Health Organization pre-qualification (a stamp of approval for global health interventions). "Man," in other words, "is capable of creating a world which he experiences as something other than a human product."[8] Social constructions become naturalized over time, as if they were invariant parts of the nature of things.

Even demonstrable scientific principles, including those established beyond doubt, are socially constructed in the sense that they remain historical products of specific questions and experiments—and of human minds, which, in an alternate history, might have asked other questions and conducted different experiments. The *Diagnostic and Statistical Manual of Mental Disorders* (DSM) is a good example of the social construction of knowledge in medicine. Given that it is an authoritative text designed to guide practice and treatment norms for psychiatry in the United States, and to some degree worldwide, one might assume that it would be immune to cultural variance. But until 1973, the *DSM* maintained that homosexuality was a psychiatric disease.[9] In this case, social biases shaped medical diagnosis. Similarly, the *DSM* has redefined and downgraded the amount of time that is considered "normal" for someone to grieve after the death of a spouse or child. In the past, a person who still felt intense symptoms of grief a year after such a personal tragedy would have been considered depressed. But in recent decades, stigma associated with depression has decreased, and the use of psychopharmaceutical drugs has become more widely accepted. According to today's *DSM,* a person is considered clinically depressed if he or she still feels grief after two weeks. This arbitrary process of *medicalization,* whereby subjective experiences are redefined as disease—such as remaking war trauma into post-traumatic stress disorder, or severe cases of premenstrual syndrome into premenstrual dysphoric disorder—illustrates the social construction of knowledge and the institutionalization of medical norms.[10]

As we grapple with the social construction of medical knowledge, a technical distinction drawn from medical anthropology might be useful. While in general parlance the terms "illness," "disease," and "sickness" are used interchangeably, medical anthropologists posit distinctions between them. Illness can be understood as the subjective experience of symptoms by laypersons and their communities,[11] disease as the reinterpretation of these symptoms as objective categories by medical practitioners, and sickness as pathology at the population level.[12] Awareness of how both knowledge and policy are socially constructed helps students and practitioners take a critically self-reflective approach to global health delivery.[13]

THE UNANTICIPATED CONSEQUENCES OF PURPOSIVE ACTION

Awareness of the social construction of knowledge, however, does not illuminate how even well-intentioned initiatives can unwittingly cost lives and resources. Robert Merton's theory about the *unanticipated consequences of purposive social action* offers insight into this phenomenon. Purposive action, according to Merton, involves motives and, consequently, a choice among alternatives; it must also have a goal and a process.[14] Nevertheless, such an action may not achieve the desired aim and may in fact result in unanticipated, and sometimes undesirable or perverse, outcomes. Unintended consequences of purposive action vary, as do their causes. One potential cause is knowledge asymmetries: for example, a doctor might misunderstand the language or cultural traditions of a patient and misdiagnose or mistreat the patient accordingly. Even with all relevant information, one can always make an error or take an action that subverts one's ultimate goal.

Merton also identifies "rigidity of habit" on the part of individuals or institutions and "the imperious immediacy of interest" as potential causes of unanticipated consequences.[15] For example, the United Nations responded to the "imperious immediacy" of the plight of refugees fleeing the 1994 Rwandan genocide by setting up refugee camps in neighboring Democratic Republic of the Congo (shown in figure 2.1). Those camps, however, became a base of operations for the perpetrators of the genocide—a devastating and unintended consequence that helped launch frequent bouts of violence that continue to this day.[16]

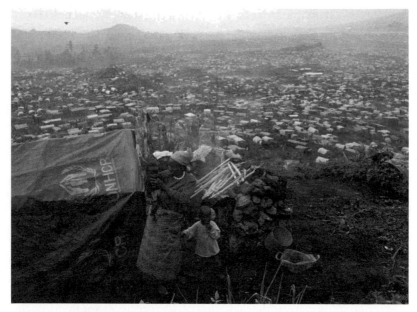

FIGURE 2.1. This Rwandan mother and her two children, refugees from the Rwandan genocide, stand in front of their sheeting shelter overlooking the Kibumba refugee camp, twenty miles northeast of Goma, Democratic Republic of the Congo, on February 13, 1996. Organized by international humanitarian organizations, such refugee camps, located along the border between Rwanda and the Democratic Republic of the Congo, unintentionally became bases of operation for Hutu militias that continued to systematically slaughter Tutsis in the camps and surrounding regions. Courtesy Associated Press/Jean-Marc Bouju.

Institutional values can also prevent us from anticipating possible outcomes. In the example of the Péligre Dam in Haiti, discussed in chapter 6, the values of international development institutions blinded the builders of the dam to the fact that the project would displace whole communities and trigger poverty and homelessness. Most large infrastructure projects, from dams to highways to power plants, have consequences both intended and unintended.

Finally, Merton explains that in some cases merely announcing one's intentions can alter the circumstances surrounding an action; even the best plans are laid on shifting ground. For example, in places where decent medical care is scarce, simply announcing plans to build a new hospital, or to upgrade an old one, can cause a surge of patient visits to the site before the new facility is ready. On-site clinical staff members, if there are any, must suddenly care for hundreds of additional patients each day, likely in outdated facilities that had previously handled only a few dozen patients each day. This is just one example. Realized and potential unintended consequences are too numerous to count, and their impact looms large in the history of global health.

THE RATIONALIZATION OF THE WORLD

Berger and Luckmann demonstrate how social institutions and legitimized knowledge shape the agency of individuals; Merton asks why purposive social actions often fail to achieve their intended result. Today, it is rare for individuals to be the sole, or even the primary, actors in an intervention. Institutions and organizations—governments, nongovernmental organizations (NGOs), corporations, and multinational organizations such as the World Bank and various United Nations agencies, including the World Health Organization—are more frequently the architects of global health practice and policy.

Embedded in the actions of institutions and some individuals are power and authority (or the lack thereof, as is the case for many of the patients this volume describes). Max Weber (pictured in figure 2.2) delineates three modes of authority.[17] *Traditional authority* such as patriarchal, patrimonial, or feudal power derives from history, custom, or (in Berger and Luckmann's words) institutionalization. It is the power passed on from generation to generation by monarchs, barons, village headmen, and tribal chiefs.

Charismatic authority is generated by extraordinary leaders capable of mobilizing large numbers of people around an idea or goal. It can be associated with religious leaders (such as Buddha, Jesus, Krishna, Muhammad, or Moses), political leaders (such as Nelson Mandela or, on the other end of the spectrum, Adolf Hitler), and leaders of moral movements (such as Mahatma Gandhi, Mother Teresa, or the Rev. Martin Luther King Jr.). Although charismatic and traditional authority are often contrasted, they can also overlap: the religious traditions inspired by charismatic leaders take on traditional authority based on custom after their founders die; many moral movements are also political in nature. Charismatic authority, though difficult to quantify, can be an important element of a successful global health endeavor. Mobilizing a team and attracting internal and external support, both critical for fledgling projects, may depend on the irreplaceable, unquantifiable attraction and effectiveness of a particular activist or leader. As Weber writes, such leadership rests "on devotion to the exceptional sanctity,

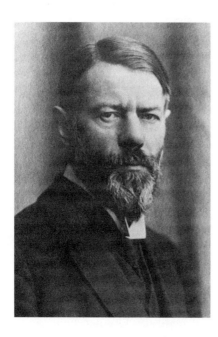

FIGURE 2.2. Max Weber, an influential social theorist who shaped our understanding of bureaucratic institutions, charismatic authority, the process of rationalization, and other social phenomena.

heroism or exemplary character of an individual person, and of the normative patterns or order revealed or ordained by [that person]."[18]

Most central to our work here is Weber's third type of power, which he called *rational-legal authority,* a category inclusive of modern law, the state, and organized institutions in which the authority of the ruler derives from laws and rules. This kind of modern authority functions in the context of what Weber terms *bureaucracy* (refer to table 2.1). Bureaucratic power, he argues, is fundamentally different from other kinds of power, deriving not from tradition or charisma, both of which are often vested in individuals, but from institutions. Bureaucrats—members of the bureaucracy—are parts of organizations that can replace them and will likely outlive them. As Weber predicted, the replaceable nature of bureaucrats resulted in an increase in programs granting certificates and degrees for specific, and increasingly specialized, jobs. Bureaucracies have a hierarchical structure of subordination: vocations and responsibilities are clearly defined and correspondingly compensated; and the individual, Weber writes, is a "single cog in an ever-moving mechanism which prescribes to him an essentially fixed route of march."[19]

Weber predicted that institutions would become the most powerful social structures in society, greater than family or community,

TABLE 2.1   MAX WEBER: MODES OF AUTHORITY

Type of Authority	Derives Its Power From
Traditional	History, custom, and habitualization over generations; accepted because "it is how things have always been"
Charismatic	Extraordinary leaders who can mobilize people around an idea or goal
Rational-legal	Consistent application of a set of rules and laws, whose execution depends on a system of bureaucracy, characterized by: • Fixed and official jurisdictional areas governed by formal rules • A hierarchy of authority composed of a system of supervision and subordination • Maintenance of files and records • Official activity distinct from private life (separation of office and officeholder) • Technically qualified personnel operating at full capacity • Specialization of tasks and division of labor

because they could both generalize and quantify. This development, he argued, would result in the technologization and bureaucratization—the *rationalization*—of everyday life. Describing "the disenchantment of the world," Weber explains how rationalization transforms the mystical and the mysterious into laws, rules, and regulations (in a manner similar to Berger and Luckmann's process of institutionalization). Protocols, technical jargon, neologisms, simplifications, standardizations, and scientific methods are all part of the rationalization that Weber believed would come to dominate the modern world and would increasingly legitimize bureaucratic power over both traditional and charismatic power. Think, for instance, of how common sense and generalized ideas of danger are now reified as specific ideas of defined risk that entail risk appraisal, categorization, management, forecasting, insurance, and prevention.

Rationalization, Weber recognized, has positive potential, yet can be very dangerous. It is unparalleled in its efficiency as a tool for administering large and complex systems because it is more generalizable and quantifiable and less ad hoc than other types of power. Although there is the ever-present possibility of corruption within bureaucracies, they are usually much more egalitarian systems than traditional or charisma-based ones. While a hereditary king or a charismatic sect leader might require certain familial connections or religious beliefs in order to allow an individual access to traveling papers or educational opportunities, bureaucracies tend to require legal—rather than ideological—authorization.[20]

Weber also presaged certain dystopian implications of the rationalization of the modern world. Bureaucracies at times function like an "iron cage," in which rules trump common sense, creative innovation, and human decency. Individuals working in bureaucracies have little incentive to change or improve the rules because their jobs are contingent on efficiently executing—not questioning—the specific tasks assigned to them. Once created, bureaucracies are thus difficult to reform or destroy: a large number of individuals have a stake in their preservation and constancy. Amid these and other observations about the modern world, Weber imagines the rising tide of rationality leading into a "polar night of icy darkness."[21]

Understanding the benefits and the dangers of bureaucratic rationality can sharpen scholarship and practice in global health. When we look at the institutions that govern international efforts in global health—such as the World Health Organization (WHO), the United Nations Children's Fund (UNICEF), and the U.S. Agency for International Development (USAID)—it is easy to spot both the tactical advantages that a bureaucratic structure gives them and instances in which rule-bound behavior leads to everything from improved outcomes (the intended consequence) to inefficiencies and even, at times, grave missteps. An example of the latter is the WHO's use of cost-effectiveness analysis to formulate policy relevant to the AIDS pandemic. Despite the existence of effective therapeutics since the mid-1990s, as we will see in chapter 5, AIDS was declared too expensive to treat among poor people until the early 2000s. Similar judgments have been made by global health policymakers about treating other chronic diseases such as multidrug-resistant tuberculosis (MDRTB), diabetes, or depression in low-income settings. Chapter 8 describes in depth how a narrow focus on cost of treatment per life-year saved has hamstrung the global response to MDRTB. Weber's notion of bureaucracy informs our discussion of global health policy and practice throughout this book, as does the brief consideration of Michel Foucault's work on disciplinary power in the next section.

DISCIPLINE AND BIOPOWER

History is written by the victor, or so the saying goes. This aphorism, and many like it, speak to the relationship between knowledge and power. Through the concept of *biopower,* French philosopher and historian Michel Foucault seeks to explain how biologic and medical data are used by the institutions of the modern world to define, count, divide, and—in a word—*discipline* populations. Biopower is another important addition to our theoretical toolkit for global health.

Foucault analyzes, among other things, the history of seventeenth- and eighteenth-century cultural and political institutions like the insane asylum, the prison system, and the clinic. He traces how these institutions constructed norms about what is considered sane and insane, licit and illicit, healthy and sick, which later generations inherited and, over time, accepted as natural. For example, the criteria for deciding whether someone is insane and should be sent to a hospital or criminal and should be sent to prison evolved from a set of institutional practices into norms, some of which became enshrined in law.

Similarly, the idea of prisons as places for reform rather than punishment evolved over time. Foucault's book *Discipline and Punish* begins with an unforgettable torture scene from eighteenth-century France. A prisoner named Damiens is taken to a scaffold, where it is ordered that "the flesh will be torn from his breasts, arms, thighs and calves with red-hot pincers, his right hand, holding the knife with which he committed the said parricide, burnt with sulphur, and, on those places where the flesh will be torn away, poured molten lead, boiling oil, burning resin, wax and sulphur melted together and then his body drawn and quartered by four horses and his limbs and body consumed by fire, reduced to ashes and his ashes thrown to the winds."[22]

According to Foucault, this gruesome punishment served a chiefly symbolic function. The king, the body of the state, had been attacked, and therefore the perpetrator's body would be attacked in return, beginning with the hand used to commit the treasonous act. Foucault terms this public display of coercive force *sovereign power,* "the right to *take* life or *let* live."[23] Weber might have classified this modality of power as traditional authority because it was reinforced by tradition and sanctified by religion.

Foucault compares this form of punishment to the prison systems that began to appear a few decades later, in which a different form of disciplinary power emerged as a tool of correction. Observing, reforming, converting, and categorizing became the mechanisms of discipline within prisons. Other institutions such as hospitals, asylums, and the bureaucracies of the state also began employing these techniques over the course of the late eighteenth and nineteenth centuries. During out-breaks of plague, for example, public health authorities developed an infrastructure of surveillance and quarantine for observing and col-lecting information about populations and individual bodies. After epi-demics of plague subsided, states continued to use this infrastructure to keep track of, and exert coercive force over, their subjects. In the mod-ern world, Foucault posits, disciplinary power is the principal means by which governments and other coercive institutions control populations.[24]

In 1785, Jeremy Bentham designed a theoretical prison called the panopticon, which illustrates the mechanisms of disciplinary power. A hexagonal prison with windowed cells around the perimeter and a dark guard tower at the center, the panopticon was designed so that inmates were always visible from the tower without knowing whether they were being watched. The possibility of being watched would lead inmates to correct their behavior automatically. The coercive force generated by the panopticon—constant self-surveillance and correction among those inside—is a form of disciplinary power. Foucault argues that the institutions of modern society exert a similar power; they discipline individuals instead of coercing them directly.

Foucault's concept of discipline helps us to understand biopower. The sovereign whom Damiens tried to kill had traditional authority, but the king's power was limited in important ways. He had the right of seizure and the right over life—that is, he could claim a certain amount of his subjects' labor or crops as tax, and he could kill a person for being a traitor or force men to die at war in his army. But the king did not know, or seek to know, what went on within the walls of people's homes, beds, prison cells, or bodies.

In the eighteenth century, however, along with the prison reform-ers came a rationalist revolution focused on quantifying and docu-menting many aspects of life—from anatomic dissection to classifica-tion to collecting census data to developing statistical analysis—often driven by the goal of consolidating power over life. Centralized bureau-cracies consolidated power in France by counting and controlling the health and social welfare of populations, moving from sovereign power to what Foucault called *governmentality*. These activities had many names and purposes, as they do today. Some employers document their employees' eating habits, for instance, in order to promote healthy liv-ing and make the workers more efficient; states require that children receive vaccinations before they attend school to improve population health and student performance. These acts carry state power and governance—the reach of governmentality—into ordinary lives and into the body itself.

Biopower, then, can be seen as the form of governmentality that deals with life. It is embedded in the processes of modern capitalism. Unlike sovereign power, biopower is diffuse and does not operate through specific visible agents. Likewise, biopower may be said to exert control over life as opposed to death: it brings "life and its mechanisms into the realm of explicit calculations and [makes] knowledge-power an agent of transformation of human life."[25]

According to Foucault, biopower emanates from two poles: first, the regulation of biologic processes (propagation, health, longevity, mortality) at the level of the population; and, second, technologies for discipline at the level of the individual (such as the panopticon) (see figure 2.3).[26] It is an essentially productive power, in that it endeavors to administer, optimize, and multiply knowledge about populations, subjecting them to precise controls and comprehensive regulations (by, for example, measuring the size and distribution of populations or categorizing populations by gender, age, race, occupation, fertility, mortality, and so on). Biopower is at work, therefore, any time quantification of life leads to categorization of life.

Manifold examples from the colonial and contemporary periods demonstrate this type of power. From anthropology, there is the history of using anthropometric measurements of the skull and a racial "science" to construct an invidious evolutionary ladder with Africans at the bottom and Europeans at the top. The colonial construction of stereotyped and institutionalized divisions between ethnic groups is a source of violence and conflict to this day. In Rwanda, Belgian colonists branded the minority Tutsis as a military and royal caste, in opposition to the Hutus, whom they categorized as peasant farmers. The distinctions the Belgians reinforced helped fuel ethnic conflict; decades later, the categories Hutu and Tutsi were the fault lines of the 1994 genocide.[27] Similarly, the British codified caste differences among the Indian population, a legacy that contributes to continued caste violence and inequality in India today.[28] There are few straight lines in history, and we must be wary of claims of causality in complex social fields like those in which ethnic violence occurs. Nonetheless, it would be naïve to disregard the long-term impacts of colonial policies, stereotypes, and hierarchies on postcolonial societies and polities today.

Biopower is not necessarily destructive, however. The two most

Biopower

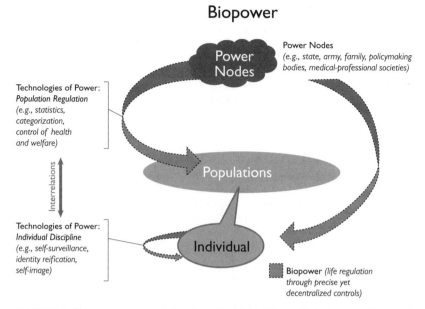

Power Nodes
(e.g., state, army, family, policymaking bodies, medical-professional societies)

Technologies of Power:
Population Regulation
(e.g., statistics, categorization, control of health and welfare)

Interrelations

Populations

Technologies of Power:
Individual Discipline
(e.g., self-surveillance, identity reification, self-image)

Individual

Biopower *(life regulation through precise yet decentralized controls)*

FIGURE 2.3. Biopower, a concept developed by Michel Foucault, helps us understand how the quantification of individuals' biology contributes to the discipline of the body and the regulation of modern life.

notorious industrial disasters of the past century, the 1984 Bhopal gas leak in India and the 1986 Chernobyl nuclear meltdown in Ukraine, illustrate how categorizing disaster-related illnesses can create new subjectivities and state policies. In Bhopal, state bureaucracies not only based disability compensation and medical care on illness categories that excluded the long-term effects of gas exposure but also demanded documents that the poor could neither access nor produce.[29] In contrast, while according to some estimates only two thousand people were affected by the Chernobyl disaster, fully one-third of Ukraine's population secured enrollment in the Chernobyl compensation scheme. The collapse of other state disability systems in the wake of Ukraine's withdrawal from the Soviet Union had created a deficit in services, which was partially remedied by the system created to care for Chernobyl survivors. Adriana Petryna calls this phenomenon "biological citizenship," a "massive demand for but selective access to a form of social welfare based on medical, scientific, and legal criteria that both acknowledge biological injury and compensate for it."[30] Hence, an important component of our toolkit is the critical examination of processes through which biopower operates in global health interventions and shapes our understanding of these interventions.

SOCIAL SUFFERING AND STRUCTURAL VIOLENCE

The study of global health consists of more than examining specific programs and interventions. At stake are the lives and livelihoods of millions of people and families. Although biopower may help identify the limits and conditions of knowledge, it may not help us understand suffering, the question of who suffers most, or why one person suffers and another does not.

Arthur Kleinman, Veena Das, and Margaret Lock developed the term *social suffering* to account for the forms of social violence that constitute inequity. "Social suffering," they write, "results from *what political, economic, and institutional power does to people* and, reciprocally, from *how these forms of power themselves influence responses to social problems.*"[31] In other words, institutions and their agents can perpetrate violence in the name of health and welfare. Social forces—including economics, politics, social institutions, social relationships, and culture—can cause pain and suffering to individuals.

Being born into poverty, facing discrimination because of the color of one's skin, or living in an abusive home are all dimensions of social suffering. The term also encompasses the interpersonal experience of suffering, the experience of chronic illness, and the ways in which society and its institutions unintentionally exacerbate social and health problems. The concept of social suffering addresses the intersection of medical and social problems—for example, the need for coordination of social and health policies in response to the clustering of inner-city violence, substance abuse, depression, and suicide.

We close with a theory that addresses the roots of global health inequities. Paul Farmer's observations of the links between poverty and ill health in Haiti informed the development of the concept of *structural violence,* which can be thought of as a form of social suffering. "Such suffering," he writes, "is 'structured' by historically given (and often economically driven) processes and forces that conspire—whether through routine, ritual, or, as is more commonly the case, the hard surfaces of life—to constrain agency. For many, including most of my patients and informants, choices both large and small are limited by racism, sexism, political violence, *and* grinding poverty."[32]

Farmer describes the plight of women living with AIDS in rural

Haiti. Without understanding the forms of structural violence at play in this setting, one might presume that these young women had contracted the disease because—to use language that casts them as free agents—they chose to be promiscuous. This conclusion, however, would be wrong on two scores. First, at the time of Farmer's research, the main difference between women in rural Haiti who had HIV and those who did not was the occupation of their primary sexual partner. With few opportunities to earn income themselves, women often partnered with drivers or soldiers, men whose mobility and status brought increased income. But these men were also more likely to have multiple girlfriends or sex partners, especially in urban areas, who in turn were more likely to have had contact with sex tourists from the United States and other countries. The rural female partners of these men, therefore, were more at risk of contracting HIV than were those women whose partners were local farmers. Neither group of women could be classified as "promiscuous." When structural violence is overlooked, agency is often overestimated, constraint underestimated. "Attentiveness to the life stories of women with AIDS," Farmer observes, "usually reveals that their illness is the latest in a string of tragedies."[33]

Structural violence helps deconstruct why for so many people suffering with disease and disability, an illness such as AIDS is but one additional misfortune piled on previous layers of hardship. At the macro level, the theory underscores the political, economic, and historical forces that pattern and link material deprivation and poor health.

CONCLUSION

This toolkit of social theories is by no means comprehensive, but its primary areas of focus—knowledge, power, institutions, and inequity—are all central to the study and practice of global health. Social theory provides an organizational framework for global health. These theories will not cure tuberculosis, bring a baby safely into the world, or care for the elderly. But illuminating some of the relationships that govern social action can help us design better programs, guide practical solutions to health challenges, and develop habits of critical self-reflection among practitioners.

Moreover, drawing on the biosocial framework that animates this textbook, we share an even more ambitious goal. We seek to show how approaches to global health problems can benefit from social theory, which helps us understand the dynamic relationships between those problems and the interventions launched to counter them. That is why theory matters. We hope, too, to convince the reader that the assortment of problems that constitutes global health can be conceptually framed in such a way as to develop global health as an interdisciplinary, academic subject.

SUGGESTED READING

Berger, Peter, and Thomas Luckmann. *The Social Construction of Reality: A Treatise in the Sociology of Knowledge.* New York: Irvington Publishers, 1966.

Farmer, Paul. *Infections and Inequalities: The Modern Plagues.* Berkeley: University of California Press, 1999.

Farmer, Paul, Margaret Connors, and Janie Simmons, eds. *Women, Poverty, and AIDS: Sex, Drugs, and Structural Violence.* Monroe, Maine: Common Courage Press, 1996.

Farmer, Paul, Bruce Nizeye, Sara Stulac, and Salmaan Keshavjee. "Structural Violence and Clinical Medicine." *PLoS Medicine* 3, no. 10 (2006): e449.

Foucault, Michel. *Discipline and Punish: The Birth of the Prison.* Translated by Alan Sheridan. London: Allen Lane, 1977.

———. *The History of Sexuality.* Translated by Robert Hurley. New York: Pantheon Books, 1978.

Kleinman, Arthur. "Four Social Theories for Global Health." *Lancet* 375, no. 9725 (2010): 1518–1519.

Kleinman, Arthur, Veena Das, and Margaret M. Lock, eds. *Social Suffering.* Berkeley: University of California Press, 1997.

Lockhart, Chris. "The Life and Death of a Street Boy in East Africa: Everyday Violence in the Time of AIDS." *Medical Anthropology Quarterly* 22, no. 1 (March 2008): 94–115.

Merton, Robert K. "The Unanticipated Consequences of Purposive Social Action." *American Sociological Review* 1, no. 6 (December 1936): 894–904.

Morgan, D., and I. Wilkinson. "The Problem of Social Suffering and the Sociological Task of Theodicy." *European Journal of Social Theory* 4, no. 2 (2001): 199–214.

Petryna, Adriana. *Life Exposed: Biological Citizens after Chernobyl.* Princeton, N.J.: Princeton University Press, 2002.

Scheper-Hughes, Nancy. *Death without Weeping: The Violence of Everyday Life in Brazil.* Berkeley: University of California Press, 1993.

Weber, Max. "'Objectivity' in Social Science and Social Policy." In *The Methodology of the Social Sciences,* by Max Weber, translated and edited by Edward A. Shils and Henry A. Finch, 49–113. Glencoe: Free Press, 1949.

———. "On Bureaucracy." In *From Max Weber: Essays in Sociology,* by Max Weber, translated and edited by H. H. Gerth and C. Wright Mills, 196–244. London: Routledge and Kegan Paul, 1948.

3

Colonial Medicine
and Its Legacies

JEREMY GREENE, MARGUERITE THORP BASILICO, HEIDI KIM,
PAUL FARMER

The groundswell of interest in global health issues over the past few
years sometimes causes observers to see the field as "new." There are
indeed many new features that characterize global health concerns in
the twenty-first century, such as the worldwide visibility of the AIDS
pandemic and the reshaping of global biosurveillance in the wake of
the SARS and H1N1 epidemics. Many of the therapeutics in the medical arsenal are also new and far better evaluated than their predecessors. But transnational and pandemic diseases are not new, even
when the ability to track them—for some, an example of biopower—
becomes more sophisticated or involves new diagnostics for previously
undescribed (or truly novel) pathogens.

The new, as always, is rooted in the old, and serious biosocial exploration of global health today would be incomplete without plumbing
history. Even a cursory evaluation of current global disparities in disease burden and access to biomedical therapeutics makes clear that
efforts to improve global health equity must navigate a landscape lit-
tered with the wreckage (and the occasional glorious monument) of
programs past. In turn, many of these failures—such as the global
malaria eradication campaign of the 1950s and 1960s (discussed in this
chapter)—may be attributed, in part, to a lack of historical reflection
and biosocial analysis. Like the social theories considered in the previous chapter, history can help us understand the intended and unintended consequences of global health interventions.[1]

The term "global health" was coined to define health problems and interventions extending beyond national boundaries, including those between developed and developing countries.[2] As noted in chapter 1, the term is distinct from "international health," used throughout the twentieth century to describe efforts to improve the health of populations transnationally—usually from global North to global South, and often grounded in development programs with diverse (and sometimes hidden) agendas. It is also distinct from "colonial medicine," the nineteenth-century term that described medicine in the days of imperial rule and colonization.[3] As this chapter explains, the legacy of colonial medicine has a long reach: both global empires and the institutions of colonial medicine persisted well into the second half of the twentieth century and, in some regards, persist today. Even the process of identifying and ranking health challenges—what historians of science call *problem choice*—demonstrates that global health priorities in the present have been patterned by social forces with roots in the colonial past.

In this chapter, we first briefly trace the relationship between global health and empire, exploring how colonial institutions exerted power over indigenous populations by adjudicating health status and care. Second, we describe how global commerce and international relations became enmeshed with global health and examine the specialized and technocratic institutions that were set up to manage public health and colonial medicine, institutions that were the predecessors of today's global public health authorities. Finally, by investigating a few key global health efforts and drawing on our framework of social theory, we reveal continuities that persist from colonial medicine and analyze the limitations of humanitarian models, old and new, of global health.

GLOBAL HEALTH AND GLOBAL EMPIRE

Notions of global health have influenced imperial ambitions, international relations, and global commerce for millennia. A concept of global health surely motivated hygienic reformers of the Roman Empire—when it constituted, at least in its own view, most of the known world—to standardize aqueducts and sewer systems and seek management of pestilential diseases across its many provinces.[4]

Since the fall of Rome, there no doubt have been countless attempts across the world to improve transregional health—and especially to stop plagues that disrupted commerce. There is no true start date for imperial medicine. There were empires in Asia and in Europe (and in the lands between them), just as there were in the continents that would later be called the Americas. But the more direct forebears of international, and thus global, health can be found among European colonialists.

It is no accident that the redefinition of public health and biomedicine as scientific professions coincided with the moment at which European powers began to build empires. Most narratives describe medical and public health advances originating in the metropoles of Europe and North America and diffusing later to the peripheries of global empires. In a few instances, however, the dynamics of knowledge transfer were more complex, as exemplified by the discovery of quinine to treat malaria. Many of the attributes of both modern medicine and public health grew out of the unintended consequences of the globalization of science, commerce, and politics in the mid- to late nineteenth century. The history of colonial medicine shows that the sites of imperial occupation often served as laboratories for medical strategies later taken up by the colonizers.

Health was a central concern for European imperial projects from the first seaborne expeditions to the New World, Africa, and Asia.[5] This was in part a result of the devastating mortality associated with the Columbian Exchange—the trade, intended and unintended, of plants, animals, and diseases between the Eastern and Western hemispheres following the voyage of Christopher Columbus. Europeans were exposed to novel pathogens and, in turn, brought many with them to the newly explored lands. Differential vulnerability to epidemic disease informed the logistics of imperial expansion, and racial ideologies were used to justify empire.

On a material level, differences in disease susceptibility between colonizer and colonized alternately aided and threatened plans for imperial expansion. Historian Alfred Crosby coined the term "ecological imperialism" to describe the exchange of organisms triggered by exploration and conquest.[6] In Haiti, for example, several hundred thousand indigenous Taíno Indians lived on the island of Hispaniola before the Spaniards arrived in 1492; by the end of the seventeenth century, when the island was divided between France and Spain, not a single native had survived. European conquest and "virgin-soil epidemics" of measles, smallpox, and tuberculosis, which spread usually by chance and sometimes by design, killed millions of American natives, from the Caribbean and across the continents and the isthmus that linked them. These sharply differentiated mortality rates were not seen as apocalyptic by the colonizers: as late as 1763, British officials were handing out blankets purposefully infected with smallpox among American Indians. European settlers had immunity, or partial immunity, to some of these diseases and therefore were able to propagate them among indigenous populations they planned to subjugate.[7]

History is rich with examples of colonial projects that undermined the health of indigenous populations. The sleeping sickness epidemics that struck East Africa at the turn of the twentieth century were linked to dramatic shifts in the movement of people and livestock that occurred under colonial management.[8] Connected along lines of intra-imperial transit, plague epidemics found new routes, such as the Indian Ocean shipping lanes of the British Empire in the first decades of the twentieth century.[9] The British colonial and military propagation of the opium trade between India and China had deleterious effects on individuals and populations—another example of the unintended consequences (addiction, an increase in piracy, overt conflict) of purposive social action (bringing vast stretches of land under British imperial sway).[10]

Early colonists from New England to Patagonia came to interpret the disparity in infectious-disease mortality as a providential sign of the rightness of the European imperial project and evidence of the frailty of "savage" bodies compared to European ones.[11] Over time, this observed disparity hardened into racial hierarchies based on embodied and seemingly unalterable biological characteristics.[12]

Colonial Medicine

And yet the European body was not universally hardy. In the second half of the nineteenth century, European cartographers elided "uncharted" territories to depict the world as the shared property of a handful of empires. In the early 1800s, European influence in many areas of Africa and Asia had been limited to fortified coastal settlements and trading zones, especially in tropical zones such as the "white man's grave" of the Gold Coast of West Africa. This sorry moniker referred to the staggering European mortality rates of 300 to 700 deaths per 1,000 population in the first year of settlement.[13] Multiple expeditions attempting to penetrate Africa's interior had failed, their members decimated by disease. As late as 1841, a missionary expedition of 150 Africans and 150 Europeans was launched up the Niger River to "civilize" the people of the interior. Forty-two of the Europeans succumbed to malaria;

none of the Africans did. In 1854, Dr. William Baikie finally led the first successful European voyage up the Niger by using quinine to treat tropical fevers.[14]

While the role of quinine in enabling the military occupation of the tropics has perhaps been overstated, the lingering narrative of the "white man's grave" is instructive on at least two levels.[15] First, it illustrates the link between colonial medicine and imperial conquest. Second, it illustrates the use of "the tropics" as a laboratory and a source of test subjects for medical and public health research and practice.[16]

Many scholars have noted the ways in which colonial medicine facilitated the expansion of European settlements in West Africa.[17] Quinine, still used today to treat certain forms of severe malaria, aided European exploits in the tropics. Perhaps one of the lesser-known products of the age of exploration was the introduction of the bark of the cinchona tree—originally known only within the area of modern-day Peru—into the pharmacopeia of European physicians. Cinchona bark had been used for centuries by South American peoples to treat fevers, but the trees were scarce. The fever-fighting bark became the object of fierce skirmishes among European powers who saw access to the cinchona tree as key to their military success within pestilential tropical zones.[18] In 1820, French chemists Pierre-Joseph Pelletier and Joseph Bienaimé Caventou isolated quinine from cinchona bark and demonstrated that it was the active ingredient against tropical fevers. The isolation of quinine from cinchona bark was an early example of biomedical therapeutics: isolating an active ingredient from a botanic source.[19]

Colonial medicine was often cited as one of the virtues of the imperial enterprise, even long after other defenses of colonialism had been discarded. One champion of colonial medicine was Hubert Lyautey, a key strategist in the French invasions of the lands they called Indochine and Madagascar and the first resident-general of the new French possession of Morocco. He famously proclaimed that "the only excuse for colonization is medicine."[20] Acknowledging the brutality of the colonial project, he nonetheless insisted that if there was one thing that "ennobles it and justifies it, it is the action of the doctor."[21] Reflecting on his long career as a colonial administrator, Lyautey noted in 1933 that "the physician, if he understands his role, is the most effective of our agents of penetration and pacification."[22]

And yet the project of colonial medicine did not merely serve the Promethean function of handing down the miracle of modern Western medicine to colonial subjects. Colonial medicine originated to support the military, before broadening to include European-born administrators and civilians, with services therefore concentrated in important ports and urban centers. Beyond that, colonial medicine expanded to protect the health of the laboring populations insofar as local labor was required to run the vast plantations and mines that extracted economic resources for colonial interests.

Britain's Colonial Medical Service, for example, was charged with building and staffing clinics in particular areas of the empire, recruiting physicians trained at home to work in the colonies. As the service slowly expanded from urban centers, where larger hospitals were likely to be located, central administrators coordinated the activities of medical officers in the outlying districts. With varying degrees of proficiency, the facilities offered curative medicine, organized public health campaigns, and collected data regarding epidemics and other health indicators (see figure 3.1). Accounts from medical officers describe extensive paperwork and recordkeeping as well as the need for "private practice" outside official duties in order to supplement their incomes.[23] Even as the mission "to develop and protect" expanded later in the colonial era, colonial medical services tended to focus heavily on particular epidemic diseases.[24]

Indeed, links between global health and global security were established early on. Colonial medicine in its military guise prompted some of the first sustained international epidemiologic investigations, which compared bodies in health and disease across all continents and led to widespread use of the term "tropical medicine" (discussed in the following section). For example, in 1835, the British Empire commissioned a statistical study of mortality rates among troops of European descent stationed throughout the world, which found that death rates ranged from 11.5 per 1,000 for soldiers stationed in the United Kingdom to nearly 500 per 1,000 for those stationed in West Africa (see map 3.1). African-born troops deployed within the same latitude—from West Africa to Jamaica, for example—did not experience significant alterations in mortality. These statistics, once tabulated and circulated broadly, helped give credence to the belief that the black body was better suited for labor in hot climates than the white body. This belief contributed to the justification of the trans-Atlantic slave trade, which had enslaved roughly 11.4 million Africans by 1870.[25]

In addition to being perceived as hardier under tropical conditions, darker bodies were also described by colonial administrators as vec-

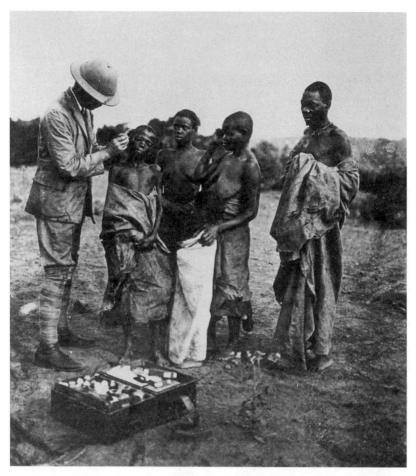

FIGURE 3.1. A colonial medical officer on Buruma Island takes a sample of blood from an individual suffering from sleeping sickness (from the 1902 Uganda Sleeping Sickness Commission). Courtesy Wellcome Library, London.

tors of disease.[26] In the late nineteenth and early twentieth centuries, the field of "imperial hygiene" focused increasingly on the "uncivilized" and "unclean" practices of nonwhite subjects, whose "primitive" state made them a menace to the civilized world. Perceptions of cholera demonstrate this rhetoric of difference as blame: its fierce waves of epidemics over the course of the nineteenth century were seen to erupt periodically from the populous centers of India's eastern seaboard and spread across Central Asia and into Europe. As British observer W. W. Hunter noted in 1872, the "over-crowded, pest-haunted dens around

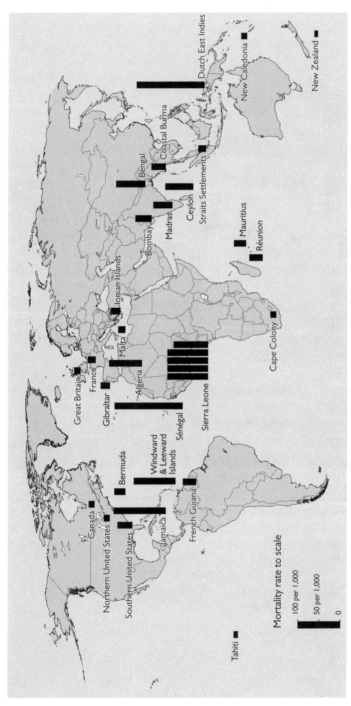

MAP 3.1. Mortality rates among troops of European descent throughout areas of colonial expansion, 1817–1838. Before medical advances made treatment of common tropical diseases possible, European troops faced major losses because of deaths from infectious diseases. Source: Philip D. Curtin, *Death by Migration: Europe's Encounter with the Tropical World in the Nineteenth Century* (Cambridge: Cambridge University Press, 1989), 12.

Jagannath" in the eastern Indian city of Orissa were "at any moment, the centre from which the disease radiates to the great manufacturing towns of France and England." Though the Indian pilgrims might "care little for life or death . . . such carelessness imperils lives far more valuable than their own." Hunter continued:

> One of man's most deadly enemies has his lair on this remote corner of Orissa, ever ready to rush out upon the world, to devastate households, to sack cities, and to mark its line of march by a broad black track across three continents. The squalid pilgrim army of Jagannath with its rags and hair and skin freighted with vermin and impregnated with infection, may any year slay thousands of the most talented and beautiful of our age in Vienna, London, or Washington.[27]

This concern with the links between distant, wealthy lands and diseased ones continues to shape conversations about global biosecurity today, including international dialogues about avian flu or SARS.[28] The recent, explosive epidemic of cholera in Haiti traces an ancient trail—from cholera-endemic regions of South Asia to the region whose natives were wiped out shortly after the arrival of Christopher Columbus and whose current inhabitants, now being felled by cholera, are the descendants of the very people held to be so resistant to tropical maladies.

The Birth of Tropical Medicine

The professionalization of colonial medicine kept pace with the development of vast empires. By the end of the century, few places remained beyond the reach of the ecological, economic, or territorial imperialism of the European, Russian, and Japanese empires.[29] No episode reflects this process as clearly as the 1884 Berlin Conference, in which European powers divided ownership of the entire "Dark Continent" among themselves with the stroke of a pen.

In addition to feeding notions of "the tropics" in the Western cultural imagination and codifying notions of racial difference, colonial health practices contributed to the construction of tropical medicine as a distinct discipline of medical research and practice. In the late nineteenth century, germ theory, elaborated by Louis Pasteur and Robert Koch, transformed notions of disease etiology by relocating the causes of illness from various "ill humors" (among other things) to microscopic agents of disease that came to infect the afflicted.[30] As cholera epidemics jeopardized European trade in North Africa, Koch, who had recently discovered the bacillus that causes tuberculosis, joined a series of expeditions to Egypt and India to identify the cholera pathogen. Through study of the intestinal tissue of cholera patients and autopsies of cholera victims, Koch ultimately succeeded in isolating *Vibrio cholerae* in 1883.[31]

By the turn of the century, Patrick Manson and other clinicians had firmly decoupled "tropical medicine" and "cosmopolitan medicine"; the latter concerned diseases like tuberculosis that could be found anywhere in the world.[32] Tropical diseases are largely associated with specific latitudes and regions; many are transmitted by insect vectors and caused by parasitic agents. Manson's principles were swiftly taken up by colleagues such as Ronald Ross, a British-trained surgeon working in the Indian Medical Service, whose description of the role of the *Anopheles* mosquito in the life cycle of the malaria parasite won him a Nobel Prize in 1902. The field of tropical medicine flourished over the course of the twentieth century and led to the identification of scores of pathogens and vectors responsible for the scourges that afflicted poor people living in hot climates. But as many have noted, temperature, humidity, and latitude are rarely, if ever, the sole determinants of the distribution of classic tropical maladies.[33] The history of tropical medicine helps explain why in rich countries the phrase "global health" connotes diseases of "elsewhere"—problems affecting an othered "them" rather than an inclusive "us."

The success of the new discipline of tropical medicine related directly to the shifting logics of imperial governance. Near the close of the nineteenth century, Joseph Chamberlain, secretary of state for the British colonies, advanced a "constructive imperialism"—the "exploitation" of vast "underdeveloped estates," which would require attending to the health needs of native and non-native laborers and British settlers. The new science of tropical medicine suggested that one could control the damaging economic effects of epidemic disease by fighting its nonhuman vectors (such as the *Anopheles* mosquito) without providing direct curative services to native populations. This logic resonated within institutions of colonial medicine that tended to deal with native subjects as populations rather than as individuals. Manson was named medical advisor to the Colonial Office and established schools for tropical medicine in London and Liverpool.[34] At the graduation of the first class from the London School of Tropical Medicine, Manson summed up the valuable contribution of tropical medicine to the continuing European presence in the tropics, noting, "I now firmly believe in the possibility of tropical colonization by the white races. . . . Heat and moisture are not in themselves the direct cause of any important tropical disease. The direct causes of 99 percent of these diseases are germs. . . . To kill them is simply a matter of knowledge and the application of this knowledge."[35]

While in theory a new paradigm of etiology—shifting the locus of disease from the "diseased native" to the microorganism—might have deracialized the discourse surrounding infectious disease, in practice the opposite was often true (as Hunter's description of Indian cholera epidemics demonstrates). Germ theory did introduce a nonhuman target for disease-control efforts, but it also introduced a new vector—the "healthy carrier"—whose hygienic practices were as important to disease control as traditional measures. The prototypical "healthy carrier" was Mary Mallon, "Typhoid Mary," a New York–based "Irish" cook known to have infected at least fifty-three people with typhoid fever in the first two decades of the twentieth century. Although she showed no symptoms of her *Salmonella typhi* infection, Mallon was branded a threat to society and spent the last twenty-three years of her life incarcerated by the State of New York.[36] Worse fates befell colonial subjects blamed (rightly or wrongly) for causing disease among white populations.

Warwick Anderson's historical research reveals the repressive public health measures used during the U.S. military occupation of the Philippines from 1898 to 1912.[37] Americans had long associated the Filipino lifestyle with backward morals and unhygienic behavior and blamed Filipinos for devastating cholera epidemics, in which more American soldiers died than in the entire Spanish-American War. When a 1902 epidemic killed two hundred thousand people in the U.S.-occupied Philippines, the U.S. Army Public Health Force declared a "cholera war" that razed villages, administered drugs—effective and (more often) ineffective—by force, imposed quarantines, and seized and cremated afflicted bodies.[38] Draconian actions such as these contributed to turning contemporary intellectuals William James and Mark Twain against American imperialism.

In this context, Anderson argues, the asymptomatic carrier of cholera microbes "recast the constitutional dangers of tropical climates into a form that stressed the hazards of a parasitic environment, a biological and social terrain in which the salients were the Filipino bodies containing invisible microbes."[39] When it was discovered that Filipinos were immune to some of the diseases that adversely affected foreigners, they were described as "microbial *insurrectos*"—an epidemiologic parallel to the armed insurgency—and as a direct threat to the health of the American residents of the Philippines.[40] The science of tropical medicine, far from extinguishing a racialized language of the "diseased native," enabled it. As one American medical officer in Manila noted, "as long as the Oriental was allowed to remain disease-ridden, he was a constant threat to the Occidental who clung to the idea that he could keep himself healthy in a small disease-ringed circle." Instead, another colonial medical officer quipped that "blonds and brunettes now had more to fear from contact with a variety of diseased native fauna than from exposure to the rays of the tropical sun."[41]

The management of cholera in the occupied Philippines provides an example of heavy-handed and racialized practices in global health—most of them completely ineffective, as far as the cholera bacterium was concerned—in the wake of germ theory. But even in less explicitly militarized encounters, a moral language of health, hygiene, and the "civilizing process" suffused colonial discourse (see, for example, figure 3.2) and was invoked to justify the continued imperial presence throughout the first half of the twentieth century. In stories, magazine articles, and advertisements, nonwhite colonial subjects were depicted as childlike or, worse, as part of the local flora and fauna that made the tropics a risky place for white bodies.[42] Physicians, social scientists, and social theorists—quite apart from the overt eugenicists—were complicit. For example, the French anthropologist Lucien Lévy-Bruhl popularized a theory of "primitive mentality" that posited structural differences between the "primitive" and "Western" minds.[43] Years later, the Martinique-born Franco-African psychiatrist Frantz Fanon used Lévy-Bruhl's metaphor as an example of how colonial medical practices perpetuate a sense of inferiority among the colonized.[44]

Fanon's writings helped to inspire a key strain of anticolonialism in twentieth-century intellectual and political history; in the wake of decolonization, his work formed the bedrock of a new canon of postcolonial theory. Yet the idea of a distinct "primitive mind" has persisted well into this century. In 2001, the head of the U.S. Agency for International Development (USAID), the lead U.S. funder of development efforts in what is now termed the developing world, decreed that antiretroviral therapy would fail in Africa because Africans "don't know what Western time is." He claimed that certain Africans would be unable to adhere to their medication courses, noting, "You say, take it at ten o'clock, they say, 'What do you mean, ten o'clock?'"[45] It is worth noting that this U.S. official was merely putting into words, and publicly, ideas that were widespread among leading voices in interna-

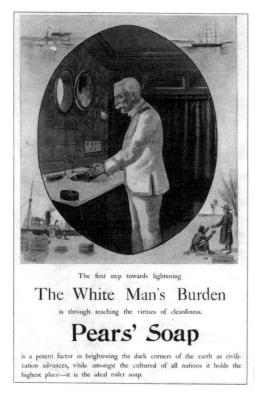

The first step towards lightening

The White Man's Burden

is through teaching the virtues of cleanliness.

Pears' Soap

is a potent factor in brightening the dark corners of the earth as civilization advances, while amongst the cultured of all nations it holds the highest place—it is the ideal toilet soap.

FIGURE 3.2. Popular culture during the colonial era often portrayed exotic, racialized visions of the colonies and the "diseased natives," as did this advertisement for Pears' Soap, which exemplifies the moral language of health and the "civilizing process." The advertisement appeared in *Harper's Weekly* in September 1899.

tional health, who also argued, in less cosmological terms, that AIDS treatment was "too difficult" or "too complex" in the very continent most afflicted by the disease (as chapter 5 describes).

Missionary Medicine

European and North American perceptions of colonized peoples typically included moral characterizations. As diverse peoples confronted each other through trade and colonization, they were also exposed to new forms of religion. Though Christian missions to foreign lands are as old as Christianity itself, imperial expansion opened new possibilities for proselytizing. These efforts included medical missions, which in turn helped to shape the history of global health. Michael Worboys points out that while colonial states concentrated their health efforts in urban areas and focused on epidemic disease, missionaries engaged more directly with local populations.[46] For people in many parts of the world, Christian medical missionaries were the sole point of contact with biomedicine. These interactions reveal that some of the roots of modern global health politics can be traced to the moral economies of missionary medicine.

Historian Megan Vaughan argues that, in addition to their different target populations, medical missionaries and colonial bureaucracies in Africa had different ideologies in approaching the "diseased native." Aligned with the colonial discourse, many missionaries believed that indigenous religions and social systems were backward, immoral, and unclean. The missionaries, however, held up Western civilization and Christianity as a solution to illness and a pathway to salvation. In contrast, the medical institutions established by the colonial state (which we refer to as colonial medicine) at times tried to limit the extent to which African communities—especially in rural areas—were disrupted by Western culture and lifestyle.[47] For example, "detribalization," or "acculturation," was frequently cited as a cause of mental illness. Vaughan describes a 1935 report by two colonial medical officers in Nyasaland (now Malawi) who argued that "the central cause of insanity was 'acculturation,' brought about, in the main, by [Western] education."[48]

Whereas colonial medicine focused on populations, missionary medicine tended to focus on individuals. To illustrate this distinction, Vaughan challenges the application of Michel Foucault's notion of biopower in the context of colonial medicine. Biopower (discussed in chapter 2) depends on the creation of active subjects who internalize and reproduce state definitions of their biologic selves. In African colonies, Vaughan argues, no real link was formed between population-level statistics and individual self-conceptions. Colonial states treated colonized peoples as collective Others—usually as tribes—rather than as productive individuals:

> In contrast to the developments [in Europe] described by Foucault, in colonial Africa group classification was a far more important construction than individualization. Indeed, there was a powerful strand in the theories of colonial psychologists which denied the possibility that Africans might be self-aware individual subjects, so bound were they supposed to be by collective identities. If modern power operates through the creation of the "speaking subject," then this colonial power cannot be the power which Foucault is describing.[49]

Missionary medicine, however, was preoccupied with the reformation of individual souls and bodies. Clinical care at mission hospitals was an individualizing force, according to Vaughan, focused on personal illness, personal hygiene, and personal sin.[50] Missionary medicine, therefore, operated through mechanisms more akin to biopower than its colonial counterpart.

Within Africa, the expansion of medical missionary work in the late nineteenth and early twentieth centuries was overwhelmingly Christian-based and generally came from Protestant churches rather than the Catholic Church. Though Catholic missions had been established around the world, the fact that Protestant missionaries were not necessarily members of the clergy probably contributed to their greater numbers and greater rate of expansion. According to historian David Hardiman, Catholic missions' ability to expand health services was hampered because the church discouraged nuns from seeking medical training; in contrast, female nurses and physicians abounded in Protestant missions.[51]

Initially, medical missionaries were not always well-trained doctors; until the professionalization of the medical field in the mid-nineteenth century, missionaries whose formal training consisted only of a few lectures often engaged in clinical care. By the end of the century, however, medical missionaries were expected to be trained physicians familiar with theology as opposed to pious people with some medical experience. This professionalization coincided with advances in medical science, including the advent of germ theory and antiseptics, anesthesia, and early vaccines. Hence, mission doctors at the turn of the century were far more effective in their clinical work than their predecessors.[52] The quality of these "deliverables"—in contrast to the imposed and ineffective attempts to stop cholera in the Philippines—began to rise even before the advent of antibiotics.

Just as disease was associated with backward morals of native peoples, traditional medicine was often linked to "heathen" religions. "Among all rude races," one missionary wrote, "magic and medicine are wedded, the priest and the doctor are one."[53] Clinical work was therefore often understood as more than treating illness; rather, many missionaries sought to convert patients both to Christianity and to their notions of modernity. On the one hand, missionaries hoped that the rational order of the clinic and the biomedical project would encourage patients to shake off traditional faiths.[54] On the other hand, extended hospital stays were seen as prime opportunities for conversion, and prayer and church services became central parts of the inpatient experience. In short, mission medicine "was not done for a purely medical purpose, but used as a beneficent means to spread Christianity."[55]

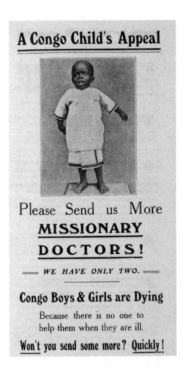

A Congo Child's Appeal

Please Send us More
**MISSIONARY
DOCTORS!**

—— *WE HAVE ONLY TWO.* ——

Congo Boys & Girls are Dying

Because there is no one to
help them when they are ill.

Won't you send some more? Quickly!

FIGURE 3.3. "A Congo Child's Appeal," an advertisement that appeared in the *Medical Missionary Journal* in 1909, requesting donations from Britons for a missionary hospital. Courtesy Bodleian Library, University of Oxford, shelfmark Per 133 d.83.

Just as missionaries were frequently the first point of contact between Europeans and non-Western peoples, the news and writings the missionaries sent back home were commonly Europeans' main source of information about the colonies.[56] Missions depended on fundraising in "home churches"; patrons who sponsored beds in the clinics learned about their occupants through missionaries' letters home (see an example of a fundraising appeal in figure 3.3).[57] The medical missionaries themselves became iconic figures in Western understandings of the colonies. The heroic image of physician-explorer David Livingstone, for example, popularized the idea of a "civilizing mission" and the role of a clinician in that process.[58] David Hardiman writes of the many young physicians inspired by Livingstone's fame and public writings to become medical missionaries.[59]

The iconography of Western physicians in developing countries persists, as those familiar with the global health movement can attest. Megan Vaughan compares colonial and missionary hero-figures to modern images of European and North American doctors working in Africa.[60] This comparison raises difficult questions: What motivates an individual to exchange comfort and familiarity for a career dedicated to improving the well-being of distant populations? To what extent does the fact that some of these providers have far more effective tools—preventatives, diagnostics, therapeutics—than their forebears dreamed possible make such comparisons misleading? What is noble in these colonial legacies, and what is perilous, for global health practitioners and the populations they seek to help? Are the answers different when the stated purpose of the so-called modern missionaries is health equity and shoring up local health systems? How important is the distinction between building up missionary health facilities and strengthening local health authorities? Students and practitioners of global health encounter these questions every day.

GLOBAL HEALTH, GLOBAL COMMERCE, AND THE FOUNDATIONS OF INTERNATIONAL HEALTH BUREAUCRACIES

In reviewing the history of global health, we find that narratives are often closely tied to specific diseases. The history of sleeping sickness, for example, is limited to the "republic of the tsetse fly," a wide belt across the waist of equatorial Africa.[61] But the understanding of global health derived from studying such a geographically delimited disease can sometimes differ from the one that emerges in the history of more distributed plagues such as tuberculosis, malaria, or pandemic influenza. Here, we consider one such disseminated disease (cholera), as well as an endemic disease (yellow fever), to illustrate the intertwined histories of global health, global commerce, and biomedicine.

Perhaps no disease exemplifies these intertwined histories as clearly as cholera. A series of major cholera epidemics over the course of the nineteenth century was communicated directly and rapidly along new trade routes. The outbreaks thus constituted significant threats to the future of global commerce. The propagation of and response to these epidemics reflected the diffusion of new transportation and communication technologies, which now define the self-consciously global character of the early twenty-first century. New modes of communication such as the telegraph and the trans-Atlantic cable warned of local cholera epidemics by bringing news of outbreaks spreading elsewhere. As new feats of engineering, such as the building of the Suez Canal, decreased the time of transit between Madras and Marseilles, for example, global commerce became an increasingly agile potentiator of the pandemic reach of infectious diseases. The Office International d'Hygiène Publique (OIHP), one of the earliest permanent international health bureaucracies, originated from a series of international sanitary conferences intended to address the vexing problem of cholera and international trade. As these conferences stretched across the late nineteenth and early twentieth centuries, almost all of them would ultimately focus on cholera.[62]

Most of these conferences produced more debate than resolution, with little agreement on the etiology of cholera. The theory of "miasma"—that exposure to unsanitary environments, in particular to "bad air" filled with noxious mists or vapors, is responsible for the spread of disease—was the most broadly accepted explanation of contagious diseases during that era. In European cities, the theory of miasma came to justify many early hygienic approaches to public health, such as the civic engineering of tenements and sewer systems designed to remove offensive odors from susceptible populations. In tropical colonies, miasmatic theory came to define the geography of social stratification in colonial settlements: European-born populations settled in the more salubrious hilltop areas, where fresh breezes kept the environment healthy, while native-born populations were relegated to the fetid, swampy lowlands associated with fevers and disease.[63]

After his now-famous investigation of a London cholera outbreak in 1854, anesthesiologist and amateur epidemiologist John Snow sought a meeting with the local health authority, the Board of Governors and Directors of the Poor. Snow presented the account of his investigation of the cholera epidemic in the neighborhood surrounding Broad Street, which suggested that the public pump was the epicenter of the epidemic and that the water it produced had likely been contaminated. Cases of cholera seemed to cluster around the pump (see Snow's drawing, map 3.2), and Snow's interviews with the families of those who were ill indicated that for most of these households, the pump provided the most accessible source of water (see figure 3.4). The meeting concluded with an order that the handle of the Broad Street pump be removed, which was carried out the very next day.[64] Though the original epidemic was already declining, the intervention may well have prevented a new outbreak. The removal of this pump handle is often considered the first successful policy recommendation supported by evidence-based infectious-disease epidemiology.[65]

The debate was far from over, however; discrepant claims of causality would be made for decades. On March 5, 1855, Snow testified before Parliament, whose members were debating the elimination of what some called the "offensive trades," defined as "trades that

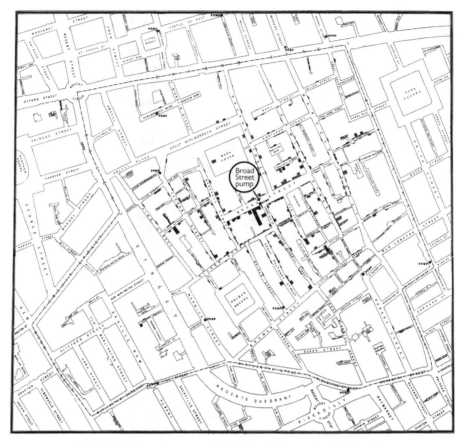

MAP 3.2. John Snow's drawing mapped the 1854 cholera outbreak in London, demonstrating that cholera cases clustered around the Broad Street pump, a water source that had become contaminated. (Scale: 30 inches to 1 mile.) Source: John Snow, "On the Mode of Communication of Cholera, 1855." Courtesy Ralph R. Frerichs, Department of Epidemiology, University of California, Los Angeles.

released foul-smelling, noxious fumes," such as bone boiling and tallow melting.[66] This sanitary reform movement was driven by the argument that "poisonous vapors, whether miasmas rising from marshes or from decomposing organic matter near human dwellings, were the main cause of disease, including epidemic cholera, which had killed tens of thousands of people in England since 1831."[67] Snow, however, had little regard for the miasma theory and said as much: "I have paid a great deal of attention to epidemic diseases, more particularly to cholera, and in fact to the public health in general; and I have arrived at the

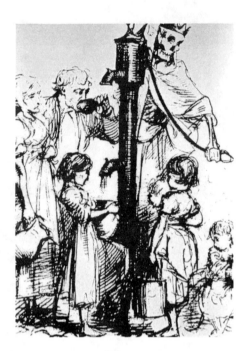

FIGURE 3.4. A contemporary image evoking the dangers of the Broad Street pump and its role in the 1854 cholera outbreak in London. Courtesy Centers for Disease Control and Prevention Image Library.

conclusion with regard to what are called offensive trades, that many of them do not assist in the propagation of epidemic diseases, and that in fact they are not injurious to the public health."[68]

Subsequent developments in the new field of medical microbiology would confirm Snow's suspicions. However, despite Snow's arguments, political interests heavily influenced international cholera regulations. The first forty years of the International Sanitary Conference (from 1851 to 1892) were stymied by debates that reflected national trade priorities rather than sound scientific evidence regarding disease transmission and prevention.

A few decades later, international deliberations over commerce and health in relation to the Panama Canal would serve as midwife to the birth of the first official international health organization, the Pan American Health Organization (PAHO), which remains an important player in the arena of global health to this day. Linking the Atlantic and Pacific oceans was a sixteenth-century dream that remained stalled until the completion of the Panama Railway in 1855. But a railroad was a modest endeavor compared to creating a passage for ships through the narrow isthmus separating two oceans. Driven by confidence and ambition, the French began construction of the Panama Canal. The cost was steep: between 1881 and 1889—the period of French activity—more than twenty-one thousand workers died, many of them from yellow fever or malaria.[69] The project foundered; the dream was defeated by epidemic disease, at least temporarily.

The idea of completing the Panama Canal regained momentum at the turn of the twentieth century. One of the chief French officials involved in the early construction began to press the U.S. government to continue the project, hiring a well-known U.S. lawyer, William Nelson Cromwell, to lobby for the cause. At the time, the United States had been considering building a canal across Nicaragua. Cromwell's job was to convince members of Congress that Nicaragua would be a dangerous place to build such a canal—a task he sought to accomplish by designing a stamp with an image of a long-dormant Nicaraguan volcano coming to life and using the stamps on informational leaflets mailed to every member of the Senate.[70] In 1902, three days after the senators received the leaflets, the United States announced its plans to complete the canal in Panama.[71]

To succeed in this project, the Americans had to accomplish what the French had not: keeping the workforce healthy.[72] Pestilential fevers were killing thousands of the laborers dispatched to build the canal, as well as their bosses, including engineers and government officials (see figure 3.5). Lingering belief in the relative immunity of black bodies to tropical fevers led to the widespread relocation of Afro-Caribbean laborers to the Canal Zone, where they were carefully segregated from white laborers and engineers but fell prey to the fevers just the same.[73]

Analogous to the work of Patrick Manson and Ronald Ross in Great Britain, Giovanni Battista Grassi in Italy, and Charles Alphonse Laveran in France, the Canal Zone soon became a public theater for the deployment of modalities of tropical medicine in the Western Hemisphere. Carlos Finlay, a Cuban physician-scientist (pictured in figure 3.6)—building on ideas set out by Pasteur, Koch, and others—sought to discover the microorganisms and vectors causing the dreaded "yellow jack" (yellow fever) that had long plagued Havana. By 1891, Finlay's research pointed to the mosquito as the responsible vector. Walter Reed, a U.S. Army physician in Cuba, confirmed the theory through a set of elegant experiments conducted at Camp Lazear in Cuba. Volunteers exposed to dirty linens and bedclothes of yellow fever victims—but protected from mosquito exposure—remained healthy in comparison to volunteers living in hygienic, well-ventilated conditions who were exposed to mosquitoes. Armed with this new evidence, General

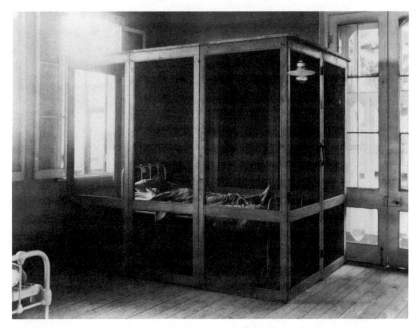

FIGURE 3.5. A yellow fever cage in Ancón Hospital, Panama, used to isolate victims of yellow fever during the construction of the Panama Canal. Courtesy CORBIS Images.

William Gorgas eliminated yellow fever from Havana through a program of mosquito control. Gorgas was then tapped to do the same in the Canal Zone.[74]

Implementing the wide-reaching yellow fever elimination project required broad institutional and international support. Shortly after announcing the U.S. initiative to complete the Panama Canal, President Theodore Roosevelt convened the First General International Sanitary Convention of the American Republics, held in Washington, D.C., in December 1902; Finlay was one of four individuals appointed to the convention's organizing committee.[75] Discussions focused on the general impact of diseases on international trade, including quarantine, prevention, and shipping regulations, and led to the creation of the International Sanitary Bureau (ISB), later to become PAHO.[76]

During the Second International Sanitary Convention, in 1905, H.L.E. Johnson, a U.S. committee member, explicitly acknowledged the strategic commercial interests driving the United States in the Panama Canal project and the subsequent Pan-American public health effort: "I feel sure that as a few months or years pass by, the diseases

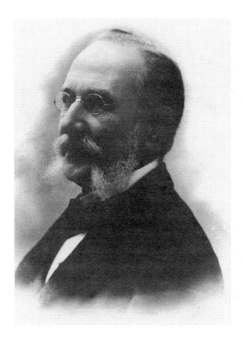

FIGURE 3.6. Cuban physician and scientist Dr. Carlos Finlay, whose research identified the mosquito as the carrier of the microorganisms causing yellow fever. Courtesy U.S. National Library of Medicine.

which have stood in the way of the completion of the Panama Canal, which we might term the ideal of the President of the United States to accomplish, will be removed and that the great good to this country which is expected in health, wealth, and prosperity will flow from it."[77] President Roosevelt himself continued to express "the greatest interest and confidence in the work of the sanitarians in the Isthmian Canal Zone."[78] These predictions and aspirations were realized in 1905, as the ISB, led by U.S. Surgeon General Walter Wyman, indeed managed to eliminate yellow fever in Panama.[79] Work continued on the Panama Canal (see figure 3.7), which was completed by 1914, beating the target by two years.

Long after the Canal Zone workers had cleared out their lockers and been repatriated (often forcibly) to their countries of origin, the ISB continued to hold international health negotiations in the Western Hemisphere. Following a Monroe Doctrine model that recognized American spheres of influence, the institution was renamed the Pan American Sanitary Bureau (PASB) in 1923. Today it exists as the Pan American Health Organization.[80] PAHO has, over time, for-

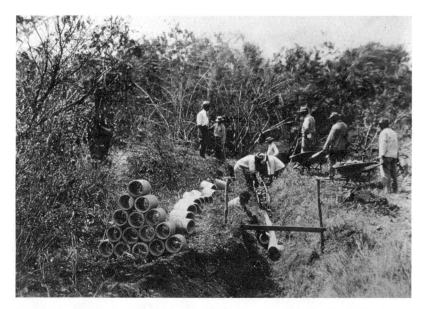

FIGURE 3.7. Sanitary engineers from the health department laying tile drains during the construction of the Panama Canal. Courtesy U.S. National Library of Medicine.

tified working relationships, shared discursive tools and vocabulary, and standardized disease definitions and methods of surveillance in an effort to serve as "a model for transnational health promotion and information sharing."[81] Although not the first organization to attempt international cooperation around public health issues, PAHO was the first permanent institution of its kind and is now the world's oldest international public health agency.[82]

The creation of the ISB was, in many ways, a realization of Max Weber's prediction that bureaucracies would come to be influential actors in modern society. In addition to PAHO, two other transnational organizations emerged in the early twentieth century: the Office International d'Hygiène Publique (OIHP), as noted earlier, and the League of Nations Health Committee. Both bodies attempted to coordinate international epidemiologic information and disseminate scientific advances. Neither organization achieved universal relevance, however, and both suffered from many of the same weaknesses as the League of Nations itself, including the overly optimistic prescriptions for global democracy that would become a hallmark of Wilsonian internationalism.

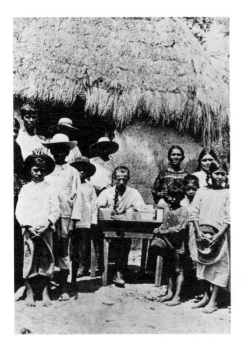

FIGURE 3.8. A Rockefeller Foundation microscopist gives local residents in Panama information about hookworm. Courtesy Rockefeller Foundation/ National Geographic Stock.

While these projects did not officially involve the U.S. government, many of them received funding from the New York–based Rockefeller Foundation, the single largest funder of global health efforts in the first half of the twentieth century.[83] The establishment of the Rockefeller Foundation followed the success of the Rockefeller Sanitary Commission in eradicating hookworm in the United States, a campaign reaching back to 1909. While the Rockefeller Foundation's focus in international health was long the eradication and prevention of infectious diseases (see figure 3.8), the early directors of Rockefeller international health programs sought to use biomedical interventions (such as antihelminthic drugs for the treatment of hookworm) as levers to build sturdier and more cost-effective public health systems (such as the creation of hygienic waste-removal systems and clean water supplies). Thus the roots of much of the terminology and practice of global health a century later—for example, using "vertical," or disease-focused, interventions to strengthen health systems—are far older than typically acknowledged.

Again we are brought back to Max Weber's work. Over time, these public and private institutions normalized transregional public health policymaking by diffusing the methodologies deemed capable of producing knowledge about health and disease. These technocratic bureaucracies created a sense of both rational-legal authority and stability that was new—a century ago—to the global health landscape. This stability allowed the organizations' assets to be passed down through time and also enabled greater specialization than had previously been possible. Facilitated by the rise of technical rationality, the emerging field of international health became more efficient and broadened in geographic scope and agenda.

At the same time, the nascent institutionalization of international health engendered the perception that centralized rules and processes were superior to local practices. Bureaucrats often found themselves trapped in Weber's famous "iron cage," finding it increasingly difficult as individuals to challenge the structures of institutional knowledge that had been shaped by social processes deemed scientific. While these institutions, from PAHO to Rockefeller, provided an opportunity to reach populations with a depth and breadth not previously possible, their power and effectiveness were sometimes limited by the values entrenched in the knowledge frameworks that colored their agenda and approach. Sometimes public health successes led to a certain "fetishization of process" that was neither nimble nor relevant. In Mexico, for example, the Rockefeller Foundation pursued a hookworm elimination campaign despite evidence of limited hookworm prevalence. The choice to embark on the hookworm program was made at upper levels of the Rockefeller Foundation bureaucracy, applying one-size-fits-all prevention and treatment techniques across Latin America.[84]

At the same time, the Rockefeller Foundation's anti-hookworm campaign also provided examples of how bureaucratization can boost efficiency. During the campaign in the Philippines (1913–1915), the target population was divided into "units of intervention," with a specialized task force assigned to each unit to systematically treat all afflicted persons in the unit. To measure progress, the foundation employed standardized recording methods, which generated detailed records kept in a centralized database. These administrative tools enabled the foundation to track the progress and impact of the campaign and allowed the transfer of this administrative efficiency across regions, from Asia to Latin America.[85]

Efficiency, however, came at the cost of comprehensiveness and, at times, the effectiveness that results from attention to local context in program design. Rockefeller Foundation records from the 1930s reveal that officers purposely avoided addressing other diseases that could clearly be attributed to socioeconomic conditions. One such example was tuberculosis, judged to be beyond the scope of the organization because of its links with poverty and other large-scale social forces.[86] At the Pan American Sanitary Conference in 1946, hosted by PAHO, a delegate from Peru described a delousing campaign among indigenous groups that was successful because of the involvement of the local population and the deep consideration that had been given to the local context. The delegate's insight, however, would not become a central focus of public health for many years.[87]

Many critical accounts have documented how the efforts of PAHO and the Rockefeller Foundation, whose programs were carried out in current and former European colonies, were vehicles for perpetuating knowledge frameworks that had taken shape within institutions of colonial medicine. Like other medical and development institutions of the early twentieth century, the Rockefeller Foundation sought to modernize "traditional," "backward," and "non-Western" cultures. It focused on problems amenable to technical interventions like vector control (for hookworm, yellow fever, and malaria, for example), pursuing a series of mass eradication campaigns against diseases. These endeavors yielded some remarkable successes. But they also relied on a narrow view of international health as a field concerned with populations rather than with individuals, devoting its energies to campaigns focused exclusively on diseases instead of achieving a comprehensive state of good health.[88] The apparent ease with which John Snow moved between his clinical practice (alleviating pain, largely) and his epidemiologic and public health efforts (protecting populations) became elusive. An emerging rigidity between clinical medicine and population-based health care efforts became readily discernible, and it would come to dominate—and ultimately undermine—international health.

Although the rise of formal global health bureaucracies in the early twentieth century was important for standardization, efficiency, and transregional cooperation, these developments left little room for consideration of community involvement or other locally specific social and economic factors. The language and concepts of global health equity were overshadowed by narrow and, in the emerging paradigm, "cost-effective" interventions that were designed to address the health problems of "backward" peoples who needed a dose of modernity. Some eradication campaigns were conducted with force, and many lacked community involvement. These trends would continue to haunt the efforts to eradicate malaria and smallpox in the 1950s and 1960s, despite the crumbling of most global empires and the introduction of more inclusive institutions during the latter half of the twentieth century.

HEALTH, DEVELOPMENT, AND THE LEGACIES OF COLONIALISM

World War I caused immense upheaval in the colonies and in Europe: as demand for raw materials skyrocketed during the war, a number of colonies experienced export booms that brought rapid (though still quite limited) industrialization and urbanization as well as a swelling of government coffers.[89] Ideologies shifted as the Allied powers used the language of self-determination to explain their motivations for war. Colonialism itself was called into question under these renewed democratic ideals, forcing colonizers to justify their presence in the colonies in new ways.[90]

The cataclysm of World War II—and the sober discussions of building a robust, rights-based international community in its aftermath (see chapter 9)—would have powerful effects on the development of global public health. Some of this great debate was quite explicit. Early in the war, the Atlantic Charter ratified the U.S. agreement to support Britain with Roosevelt's understanding that the end of the conflict would also spell the end of Britain's global empire.[91]

As the political realities of the postwar, and increasingly postcolonial, world became clear, the political, military, and economic power asymmetries between the global North and South were reorganized around emerging languages of "development," replete with a set of practices deeply rooted in colonial disparities. Development redefined the relationship between rich and poor countries, the colonizers and their former colonies. Although the war itself raised the key issues— and in part catalyzed the wave of independence movements across Africa, Asia, and Latin America—the language of technocracy and science was more explicitly harnessed than that of equity. Arturo Escobar, Wolfgang Sachs, and others from the academic field of development studies have traced the origins of modern development ideology to President Harry Truman's inaugural address in 1949, during which Truman introduced his vision of a "fair deal" for the postwar world:[92]

> We must embark on a bold new program for making the benefits of our scientific advances and industrial progress available for the improvement and growth of underdeveloped areas. . . . The old imperialism—exploitation for

foreign profit—has no place in our plans. What we envisage is a program of development based on the concept of democratic fair dealing. . . . Greater production is the key to prosperity and peace. And the key to greater production is a wider and more vigorous application of modern scientific and technical knowledge.[93]

The commitment to the welfare of the former colonies was reflected in the scale of the projects, which were often financed through official state policies, including export taxes and state control of exporting industries. The projects under this development framework were, however, heavily shaped by the legacies of colonial medicine. Given limited resources, administrators of development projects were frequently forced to choose between immediate provision of services and long-term investment in infrastructure. "Socialization for scarcity"— the assumption that resources for poverty reduction and international health initiatives will be in perpetually short supply—would come to be the dominant logic of international health, whether acknowledged or not. For example, tension arose between officials in the colonies and those in the British legislature, with the former pushing for spending on social services such as health and educational projects, and the latter asserting the importance of roads and communications (projects that would not require continuing expenditures in future years).[94] Colonial state institutions rarely extended their reach beyond a few urban centers, often on the coast.[95] As a result, development usually lagged far behind expectations and need. Moreover, when colonies gained their independence, these nascent nations were often left with incomplete infrastructures, very small national budgets based almost entirely on export crops, and enormous fiscal responsibilities to their populations.[96]

Flush with the optimism of independence in the 1950s and 1960s, some new states embarked on ambitious development projects similar to those run by the colonial forces that preceded them. Because state tax revenues were generally determined by money brought in from one or two export crops or commodities—for example, cocoa in Ghana, oil in Nigeria, and tea and coffee in Kenya—the success of these projects depended on global commodity prices. Postcolonial states thus achieved varying levels of "development" at different times, but few national health systems were consistently successful and comprehensive. Throughout the 1970s and 1980s, health systems, education, and infrastructure development suffered greatly as a result of conflicts, natural disasters, declines in export prices and access to credit, sharp political pressures, and heavy-handed postcolonial policies (discussed in the next chapter).

In addition to introducing new development frameworks globally, the end of World War II ushered in a different era of international cooperation. The new United Nations and its affiliated agencies strove to succeed where the League of Nations had failed. One of the first declarations of the United Nations, proposed by Brazil and China, requested the formation of a single agency responsible for international health cooperation. PAHO, the OIHP, the League of Nations Health Committee, and others were given the task of drafting the constitution for a unified global health body.[97] By 1948, the World Health Organization (WHO) had been formed and the first World Health Assembly had been convened, bringing together representatives from nearly seventy nations.

At its formation, two primary aims set the WHO apart from its predecessors: universal membership and decentralization.[98] The organization actively sought to engage states even before they became members of the United Nations: as of 2010, 193 countries were included in the member roster. Due in large part to the preexistence of PAHO and the OIHP, its European counterpart, and to the pressure imposed by the United States to maintain the strength of PAHO, the WHO chose a decentralized structure. It created regional offices that would carry out most of the responsibilities of the organization and a central office in Geneva to serve as a coordinating body. PAHO became the regional office for the Americas, while the OIHP was subsumed into WHO headquarters in Geneva. Integrating PAHO served to engage the United States in the WHO, which was especially important given its new role as a global superpower.

When cholera broke out in Egypt in 1947, the WHO took on its first international health crisis. The organization stepped in with both diplomatic efforts—WHO epidemiologists discouraged neighboring countries from enacting unnecessary quarantine regulations—and technical help, providing supplies for rehydration treatment, sanitation, and extensive vaccination.[99] The campaign was a remarkable success, and the WHO gained international legitimacy as an advisory and coordinating body. Nevertheless, its role as the principal funder and implementer of international health programs was not well defined until 1955, when the organization announced the most ambitious goal in its history: the global eradication of malaria.

The Malaria Eradication Programme

The parasite that causes malaria has a complex life cycle with two points of vulnerability: as a breeding parasite in the human host and as a latent source of infection carried by *Anopheles* mosquitoes. Although most effective malaria campaigns have included attempts to exploit both vulnerabilities, debate continues regarding the best way to protect humans from the illness. Again, socialization for scarcity has pitched this as an either-or debate. Those who advocate vector control encourage drainage of potential mosquito breeding sites, the use of insecticides in homes and fields, and widespread distribution of insecticide-treated bed nets. Many argue that vector control can take place even in areas without robust health services and that the full cooperation of at-risk populations is not required, a feature of the approach that was also attractive to colonial officials in the early twentieth century.

Parasite control, in contrast, relies on medicinal intervention in the form of malaria prophylaxis and treatment with such medications as quinine and, more recently, artemisinin. Proponents of this strategy cite the immense and prohibitive cost of draining all mosquito breeding sites. A third perspective, typically less popular within the medical community, argues that malaria will never be effectively controlled without transformation of living conditions and land tenancy agreements that keep peasant farmers poor—and thus less likely to invest in land improvements such as drainage.[100]

In the postwar period, such debates took place in a rapidly changing social and political environment, as a properly biosocial analysis reveals. But changes were also occurring in the pathogens, vectors, and tools to fight them. The years following World War II saw not only the end of colonization and an increase in international cooperation but also the development of new antibiotics and the pesticide DDT. These powerful compounds transformed the public's opinion of science in general and medicine in particular: that technological tools could be so effective against great scourges gave the world a strong belief in the power of science and technology.[101] Skepticism over the role of these technical fixes would arise later, but general faith in technology boomed in the immediate postwar years.

The WHO's Malaria Eradication Programme (MEP) can be viewed as a direct result of the success of DDT and vector control as well as a result of donors' preferences for narrow, top-down approaches to health. DDT had been used during World War II to protect troops from mosquitoes and afterward to control disease among displaced populations in Europe. Reflecting a global faith in the power of DDT, which silenced much potential debate about vector versus parasite control, the WHO announced in 1955 that it would coordinate and fund a program designed to completely eradicate malaria around the world.[102] Success in several small-scale campaigns, including the Panama Canal sanitation efforts, had strengthened belief in vector control. The Cold

---

The McKeown Hypothesis

Thomas McKeown, a physician and influential demographic historian, has challenged the extent to which medical interventions have contributed to improvements in health outcomes. In his research, published from the 1950s to the 1980s, McKeown classifies the variables contributing to the control of infectious disease into three categories: "medical measures (specific therapies and immunization), reduced exposure to infection, and improved nutrition." He argues that declining mortality can be attributed mainly to improved standards of living, which lead to reduced exposure to disease and, more important, advancement in nutrition. Contrary to the widely held belief that advances in medicine have been a main cause of population growth, McKeown suggests that medical measures played only a part, perhaps a small one, in improving health outcomes (see figures 3.9 and 3.10, which show steep declines in mortality rates before the introduction of medical measures to combat several diseases).[1]

McKeown's thesis has since been criticized for its methodology and for the political biases that may have influenced his argument.[2] Despite the technical flaws of McKeown's study, however, his ideas continue to resonate. McKeown forces us to think about the limitations of relying too heavily on targeted medical interventions, and he asks us, albeit indirectly, to examine broader approaches that consider the social, political, and economic factors of the local context. From this perspective, one can better understand the failure of the malaria eradication campaign and others that have ignored crucial dimensions that pattern disease persistence.

McKeown's work has remained relevant, but it was challenged significantly by the course of the response to the AIDS epidemic (see figure 3.11). In the span of three decades, scientists developed preventative tools, diagnostics, and powerful therapeutics that directly led to substantial and observable reductions in AIDS mortality in a wide variety of contexts.

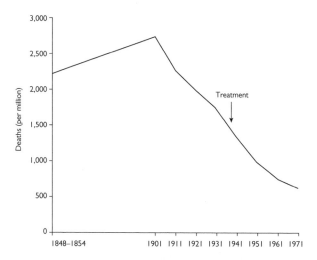

FIGURE 3.9. For bronchitis, pneumonia, and influenza in England and Wales from 1848 to 1971, McKeown and colleagues present data showing that dramatic declines in the mortality rate preceded major biomedical interventions. (These death rates are standardized to the age-sex distribution of the 1901 population.) Source: Thomas McKeown, R. G. Record, and R. D. Turner, "An Interpretation of the Decline of Mortality in England and Wales during the Twentieth Century," *Population Studies* 29, no. 3 (1975): 391-422.

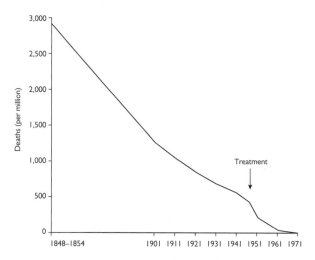

FIGURE 3.10. For cases of respiratory tuberculosis in England and Wales from 1848 to 1971, McKeown and colleagues present data showing a precipitous decline in the mortality rate well before major biomedical interventions were available. (These death rates are standardized to the age-sex distribution of the 1901 population.) Source: Thomas McKeown, R. G. Record, and R. D. Turner, "An Interpretation of the Decline of Mortality in England and Wales during the Twentieth Century," *Population Studies* 29, no. 3 (1975): 391-422.

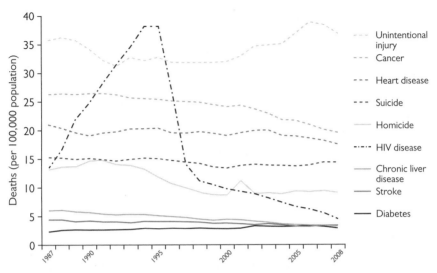

FIGURE 3.11. The case of HIV can be taken as a direct challenge to the McKeown hypothesis: AIDS mortality rates in the United States declined dramatically after the development of Highly Active Antiretroviral Therapy (HAART) in 1995. Source: Centers for Disease Control and Prevention, *HIV Mortality: Trends (1987–2008),* "Slide 18: Trends in Annual Rates of Death Due to the 9 Leading Causes among Persons 25–44 Years Old, United States, 1987–2008," www.cdc.gov/hiv/topics/surveillance/resources/slides/mortality/slides/mortality.pdf. Courtesy Centers for Disease Control and Prevention.

War may have also played a role in favoring an eradication campaign over a more comprehensive rural development plan that would have facilitated malaria control: wary of the ideologies underpinning a program seeking to organize and serve rural masses, political leaders in the United States and other Western powers tended to prefer a more vertical, disease-specific approach.[103]

Although the Malaria Eradication Programme included some distribution of chloroquine, an antimalarial, the MEP favored the tactic of spraying DDT inside homes. Every home in malaria-stricken regions was to be sprayed at least once a year until the disease was eradicated. Even considering DDT's effectiveness and ease of application, this program was slated to be an enormous undertaking. Spraying teams around the world faced tremendous obstacles, including accessing very remote areas, earning the cooperation of residents, anticipating the possible reintroduction of the parasite from neighboring regions that lacked robust malaria eradication programs, and paying the skyrocketing costs of personnel and supplies. The program was essentially top-down in nature. Local teams received orders from the WHO and did not have the flexibility to adapt them to local social or geographic conditions or to address problems that arose during the campaign, such as distrust between local populations and spray teams, or labor migration patterns that periodically reintroduced the parasite into previously malaria-free areas.[104] There were other forms of resistance, too. By the mid-1960s, mosquitoes and the malaria parasite were demonstrating resistance (to DDT and chloroquine, respectively), and the future of malaria eradication began to look extremely expensive, if not outright impossible.

When the WHO abandoned the Malaria Eradication Programme in 1969, opting for a less ambitious program of malaria control, eighteen countries that had participated declared eradication, and eight more followed in the next few years. As historian Randall Packard points out, however, every one of these countries was either developed (such as the United States and Spain), an island (including much of the Caribbean), or socialist (primarily Eastern European nations).[105] He argues that the primary reason for the failure of the MEP was not lack of resources or mosquito resistance to DDT, nor was it the calls from environmentalists to end the use of DDT, which were not heeded until well after the WHO had abandoned the MEP. Rather, the campaign failed, writes Packard, because of overwhelming belief in technological fixes. The WHO eradication campaign underestimated the biosocial fact that malaria is a disease deeply embedded in social factors like agricultural traditions (including the use of irrigation reservoirs) and labor migration patterns; a campaign like the MEP could succeed only when effective diagnostic, preventative, and therapeutic tools were linked to a transformation of living conditions in the poor countries in which malaria remains, to this day, a leading killer of children and adults.

Smallpox Eradication

Not all eradication campaigns were doomed to fail. The WHO initiated the smallpox eradication campaign in 1967 as its efforts against malaria were winding down. The smallpox program focused on two main activities: large-scale vaccination, and surveillance and containment. The vaccination campaigns aimed to reach 80 percent of the population of endemic areas, both by convening large gatherings of local residents at a single vaccination point and by sending vaccination teams from house to house. For surveillance and containment, a strong reporting infrastructure was necessary to enable local health workers to notify a country's smallpox-control program when ill residents were identified.[106] Once a case was discovered, health workers were expected to isolate the sick, quarantine those who had come into contact with infected people, ensure vaccination of the whole community, and disinfect all surfaces that might have been contaminated with the virus.[107] This system required large numbers of health workers, but not necessarily professionals with advanced training. In fact, the vast majority of people engaged in this campaign were trained quickly and paid very little.[108]

The eradication of smallpox is lauded as a triumph of modern public health efforts, in part because of superior program management and design. There were significant obstacles, such as detecting smallpox sufferers in rural areas, where cases often went unreported. Patients would frequently not seek care even after symptoms developed, primarily because no known treatment for the disease existed (and of course because modern biomedical care, with little to offer, was only scantily available in smallpox-affected regions). As with malaria, migration created the risk of reimporting the disease into previously eradicated areas. Distributing vaccines and training health workers across broad swaths of the developing world also posed major logistical challenges for implementers to overcome. In addition to remarkable program design and management, several external factors enabled success as well: smallpox is easily identifiable, symptoms appear quickly, transmission is easily tracked, and the vaccine is effective and easy to administer (see table 3.1).[109] In 1977, it was announced that smallpox had been eradicated globally (see map 3.3).

Despite its success, the campaign was not without controversy. In three of the last countries to declare eradication—India, Bangladesh, and Ethiopia—health workers met strong resistance from local populations. In fact, multiple incidents of coercion, sometimes violent and often under the auspices of expatriate health officials commissioned by the WHO to coordinate campaigns, were reported during the end of the campaign in South Asia. Besides being a human rights concern, forced vaccinations left a residue of resentment in rural communities, potentially hampering future public health efforts.[110]

TABLE 3.1   FACTORS AFFECTING THE SUCCESS OF ERADICATION EFFORTS:
MALARIA VERSUS SMALLPOX

	Malaria	Smallpox
Transmission	Vector-borne: *Anopheles* mosquitoes	Direct personal contact
Recurrence	Patients may experience recurrent bouts throughout their lifetime	No recurrence; immunity is acquired after a single infection or vaccination
Latency	Can remain in the body without symptoms for several months	Symptoms appear within ten to fourteen days
Case-Finding	Diagnosis can be challenging; presentation mirrors other diseases	Infection is marked by obvious and distinctive sores on the body
Prevention	Either vector control (bed nets, DDT spraying) or parasite control (chemoprophylaxis)	Vaccine is extremely effective

Nevertheless, the success of the WHO's campaign against small-pox restored the agency's political stature, which had been damaged by the failure of malaria eradication. Historical reflection suggests that the smallpox campaign may, in the eyes of some, be considered insufficient, since in many regions it failed to build infrastructure for long-term impact, as demonstrated in subsequent vaccination drives and other public health efforts. The top-down approach of the campaign, which prioritized technological fixes over consideration of local context and broader infrastructure, and which at times compromised the agency of the populations targeted for intervention, would later be critiqued by advocates of community-based primary health care. To some extent, the smallpox campaign allowed a continuation of the discourses of colonial medicine, such as underlying notions of the diseased native, a pathologized collective, and faith in technological fixes. All of that said, however, the world had been freed of a terrible scourge. Program implementers achieved a goal that many critics believed would be unattainable and overcame numerous logistical and political challenges at each stage. Smallpox had been responsible for 300 million to 500 million deaths in the twentieth century, and the last naturally occurring outbreak occurred on October 27, 1977.[111] For many, the eradication of smallpox remains the high-water mark of twentieth-century global health efforts.

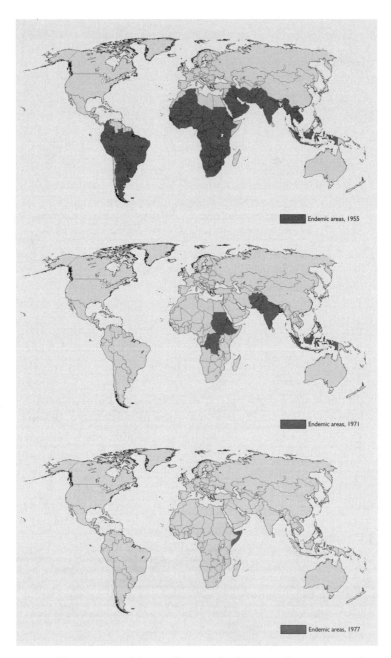

MAP 3.3. The progress of the smallpox eradication campaign, 1955–1977. In 1955, much of the global South faced a heavy smallpox burden. The WHO's eradication campaign began in 1967, and by 1971 the disease had been eliminated from many countries. Somalia was the last country to eliminate smallpox before global eradication was declared in 1977. Courtesy Centers for Disease Control and Prevention Image Library.

CONCLUSION

To discern the persistence of colonial health structures in modern-day global health practices is to understand the importance of historical analysis in tracing both the continuities and ruptures between present and past public health practices. Throughout this book, we argue that the resocializing disciplines can illuminate—and improve—global health practice. History provides a vital, easily available, yet frequently overlooked method of critical social analysis, which can shed important light on the political, economic, cultural, intellectual, and material specificity of the global health problems we now face. Historical consciousness of the colonial roots of global health challenges us to question the knowledge frameworks that constitute the emerging field of global health today.

If there is one message to retain from this chapter, it is that history offers many lessons for modern global health initiatives. Critical social history seeks to accomplish three goals: to render the present unfamiliar, and therefore open to social critique; to emphasize the role of *continuity* between, for example, current global health efforts and former colonial rule; and to work to understand the rifts and discontinuities that account for meaningful social change.

The knowledge frameworks carried forward from colonial times continue to influence both who is invited to the policymaking table and how global health agendas are then prioritized. As the next chapter argues, such frameworks often put a premium on vertical programs, such as eradication campaigns, at the expense of long-term efforts to strengthen health systems; they also may have little regard for the social and economic roots of disease or for interventions designed to address them.

Chapter 4 details a series of crises that arose in the 1970s. In light of the changing international politics of the postcolonial era and the failure of large-scale interventions like the Malaria Eradication Programme, the dominant models of international health and international development were called into question. The reformulation of global public health priorities in the 1970s led to broader international discussions of "horizontal" health interventions and the birth of the primary health care movement. [112]

SUGGESTED READING

Anderson, Warwick. *Colonial Pathologies: American Tropical Medicine, Race, and Hygiene in the Philippines.* Durham, N.C.: Duke University Press, 2006.

———. "Postcolonial Histories of Medicine." In *Locating Medical History: The Stories and Their Meanings,* edited by John Harley Warner and Frank Huisman, 285–308. Baltimore: Johns Hopkins University Press, 2004.

Armelagos, George, Peter Brown, and Bethany Turner. "Evolutionary, Historical, and Political Economic Perspectives on Health and Disease." *Social Science and Medicine* 61, no. 4 (2005): 755–765.

Arnold, David. "Introduction: Disease, Medicine, and Empire." In *Imperial Medicine and Indigenous Societies,* edited by David Arnold, 1–26. Manchester, U.K.: Manchester University Press, 1988.

Biehl, João, and Adriana Petryna. *When People Come First: Critical Studies in Global Health.* Princeton, N.J.: Princeton University Press, 2013.

Birn, Anne-Emanuelle, Yogun Pillay, and Timothy H. Holtz. "The Historical Origins of Modern International Health." In *Textbook of International Health: Global Health in a Dynamic World,* 3rd ed., by Anne-Emanuelle Birn, Yogun Pillay, and Timothy H. Holtz, 17–60. New York: Oxford University Press, 2009.

Birn, Anne-Emanuelle, and Armando Solórzano. "Public Health Policy Paradoxes: Science and Politics in the Rockefeller Foundation's Hookworm Campaign in Mexico in the 1920s." *Social Science and Medicine* 49, no. 9 (1999): 1197–1213.

Colgrove, James. "The McKeown Thesis: A Historical Controversy and Its Enduring Influence." *American Journal of Public Health* 92, no. 5 (2002): 725–729.

Cueto, Marcos, ed. *Missionaries of Science: The Rockefeller Foundation and Latin America.* Bloomington: Indiana University Press, 1994.

———. *The Value of Health: A History of the Pan American Health Organization.* Washington, D.C.: PAHO, 2007.

Escobar, Arturo. *Encountering Development: The Making and Unmaking of the Third World.* Princeton, N.J.: Princeton University Press, 1995.

Fanon, Frantz. "Medicine and Colonialism." In *A Dying Colonialism,* by Frantz Fanon, 121–147. New York: Grove Press, 1967.

Gish, Oscar. "The Legacy of Colonial Medicine." In *Sickness and Wealth: The Corporate Assault on Global Health,* edited by Meredith P. Fort, Mary Anne Mercer, and Oscar Gish, 19–26. Cambridge, Mass.: South End Press, 2004.

Greene, Jeremy A. *Prescribing by Numbers: Drugs and the Definition of Disease.* Baltimore: Johns Hopkins University Press, 2007.

Greenough, Paul. "Intimidation, Coercion, and Resistance in the Final Stages of the South Asian Smallpox Eradication Campaign, 1973–1975." *Social Science and Medicine* 41, no. 5 (1995): 633–645.

Hardiman, David, ed. *Healing Bodies, Saving Souls: Medical Missions in Asia and Africa.* New York: Editions Rodopi B.V., 2006.

Jones, David Shumway. *Rationalizing Epidemics: Meanings and Uses of American Indian Mortality since 1600.* Cambridge, Mass.: Harvard University Press, 2004.

Packard, Randall M. *The Making of a Tropical Disease: A Short History of Malaria.* Baltimore: Johns Hopkins University Press, 2007.

————. *White Plague, Black Labor: Tuberculosis and the Political Economy of Health and Disease in South Africa.* Berkeley: University of California Press, 1989.

Starn, Orin. "Missing the Revolution: Anthropologists and the War in Peru." *Cultural Anthropology* 6, no. 1 (1991): 63–91.

Vaughan, Megan. *Curing Their Ills: Colonial Power and African Illness.* Stanford, Calif.: Stanford University Press, 1991.

Worboys, Michael. "Colonial Medicine." In *Medicine in the Twentieth Century,* edited by Roger Cooter and John Pickstone, 67–80. Amsterdam: Harwood Academic, 2000.

4

Health for All?

Competing Theories and Geopolitics

MATTHEW BASILICO, JONATHAN WEIGEL, ANJALI MOTGI,
JACOB BOR, SALMAAN KESHAVJEE

The final quarter of the twentieth century was, to borrow historian Eric Hobsbawm's phrase, an "age of extremes" for global health.[1] The notion that all people deserve access to health care gained substantial support at a 1978 international conference in Alma-Ata, Kazakhstan—but it was soon eclipsed by neoliberalism, a different type of idealism that put faith in markets to efficiently deliver health care services. This history shapes the landscape of global health today. Analyzing the rise and fall of the primary health care movement in the 1970s and 1980s sheds light on current discussions of strengthening health systems; the ascendance of neoliberalism in the 1980s offers insight into the institutional development of many key global health bureaucracies, including the World Health Organization (WHO), the United Nations Children's Fund (UNICEF), the International Monetary Fund (IMF), and the World Bank.

The WHO's 2008 report *Primary Health Care, Now More Than Ever* attempted to reinvigorate the vision of "health for all" articulated thirty years earlier at Alma-Ata.[2] Universal access to primary health care remains a core aspiration for many practitioners and students of global health today. But the interplay of economic ideology, geopolitics, and institutional agendas during the roughly two decades considered in this chapter—the mid-1970s to the mid-1990s—continues to inform global health policy and practice. In describing these decades, this chapter details four major topics: Alma-Ata and the primary health care movement; the ascendance of structural adjustment;

UNICEF's selective primary health care campaign; and the emergence of the World Bank as a key player in global health.

PRIMARY HEALTH CARE AND SELECTIVE PRIMARY HEALTH CARE

In 1978, thousands of conference delegates from all corners of the planet rallied behind the goal of universal primary health care. "Health for all by the year 2000" was the audacious slogan of the day. But 2000 has come and gone, and the world is only marginally closer to universal health care than it was in 1978: billions of people across the globe still lack access to basic medical services. The global health discourse today is dominated by concepts like "cost-effectiveness" and "absorptive capacity"; "health for all" will sound utopian to some. What happened to the idealism of 1978? This section examines the origins and course of the primary health care movement—and its promise of equity and a human right to health.

Roots of the Primary Health Care Movement

The primary health care (PHC) movement was a child of the hopeful but tumultuous 1970s. Divergent economic and political ideologies, driven by the interests of Cold War superpowers, influenced the discourse of international health: most Soviet health ministers favored state-led health programs, while U.S. policymakers tended to promote market-based programs. This was also the era of decolonization: liberation struggles in the third world fueled grand visions of self-determination and grassroots community mobilization. This heady atmosphere was tempered by growing global awareness of the lack of access to modern health services across the developing world.

Momentum behind a global primary health care campaign emerged after "vertical" (disease-specific) eradication programs of the 1960s and 1970s achieved mixed results. While the WHO's Malaria Eradication Programme (1955–1969) failed to reach its goal, the subsequent campaign to eradicate smallpox (1967–1979) showcased the fruits of modern medicine, as detailed in chapter 3. The delivery of the last doses of smallpox vaccine in Somalia on October 26, 1979, represented a coup for international health. But the existence of a single-dose, field-deployable vaccine made smallpox eradication uniquely feasible. Similar "magic bullet" interventions did not exist for scores of other diseases that caused untold suffering and death in poor countries, and

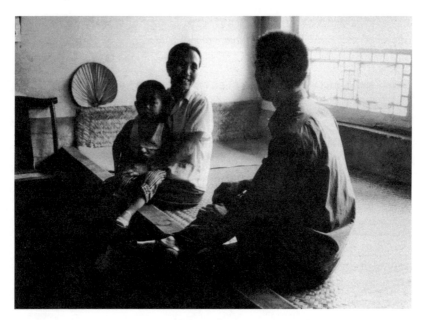

FIGURE 4.1. A clinician in northern China, a "barefoot doctor" who is part of the community-based Cooperative Medical System, speaks with a patient. Courtesy World Health Organization, photo by D. Henrioud.

significant delivery challenges complicated any intervention attempted in the absence of robust health systems. Memories of malaria eradication efforts led many international health policymakers to believe that tackling diseases that had no quick fix would require a more comprehensive—or "horizontal," in the jargon of the day—approach, namely, primary health care.

Health scholars and policymakers began looking for models of primary health care delivery in the developing world. Public health expert Kenneth Newell praised rural doctors in India, for example, for integrating local ayurvedic and biomedical practices and drawing on community participation to deliver care. A similar "health by the people" approach could, he argued, be adopted elsewhere.[3] For instance, the Cooperative Medical System, or "barefoot doctor" movement, in the People's Republic of China demonstrated the strengths of community-based medicine (see figure 4.1). In almost 90 percent of Chinese villages, the Cooperative Medical System built networks of health workers capable of handling public health interventions such as immunizations and sanitation and attending to basic needs.[4] Like the rural Indian doctors whom Newell admired, the barefoot doctors combined Western and local medical traditions—in this case, Chinese acupuncture and herbal medicine practices. Their efforts to control parasitic diseases, such as malaria, lymphatic filariasis, and schistosomiasis,[5] achieved impressive results and contributed to a significant rise in average life expectancy—from thirty-five years to sixty-eight years between 1952 and 1982.[6]

Some accounts have found that the Indian and Chinese programs—which relied on grassroots participation—cost less than concurrent top-down health initiatives.[7] Although these and other community-based programs have been romanticized—their successes, at times, exaggerated—by proponents of horizontal interventions, barefoot doctors in China and rural doctors in India demonstrate that basic health care services are deliverable at low cost by encouraging community participation and integrating Western and local medical practices.

Halfdan Mahler

Halfdan Mahler, born in 1923, is one of the most forceful leaders in the history of global health, and he is widely regarded as a founder of the primary health care movement. Raised in Denmark, where his father was a Baptist minister, Mahler (pictured in figure 4.2) has long been a champion of health equity and social justice; in fact, he once called "social justice" a "holy phrase."[1] Mahler's charisma and religious conviction explain, in part, his substantial impact on international health policy in the 1970s. One religious activist who worked with Mahler said of meeting him, "I felt like a church mouse in front of an archbishop."[2]

In the 1950s, Mahler ran a Red Cross tuberculosis-control program in Ecuador before serving as the WHO officer of India's National Tuberculosis Program. He was appointed chief of the WHO Tuberculosis Unit in Geneva in 1962 and worked on the WHO Project on Systems Analysis, which focused on national health planning. He was first elected director-general of the WHO in 1973 and was reelected in 1978 and 1983. Eager to find middle ground between the state-led Soviet model and the market-based U.S. model, Mahler looked to community-based initiatives capable of strengthening health systems in the developing world. He coined the phrase "health for all by the year 2000," the slogan of the primary health care movement. Today, Mahler remains a vocal champion of strengthening primary health care systems. In a 2008 speech to the World Health Assembly, he called for a new vision of health that would shed the "tyranny" of the health consumer industry and discover renewed value in primary health care.[3]

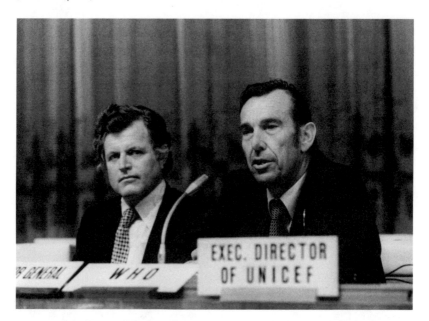

FIGURE 4.2. Halfdan Mahler (right), director-general of the World Health
Organization from 1973 to 1988, pictured at Alma-Ata in 1978, seated beside U.S.
Senator Edward Kennedy. Courtesy of the Pan American Health Organization/World
Health Organization.

The rising tide of the PHC movement had diverse roots. In the early
1970s, the Soviet minister of health, D. D. Venediktov, began calling for
an international conference on "national health services."[8] The USSR
was proud of its public health services and eager to showcase them
globally. However, Halfdan Mahler, director-general of the World
Health Organization from 1973 to 1988, was wary of hosting a PHC
conference. A champion of community-based health programs, Mahler
disagreed with Venediktov's emphasis on state-led health systems; he
also wished to prevent the devolution of international health policy discussions into a spectacle of dueling Cold War ideologies.[9] When China
also suggested a conference on PHC, however, Mahler conceded. The
stage was set for Alma-Ata.

Alma-Ata

The Alma-Ata International Conference on Primary Health Care, September 6–12, 1978, remains a landmark event in the history of global
health (see figure 4.3). Some three thousand representatives from 134

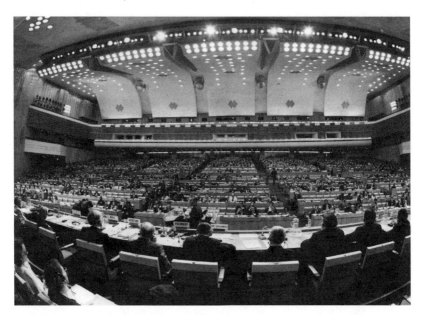

FIGURE 4.3. The Alma-Ata International Conference on Primary Health Care, September 6–12, 1978, in Alma-Ata, Kazakhstan. Courtesy of the Pan American Health Organization/World Health Organization.

countries and 67 international organizations affirmed a commitment to achieving universal primary health care by the year 2000.

Historian Marcos Cueto identifies three key themes in the Declaration of Alma-Ata, the document issued by the conference.[10] First, it introduces the concept of "appropriate technology" to describe medical and public health tools that are readily deployable in resource-poor settings. The concept was developed as a way to address the concentration of international health resources in urban hospitals, which often left rural dwellers—the majority of people in the developing world—without access to medical care. Mahler, for example, had decried the substantial investments in Kenyatta Hospital in Nairobi, while the majority of Kenya's population endured shoddy health infrastructure and low-quality care. He suggested prioritizing "appropriate health technologies" to strengthen rural primary health care systems. The second theme Cueto identifies in the Declaration of Alma-Ata is a critique of "medical elitism."[11] The declaration lambastes top-down health initiatives steered by highly trained doctors in urban (and often Western) centers and calls for increased community participation in health care delivery as well as integration of Western and traditional medical practices. Third, the declaration frames health as an avenue for social and economic development. Delegates at Alma-Ata argued that expanding access to primary health care services would improve education and nutrition, thereby bolstering the workforce. They conceived of health as an end in itself and also as a tool for development.

Perhaps most notable, however, is the declaration's all-encompassing definition of primary health care, which includes "education concerning prevailing health problems and the methods of preventing and controlling them; promotion of food supply and proper nutrition; an adequate supply of safe water and basic sanitation; maternal and child health care, including family planning; immunization against the major infectious diseases; prevention and control of locally endemic diseases; appropriate treatment of common diseases and injuries; and provision of essential drugs." (The full text of the Declaration of Alma-Ata can be found in the appendix.)

This broad interpretation of health care, and the conference that had conceived it, satisfied the major players at Alma-Ata. Venediktov was content that health policymakers around the globe had convened in the USSR; Mahler convinced delegates of his vision of grassroots health scale-up. Finally, despite ideological discomfort with the Soviet emphasis on nationalized health care, the U.S. delegation was also willing to sign the declaration because it resonated with Surgeon General Julius Richmond's new emphasis on prevention and basic health services.[12] The support of the United States was seen as a victory for advocates of international health equity, especially given that the statement reaffirmed the notion of health care as a human right.

The Alma-Ata Conference generated support for the primary health care movement among policymakers around the globe, but lack of access to medical care remained the status quo in the great majority of poor countries. A handful of governments, including those of Cuba and Tanzania, built new health centers and began improving rural health infrastructure in the early 1980s.[13] But even these few examples had more in common with Soviet-style statist health reform than the community-participation model enshrined in the Alma-Ata Declaration. The fate of the Alma-Ata goals recapitulates an unfortunate theme in the history of global health: ambitious plans can fail to be translated into action.

The bold vision of Alma-Ata foundered for several reasons. Of great importance, the Alma-Ata Declaration did not specify who would pay for or implement primary health care scale-up worldwide. Signers pledged support for the abstract principles of PHC without a parallel commitment to implementation. In the eighty-page *Report on the International Conference on Primary Health Care,* only a single paragraph discusses financing. One telling sentence reads, "The affluent countries would do well to increase substantially the transfer of funds to the developing countries for primary health care."[14] Critics who wrote off the primary health care movement as idealistic had reason to do so.

Furthermore, the early 1980s brought a sovereign debt crisis that left many developing countries unable to provide comprehensive social services and dried up international development aid; "health for all" was shelved, as it remains more than a decade after the year 2000. The final nail in the coffin was the emergence of an alternate international health agenda that found more support among decision-makers in the battered global economy and shifting ideological climate: selective primary health care.

Selective Primary Health Care: An Interim Strategy

Mere months after the Alma-Ata Conference, a group of policymakers from wealthy nations convened a meeting at the Rockefeller Foundation's Bellagio conference center in Italy (shown in figure 4.4) to discuss the future of world health. The Rockefeller Foundation intended the conference to focus on the impact of population growth on health, a topic that concerned many international development agencies.[15] Instead, the Bellagio Conference gave birth to a new plan—one with clear action steps and funding commitments—to improve health around the globe.

In preparation for the Bellagio meeting, researchers Julia Walsh and Kenneth Warren published an article titled "Selective Primary Health Care: An Interim Strategy for Disease Control in Developing Countries," which synthesized the major critiques of the primary health care movement and offered a different approach. Walsh and Warren paid homage to the "comprehensive primary health care" platform of Alma-Ata but argued that "its very scope makes it unattainable because of the cost and numbers of trained personnel required."[16] By estimating the costs and benefits of specific health interventions—that is, by doing cost-effectiveness analysis—Walsh and Warren sought to identify a package of health care services that would offer a high return in lives saved per dollar spent. For example, they included measles and diphtheria-pertussis-tetanus (DPT) vaccinations, febrile malaria treatment, oral rehydration therapy for children with diarrhea, and promo-

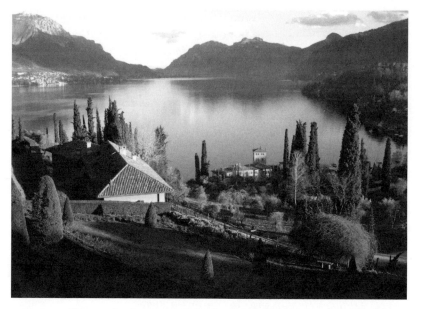

FIGURE 4.4. The 1979 Conference on Selective Primary Health Care was held at the Rockefeller Foundation's conference center in Bellagio, Italy. Courtesy League for Pastoral Peoples.

tion of breastfeeding as examples of cost-effective interventions. Walsh and Warren introduced "selective primary health care" (SPHC) not as the holy grail of international health but as an "interim strategy" for "an age of diminishing resources."[17]

This cost-effectiveness framework appealed to those convened in Bellagio and to many thought leaders in the aid enterprise. Over time, selective primary health care crystalized into four interventions, which came to be represented by the acronym GOBI:

Growth monitoring

Oral rehydration therapy (use of a simple solution of salt and sugar effective for treating diarrheal diseases)

Breastfeeding

Immunizations

In theory, GOBI offered a low-cost, high-impact platform for international health. GOBI interventions (discussed in greater detail later in this chapter) were also easy to monitor and measure, which attracted donors anxious to evaluate the effects of their aid dollars.

Although introduced as an interim strategy to complement the Alma-Ata Declaration, SPHC offered an alternate and incompatible vision of international health. Critics argued that GOBI excluded leading causes of death in poor countries, such as acute respiratory infections, and was merely a Band-Aid covering the real problem of deficient health systems.[18] The principal question was whether more suffering and death could be eliminated by boosting basic health care services or by delivering a limited package of cost-effective interventions through mechanisms that bypass many components of typical health systems. Thus continued the vertical versus horizontal debate, another all-too-familiar theme in the history of global health.

The major international health institutions clustered around the different poles of the debate between PHC and SPHC. The WHO, under the leadership of Mahler until 1988, continued to endorse the Alma-Ata Declaration. With Kenneth Warren directing its health program, the Rockefeller Foundation dedicated $20 million to SPHC. But it was UNICEF that soon emerged as perhaps the greatest champion of GOBI. James Grant, executive director of UNICEF from 1980 to 1995, led the selective primary health care movement to global prominence. A lawyer who had been raised by medical missionaries in China, Grant was a charismatic leader like Halfdan Mahler but had contrasting views about international health reform: instead of Mahler's community-based primary health care approach, Grant sought to deliver disease-specific technical fixes, given constrained resources. He fought for a "child survival revolution" that would cut the number of child deaths in half by raising immunization rates in developing countries to 80 percent. At the World Summit for Children in September 1990, UNICEF announced that the 80 percent immunization target had been met.[19]

The selective primary health care coalition obtained the support of the International Bank for Reconstruction and Development (the World Bank), where Grant's lifelong friend Robert McNamara had served as president since 1968. This was a break from the bank's policy of the previous decade. In the 1970s, the bank had focused its development aid on social services like education and health.[20] A 1975 *Health Sector Policy Report* explained the poor quality of health care in low-income settings as a market failure that demanded significant investment by the public sector.[21] Another World Bank policy paper stated that "the use of prices and markets to allocate health care is generally not desirable."[22] The 1980 *World Development Report* suggested further social-sector expenditures and embraced a conception of health, and of health care reform, not unlike that guiding Alma-Ata.[23]

As recession dragged on, however, the World Bank became cautious about public spending and moved toward a narrower approach comprising targeted interventions. In 1981, economist David de Ferranti took a leading role in the Health, Nutrition, and Population Division of the bank and began reorienting policy around neoclassical economic principles. By the time de Ferranti's working paper "Paying for Health Services in Developing Countries: An Overview" was published in 1985,[24] the bank had reversed its policy. De Ferranti's title is revealing: "*Paying* for Health Services" (emphasis added). Instead of focusing on health care quality and equity, the new paradigm reoriented the debate as a problem of cost containment for governments, best addressed by the market system.[25] The cost-effectiveness and optimization discourse of SPHC appealed to the economist base at the bank. McNamara advised Grant to create a strategy that would be easy to roll out and measure. Thus, after settling on GOBI, UNICEF counted the World Bank as a powerful ally in debates over international health policy.[26]

In 1982, Mexico defaulted on its loans, triggering a debt crisis across the developing world—which in turn supported the triumph of selective primary health care among policy circles. Facing the troubled balance sheets of poor countries and fearful of wasteful development aid, donor nations scaled back funding for global public health. Health ministries took up GOBI as an "interim strategy" until the economic climate improved.[27] Meanwhile, the debt crisis ushered in a new ideology that soon supplanted the primary health care movement altogether.

THE RISE OF NEOLIBERALISM

The champions of the primary health care movement at Alma-Ata soon discovered that even if they could forge consensus in the international health arena, their proposal was sailing against the winds of global politics. The "health for all" vision—which had drawn support from hundreds of policymakers in 1978—became almost unthinkable in the early 1980s.

Antecedents of Structural Adjustment

The 1979 election of Margaret Thatcher as prime minister of the United Kingdom and the 1980 election of Ronald Reagan as president of the

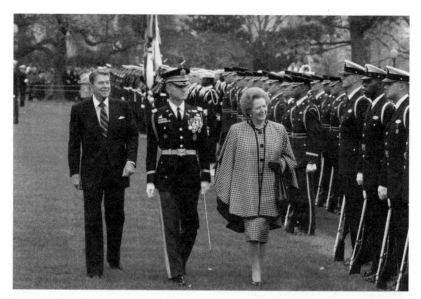

FIGURE 4.5. Prime Minister Margaret Thatcher of the United Kingdom and President Ronald Reagan of the United States, whose administrations assisted in establishing the dominance of neoliberalism in the West during the 1980s. Courtesy Bettman Collection/Corbis.

United States (see figure 4.5) ushered in a new era of conservative politics in the West. The theoretical framework of "neoliberalism," one component of their conservatism, drew on the work of Nobel laureate economists Friedrich von Hayek and Milton Friedman (pictured in figure 4.6), who argued that free markets distribute society's resources in an optimal way and to view with skepticism the efficiency of most forms of government intervention. This framework stood in opposition to prevailing economic theory—influenced by John Maynard Keynes—which promoted a larger role for the state in macroeconomic stabilization, market failure, and social welfare.

Armed with neoliberal approaches, which some would later term "market fundamentalism," economic advisors in the Reagan and Thatcher administrations argued that many components of social safety nets, including public-sector health care and education, were preventing markets from achieving efficient social equilibria.[28] Accordingly, by late 1981, the Thatcher and Reagan administrations had appointed policymakers with neoliberal orientations to the World Bank and the International Monetary Fund. Over the next decades, these two insti-

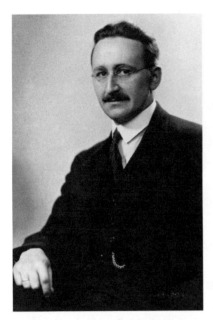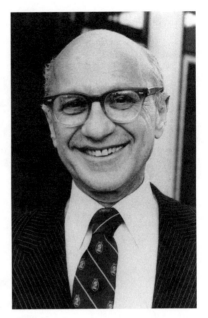

FIGURE 4.6. The ideas of Austrian economist Friedrich von Hayek (left) and University of Chicago economist Milton Friedman, both Nobel laureates in economics, were a vital part of the intellectual foundation of neoliberalism. Von Hayek photograph courtesy Hulton-Deutsch Collection/CORBIS; Friedman photograph courtesy University of Chicago.

tutions, guided by market-based approaches to development and health reform, had a far-reaching impact on the structure of health care in the developing world. The ideas of neoliberalism would also come to shape the way many policymakers thought about health and health services. The economic theory supported the notion that health was a commodity delivered within a market context instead of a right for all people as proclaimed at Alma-Ata.

As we have seen, the late 1970s and early 1980s were a tumultuous time for the world economy. High oil prices in the mid-1970s, followed by soaring interest rates, caused an economic contraction throughout the developed world, lowering demand for products exported from the developing world. The governments of the developing countries, many of which were highly extractive, nondemocratic, and unaccountable to their citizens, had taken out significant loans at flexible interest rates and were now squeezed by growing debt service on the one hand and declining demand for their exports on the other. In many cases, the situation was exacerbated by hyperinflation, fueled in part by expansion-ary monetary policies aiming to abate the initial crisis. The levee broke on August 18, 1982, when the Mexican government defaulted on its loans, damaging Mexico's creditors and signaling systemic debt problems across the developing world.[29] Within months, dozens of developing countries, especially in Latin America, were also nearing default. Commercial lenders panicked, drawing significant amounts of capital out of developing countries and pressuring Western governments to intervene on their behalf to increase debt repayment.

The "Washington Consensus"

The Reagan and Thatcher administrations urged the IMF and the World Bank to respond to the debt crisis forcefully. The 1981 Berg Report marks the World Bank's shift toward neoliberalism.[30] This controversial study argued that excessive government intervention had driven sub-Saharan Africa's economic stagnation and suggested significant limitations on public spending as a cornerstone strategy for development policy. By 1982, these prescriptions had become mainstream in discussions of economic policy in developing countries.[31] The IMF, created in 1944 to foster macroeconomic stability and avert a second Great Depression, was expanding its lending program to the governments of developing countries in the early 1980s.[32] Like the World Bank, the IMF issued loans with conditions: recipient countries had to agree to significant reforms on government intervention in the market, including shrinking public deficits, opening economies to free trade, and establishing rigid benchmarks for macroeconomic policy. "Stabilize, liberalize, privatize"—the "Washington Consensus"—became the mantra of IMF and World Bank policy.[33]

For developing countries across the globe, meeting the conditions of these "structural adjustment" loans—as they were called by the IMF—generally entailed contracting government expenditures, including outlays for social services. Scores of countries cut funding to their health sectors to meet the conditions for deficit reduction demanded by the new loan requirements. The scale of lending was enormous: during the 1980s, the IMF or the World Bank issued six structural adjustment loans to the average country in sub-Saharan Africa, five to those in Latin America, and four to those in Asia.[34] In addition to the impact of structural adjustment loans, the IMF and the World Bank—governed by representatives of powerful Western nations—exerted "soft power" over other development aid transactions, as donor agencies and official creditors followed the lead of these two institutions in conditional lending practices.[35]

Structural adjustment policies were a radical departure from the former lending conventions of the IMF and the World Bank. The IMF, for example, had been chartered as a lender of last resort for the global economy, charged with monitoring monetary crises. The World Bank had a tradition of making loans to poor countries, but these were generally for individual projects and often limited to infrastructure development. With the ascendance of the Washington Consensus, however, both agencies began lending unparalleled sums of money directly and repeatedly to the governments of developing countries.[36] In exchange for loans, the IMF and the World Bank demanded adherence to provisions regarding government outlays and economic policy, two building blocks of national sovereignty and self-determination. When the initial loans and the reforms they required failed to produce economic growth, countries were generally left with no other option but to borrow additional funds from the only available lenders, the IMF and the World Bank, which added to their debt burden and further weakened their economies. The debt crisis thus ushered in cycles of borrowing and lending with punitive conditions.

The Commodification of Health

The Washington Consensus emphasized market-oriented policy reforms and a diminished role for the state as a direct service provider. In line with these prescriptions, the World Bank promoted a new vision of health reform, resting on the notion that health care is a commodity—not a right—that can be efficiently allocated by the market. "Greater reliance on the private sector to deliver clinical services," reads a 1993 World Bank report, "both those that are included by a country in its essential package and those that are discretionary, can help raise efficiency."[37] The bank also promoted privatizing public health services:

> To help the poor improve their household environments, governments can provide a regulatory and administrative framework within which efficient and accountable providers (often in the private sector) have an incentive to offer households the services they want and are willing to pay for, including water supply, sanitation, garbage collection. . . . The government has a vital role in disseminating information about hygienic practices. It can also improve the use of public resources by eliminating widespread subsidies for water and sanitation that benefit the middle class.[38]

Predictably, neoliberal policies had a substantial impact on health care delivery in the developing world. In a study that analyzed the impact of the IMF on tuberculosis control in post-communist countries, David Stuckler and colleagues found that participating in an IMF structural adjustment program was associated with an 8 percent drop in government spending as a percentage of gross domestic product, a 7 percent drop in the number of physicians per capita, and a 42 percent drop in the percentage of the population covered by directly observed therapy for tuberculosis control. These figures were calculated after correcting for economic growth, level of economic development, surveillance infrastructure, past tuberculosis trends, and several other possible explanations.[39]

One pillar of the World Bank's privatization of the health sector was user fees—charging patients for utilizing health services. The bank's 1987 report *Financing Health Services in Developing Countries* reasoned that user fees would accomplish three aims: generate revenues for health services; increase the efficiency of health services by reducing "overconsumption" from patients and by encouraging people to seek care at low-cost primary care facilities instead of expensive hospitals; and subsidize rural health care with revenue collected from urban user fees.[40] The 1987 Bamako Initiative, led by a number of African ministers of health, embraced the World Bank's arguments, proposing to close the health-resource gap in poor countries by instituting user fees to boost household and community-based financing. Participants in the Bamako Initiative argued that universal access to primary health care would require "substantial decentralization of health decision making to the district level" and "user-financing under community control" to promote the sustainability of such care.[41] By the 1990s, more than thirty African countries had implemented user fees at health clinics.[42]

Though the results of user fees varied from country to country, the arguments made for introducing the fees by the World Bank and in the Bamako Initiative did not prove to be applicable in many countries that adopted such fees. First, user fees tended to produce underconsumption of health care, since even nominal fees prevented poor populations from seeking health services.[43] With little to no income to spend on health care, people living in extreme poverty either went without care or sought out alternative healers.[44] Evidence is found in reports that the abolition of user fees in South Africa, Uganda, and Zambia resulted in sustained increases in health center visits. In Uganda, the poorest quintile of the population disproportionately benefited when the fees were lifted. Eliminating user fees also had pronounced effects on access to typically free vertical health programs: for example, the immunization uptake for DPT (the percentage of the eligible population using the service) nearly doubled, from 48 percent to 89 percent, in Uganda in the five years after user fees were abolished in 2001.[45] Conversely, studies in Kenya have demonstrated that charging pregnant mothers even an amount as small as US $0.75 for an insecticide-treated bed net reduced demand by as much as 75 percent.[46]

Second, though the World Bank predicted that user fees would recover 15–20 percent of operating costs,[47] in actuality such fees did not raise substantial revenues—averaging about 5 percent of total health expenditures—for countries that implemented them.[48] In fact, in some countries, such as Zambia, the cost of administering user fees actually *exceeded* the revenue generated; thus, eliminating the fees would have increased funds available for health care.[49] The underlying goal, however, was not cost recovery, but privatization. By raising the cost of government care, proponents of user fees hoped that more private providers would enter the health care market. "User fees are a necessary precondition for self-financing," asserts a World Bank report, "as otherwise the public would lack an incentive to participate [in markets for private health care] when no- or low-cost health care is available through government facilities."[50] In reality, user fees in many resource-poor settings deterred the poor from accessing any health services.

To some degree, the World Bank did anticipate that user fees would be unaffordable for some, especially rural populations. Though the bank's recommendations included exempting impoverished patients who were too poor to pay the fees, in countries such as Kenya patient surveys reveal that poor patients were no more likely to be exempted from fees than those who had higher incomes.[51] User fees might have had appeal on multiple theoretical grounds, but their implementation in countries with limited administrative capacity proved difficult.

By the late 1980s, voices across the globe began calling attention to the unintended (and at times perverse) health effects of structural adjustment programs. In 1987, UNICEF backed a seminal report titled *Adjustment with a Human Face,* which documented some of the harmful consequences of IMF and World Bank policies on health systems across the developing world.[52] The report drew attention to several cases of supposedly successful policy adjustment (in compliance with IMF conditions) that undermined health outcomes. Frances Stewart found that among countries that accepted World Bank loans, interest payments increased from an average of 9 percent to 19.3 percent of budgets across Latin America and from 7.7 percent to 12.5 percent in Africa between 1980 and 1987. The increase in interest payments on debt came at the expense of per capita social spending on health and education, which declined by an average of 26 percent in African countries and 18 percent in Latin America between 1980 and 1985.[53] Though it is difficult to determine the extent to which structural adjustment, rather than preexisting economic and political conditions, was responsible for declines in social service funding, the "stabilize, liberalize, privatize" platform of the World Bank did little to strengthen the public delivery and accessibility of social services.

Dissatisfaction with the Washington Consensus arose outside the health arena as well. The United Nations Development Programme (UNDP) launched its annual publication of the *Human Development Report* in 1990 to refocus the debate from the application of neoliberal theories to the human realities of antipoverty policy. For example, the report emphasizes indicators for health and education—sectors in which government services can help mitigate the effects of poverty—rather than focusing narrowly on gross domestic product (GDP) per capita as a measure of development.

Despite increasing evidence about the harmful consequences of structural adjustment, such lending continued throughout the 1990s. Indeed, one of the best-known applications of the Washington Consensus came after the fall of the Berlin Wall in 1989: Western economic advisors recommended "shock therapy"—an aggressive approach to guiding former Soviet states that were transitioning to capitalism, which endorsed hardline free-market reforms mirroring those used in structural adjustment programs.

Viewed historically, the ascendancy of neoliberalism sounded the death knell of the primary health care movement. Calls for expanding primary health care systems ran counter to IMF and World Bank policies of shrinking government budgets. Leaders from different fields began advocating "health exceptionalism," exempting the expansion of health services from the constraints of structural adjustment reforms. In 1990, World Bank economist John Williamson, who coined the term "Washington Consensus," stated that "education and health, in contrast, are regarded as quintessentially proper objects of government expenditure."[54] However, these proposals remained overshadowed by market fundamentalism.[55] Only limited and "cost-effective" interventions, such as those recommended by selective primary health care proponents, found traction on the global political stage.

It is now widely acknowledged that structural adjustment, as implemented, often did little to achieve growth, reduce poverty, or improve health. Aggregate economic growth was negative across sub-Saharan Africa, Latin America, Eastern Europe, the Middle East, and North Africa during the 1980s and 1990s.[56] There are many competing claims of causality about these two decades of stagnation, most of them oversimplified. Some blame structural adjustment for the lack of growth; others argue that this approach didn't go far enough in addressing underlying structural weaknesses. Still others claim that leaders of developing countries mostly managed to dodge the strictures of structural adjustment, allowing business to go on as usual.[57]

IMF-supported countries in Latin America and Southeast Asia experienced repeated crises, which may have been linked to the severe conditions imposed by the structural adjustment loans. Some scholars believe that the deregulation of capital markets under structural adjustment helped trigger the East Asian financial crisis of 1998. In comparison, certain countries that undertook economic reform independent from the IMF and the World Bank, most notably China and India, performed significantly better during this period. But there are complex historical, political, and economic reasons for the growth of these two emerging economies. On one score, at least, humble conclusions can be drawn: structural adjustment eroded public financing of health services in many developing countries.[58]

In sum, more often than not, structural adjustment failed to fix the systemic problems—inefficient and inequitable allocation of resources, ballooning government deficits, graft and cronyism—it was designed to address; the 1980s and 1990s were characterized by sluggish economic performance and deterioration of health systems. Sub-Saharan Africa was hit particularly hard both because of low economic growth and the spread of HIV, which substantially increased the need for health services just as health budgets were being trimmed. For instance, in the late 1990s in heavily AIDS-afflicted countries such as Zambia, nurses and teachers died of AIDS almost as fast as they were trained.[59]

As the appraisals of these trends finally caught up to policymakers, one leading development economist stated in 2005 that "nobody really believes in the Washington Consensus anymore."[60] By the early 2000s, even the World Bank had begun supporting AIDS programs in Africa, and two different theories—geography-related poverty traps and the importance of nonmarket institutions—were being used to explain poor growth in the developing world. Although some leading development economists have reconceived the complex linkage between government and pro-growth economic policies[61]—arriving at far different prescriptions than structural adjustment—other scholars and policymakers continue to think that a variation on the Washington Consensus approach, with better implementation, is still the best hope for long-run growth in developing countries. The debate continues, as chapter 10 explores.[62]

It's a long way from "health for all" to "stabilize, liberalize, privatize." How did "consensus" move so rapidly from the principles of the primary health care movement in 1978 to those of neoliberalism in 1982? One answer draws on the theory of institutionalization articulated by Peter Berger and Thomas Luckmann (introduced in chapter 2). Radical change often follows moments of crisis, such as the 1982 debt crisis. Because the roots of that crisis involved global economic forces (high oil prices, decreasing demand for exports from the developing world), economists stepped in to "fix" the problem. A premium was thus placed on *economic knowledge* (interest rates, public spending, inflation), which supplanted other types of knowledge (political, medical, ecological, local) as new habits and norms crystalized around an assessment of what went wrong and what needed to change. The consolidation of conservatism in the governments of Reagan and Thatcher—who led two of the world's largest economies—supported the ascendance of this economic thinking. Voices like Milton Friedman's gained prominence, while others—like those of Halfdan Mahler, leaders of heavily indebted countries, and people affected by the closing of their local health clinics—faded from discussions of global development policy.

Global policies are imagined, developed, and implemented in complex social worlds; when new norms are institutionalized, and "relevant" knowledge reshuffled, the effects are widespread and unpredictable. Structural adjustment programs and their adverse effects on the health of poor populations demonstrate the unintended consequences that Robert Merton deemed inherent in social action. These effects can be magnified when decision-making is divorced from the lived experience of individuals. Although there is no way to eliminate unintended consequences, Arthur Kleinman suggests that by adopting habits of "critical self-reflection," global health actors may be able to respond more nimbly to harmful consequences and thus mitigate some of their ill effects, as we explore in chapter 9.

SELECTIVE PRIMARY HEALTH CARE AND THE RISE OF UNICEF

Following the 1978 Declaration of Alma-Ata and the adoption of the goal "health for all by the year 2000," the primary health care movement gained ground over disease-specific eradication campaigns in global health policy circles. But without resources and a clear plan of action, the principles outlined at Alma-Ata were never realized. The dominance of neoliberalism and structural adjustment programs in the early 1980s diminished public-sector budgets—and ambitions for global public health. Though UNICEF was a vocal critic of structural adjustment, its strategy of selective primary health care meshed with the approach of the World Bank and the International Monetary Fund, which prioritized efficiency and cost-effectiveness. Thus, after structural adjustment policies failed to improve health outcomes in developing nations, many policymakers turned hopefully to SPHC. Many economists also viewed good health as a precondition of economic development and therefore considered health interventions an important feature of country-level development programs. This section considers the most visible SPHC campaign, GOBI-FFF, and the emergence of UNICEF as a major player in global health during the 1980s.

UNICEF Takes the Lead

In the early 1980s, an estimated 15 million children under the age of five died each year in the developing world. UNICEF's GOBI-FFF program, launched in 1982, had the ambitious goal of halving that mortality rate. UNICEF identified the reduction of child and infant mortality and the improvement of maternal health as its chief health priorities. It began by focusing on the four interventions that made up the GOBI package: growth monitoring; oral rehydration therapy, or ORT (see figure 4.7); promotion of breastfeeding; and universal childhood immunization. The four interventions were extremely cost-effective, estimated at less than $10 per child.

In 1983, three more interventions, known as FFF, were added to the campaign in an effort to improve maternal health:

Family planning and birth spacing

Female literacy campaigns

Food supplementation

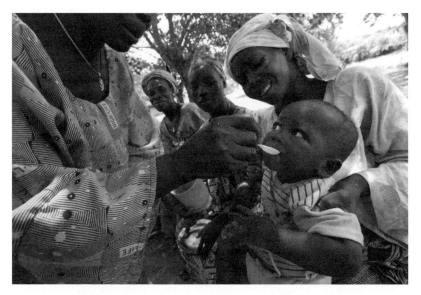

FIGURE 4.7. A woman gives a toddler a spoonful of oral rehydration therapy, a staple of UNICEF's GOBI-FFF campaign. Courtesy UNICEF/NYHQ2007–1583/Olivier Asselin.

Observers considered these interventions "universal in relevance and synergistic in their relationships, and . . . not dependent on profound changes in values or priorities."[63] Although alternatives were considered—most notably malaria and rotavirus control, interventions targeting vitamin D deficiency, and treatments for acute respiratory conditions—the architects of the program felt that the GOBI-FFF program was most likely to result in "a major decrease in observed mortality" at the individual, household, and community levels.[64] Most important, the GOBI-FFF interventions required minimal health care infrastructure and capitalized on existing cost-effective advancements in medical technology, such as ORT and the Sabin polio vaccine, which did not require a cold chain and could be administered orally.[65]

The GOBI-FFF campaign appealed to a wide range of stakeholders—from policymakers to families seeking care—and its programs were quickly rolled out. Richard Cash and colleagues note that while public health experts continued to debate which interventions should be included in an ideal SPHC package, the concept of a package of discrete interventions was uncontested. The "menu of interventions selected is not as important," they write, "as the need to address several of the steps in the 'pathogenesis' of infant and child mortality."[66]

One of UNICEF's greatest challenges was drumming up support for the target of universal child immunization set by the World Health Assembly in 1977. By the early 1980s, little progress had been made; few developing nations could claim immunization rates above 20 percent. After a 1984 conference in Bellagio, the Task Force for Child Survival—composed of UNICEF, the Rockefeller Foundation, the

---

James P. Grant

Jim Grant (1922–1995), pictured in figure 4.8, was born in Peking. During his childhood in China, he learned to speak Mandarin fluently and spent years closely watching the work of his father, John Grant, a missionary doctor who worked for the Rockefeller Foundation. John was himself a pioneer in the field of public health, providing basic medical training in rural Chinese communities for many years. He had followed in the footsteps of his own father, Jim's grandfather, also a medical missionary.

Jim Grant's path to becoming a public health visionary involved years of international humanitarian work. After earning an undergraduate degree from the University of California, Berkeley, and a law degree from Harvard, he began working for the UN Relief and Rehabilitation Administration in China in the 1940s. He later helped lead aid missions for the U.S. State Department in East and South Asia and in Turkey; and in the 1960s, he became an assistant administrator of the U.S. Agency for International Development. In 1969, he left USAID to found the Overseas Development Council, a think tank where he served as president and chief executive officer for nearly a decade.

In 1980, President Jimmy Carter urged the United Nations to appoint Grant executive director of UNICEF, a position Grant held until his death in 1995. Grant was praised by his supporters for being a political realist who was nevertheless unafraid to make unpopular policy decisions. Many critics at the WHO, the United Nations, and within UNICEF itself were skeptical of the GOBI-FFF initiative. But Grant forged ahead; his enthusiasm and relentless campaigning were no small part of its success. Grant considered the announcement made at the 1990 World Summit for Children—that UNICEF had achieved its goal of vaccinating 80 percent of the world's children—his greatest achievement at UNICEF. In 1994, President Clinton awarded Grant the Presidential Medal of Freedom, praising him for his "compassion and courage in his crusade for the world's children."[1]

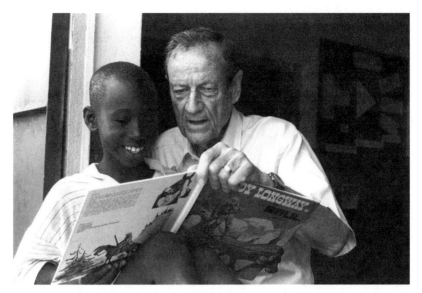

FIGURE 4.8. Jim Grant, executive director of UNICEF from 1980 to 1995. Courtesy UNICEF/NYHQ1994–0093/Giacomo Pirozzi.

WHO, the UNDP, and the World Bank—declared immunization the most important of the seven interventions of the GOBI-FFF campaign and the selective primary health care movement generally.

Jim Grant and other UN officials urged heads of state to hold "national immunization days," during which large segments of the infant and child populations could be vaccinated against polio and other preventable diseases. The UN leaders even called for states engaged in civil wars to cease fire for "days of tranquility" so that children could be immunized. On national immunization days, clinics and health care providers, often aided by support teams from UNICEF or the WHO, provided basic vaccinations—usually for smallpox, polio, and measles—free of charge. The first immunization days were carried out in Colombia, Burkina Faso, Senegal, parts of India and Nigeria, and, most successfully, in Turkey.

For the first national immunization day in Turkey in 1985, UNICEF set up 45,000 vaccination posts, trained 12,000 health personnel and 65,000 helpers, and persuaded the parents of 5 million children to participate. The campaign worked to secure the support of "opinion-formers at every level of society and in every geographical area" so that the vaccination day became "a truly national event."[67] Radio and television networks publicized the dates of the immunization days and the locations of the vaccination posts. Participation was promoted by 200,000 school-teachers, 54,000 imams, 40,000 village leaders, and countless doctors, pharmacists, and health workers. In her book *Children First: The Story of UNICEF Past and Present,* UN historian Maggie Black writes that vaccines were transported "from stores and corner shop refrigerators . . . by car, truck, on horseback or on foot."[68] Two months after the campaign was launched, UNICEF and the national government of Turkey reported that 84 percent of the target group had been immunized.

Turkey's celebrated national immunization days encouraged other countries in the region to hold similar days and helped convince the international community that the target of universal child immunization was within reach. By demonstrating the efficacy of matching service delivery with mobilization of targeted populations, the campaign also informed large-scale UNICEF interventions in other countries in the Middle East and North Africa. Although these national immunization days were primarily used to vaccinate children against polio, they were later used to distribute vitamin A supplements and, in the case of countries such as Zimbabwe, to distribute insecticide-treated bed nets to decrease pediatric malaria infections. The strategy of enlisting a cadre of volunteers and establishing temporary vaccination sites to facilitate widespread immunization in a short time is still employed by countries around the world today.

The child survival revolution culminated in the 1990 World Summit for Children, when UNICEF proudly announced that it had met its goal of vaccinating 80 percent of children in the developing world. (Eighty percent is an important threshold because it is thought to confer "herd immunity," inhibiting disease transmission within a population.) The World Summit was sponsored by UNICEF and attended by seventy-one heads of state and eighty-eight additional senior officials who publicly pledged to continue efforts to reduce child and infant mortality. UNICEF employees also headed up many polio vaccination efforts in the Americas, which accelerated the eradication of polio in the region (announced officially in 1994).

In addition, the GOBI-FFF campaign is credited with expanding the use of oral rehydration therapy and nutritional supplementation worldwide.[69] UNICEF called on nations to increase access—through local health clinics and pharmacies—to oral rehydration therapy, which has saved the lives of more than 40 million children in developing countries since 1970. The World Health Organization reports that ORT has

Days of Tranquility, El Salvador, 1985

For some nations, the goal of universal child immunization seemed beyond the realm of possibility. In 1985, El Salvador was engulfed in a bitter civil war between the military government and the Farabundo Martí National Liberation Front, a coalition of left-leaning militias. The conflict began in 1980 and dragged on for twelve years, claiming some seventy-five thousand lives. Many health clinics closed, and the government's efforts to deliver health services—including vaccinations—were severely disrupted.

But in 1985, while meeting with El Salvador's president José Napoleón Duarte and UN Secretary-General Javier Pérez de Cuéllar, Jim Grant noted that more Salvadoran children were dying each year of measles and other vaccine-preventable illnesses than had died in the war up to that point. Grant suggested that Duarte call for a "day of tranquility" on a Sunday, when children across the country could be vaccinated against these illnesses.[1] At the urging of the United Nations, both sides agreed to temporary ceasefires on three separate occasions, which allowed the immunization of a quarter-million children across El Salvador. The success of El Salvador's days of tranquility illustrated that simple health interventions could be implemented even in unstable political climates and that the needs of children could be used to initiate "zones of peace" in conflict settings.

The days of tranquility long outlasted the GOBI-FFF program. Since 1985, the United Nations has continued to call on warring factions to lay down their weapons to allow childhood vaccinations. In Lebanon, Sudan, Uganda, Yugoslavia, and the Democratic Republic of the Congo, the United Nations successfully negotiated temporary pauses in fighting to facilitate widespread immunization of children in "corridors of peace," conflict-free zones dedicated to public health.[2] In 1999, the rebel group known as the Tamil Tigers halted its armed struggle against the Sri Lankan government for four days of tranquility at UNICEF's request. In 2002, the Burundian civil war was suspended so that children could be vaccinated for polio and measles and receive vitamin A supplements.[3] In 2004, combatants in a civil war in Sierra Leone allowed UN officials to vaccinate children in rebel-held areas and hard-to-reach conflict zones; a Sierra Leonean delegate to the United Nations recounted that to reach these children, "we used relatives of the rebels who were in government areas to take the message to them, we used women's groups, we did advocacy."[4] In 2006, more than forty-four thousand children were safely vaccinated during a November 26 day of tranquility in war-torn Sudan.

reduced fatalities from diarrhea by an estimated 36 percent.[70] Until the widespread introduction of ORT—one of the most important public health advancements of the twentieth century—diarrhea was the leading cause of infant mortality in the developing world.

GOBI-FFF's successes contain important lessons about global health leadership and political advocacy. To realize these gains in child and maternal survival, UNICEF had to mobilize enormous political will. Early on, the GOBI-FFF campaign benefited from existing interest in these issues: stakeholders in many countries were already concerned with high infant mortality. In 1980, under Grant's supervision, UNICEF launched its annual *State of the World's Children* report to document the activity of the organization and create a platform to advocate for children's rights. These reports ranked nations according to child survival indicators, thereby creating constructive competition among them and fostering political will for the GOBI-FFF agenda. The publication implied that a country's progress toward achieving the goals outlined by GOBI-FFF could be read as a proxy for its economic and political development.

Of course, Grant's charismatic leadership was instrumental to UNICEF's rise and the accomplishments of GOBI-FFF. Grant "cajoled and persuaded and flattered and shamed and praised" and eventually generated more political capital for the child survival revolution than anyone at UNICEF had believed possible.[71] By 1985, Grant had met personally with nearly forty heads of state and other key national leaders to discuss the "silent emergency" of child and infant mortality, encouraging widespread adoption of ORT and other GOBI-FFF interventions. He supposedly attended official banquets armed with oral rehydration salt packets, proclaiming their virtues—including the benefits of iodized salt for decreasing iodine deficiency, a condition that increases the risk of physical and mental retardation—to those seated nearby. He convinced Audrey Hepburn and a number of other actors to serve as "goodwill ambassadors" for the campaign.[72]

Another of Grant's tactics was emphasizing that the benefits from the seven GOBI-FFF interventions would be magnified by synergies and the momentum created by successful programs. In the 1995 *Progress of Nations* report, Richard Jolly, former deputy executive director of UNICEF, observed: "Jim Grant believed that the struggle to set and achieve these specific targets was part and parcel of a historic struggle to improve the human condition. In the face of all the bad news which daily assaults our hope and optimism, he insisted on lifting our eyes from the headlines of the day to the horizons of our history."[73] Although Grant is not solely responsible for the success of the GOBI-FFF campaign, his galvanizing presence and dogged pursuit of UNICEF's goals offer a model for mobilizing political will to support health initiatives on a global scale.

The Limits of GOBI-FFF

Financed largely by the Rockefeller Foundation, the GOBI-FFF campaign met a number of its child survival targets. Average immunization rates in the developing world jumped from 20 to 40 percent in the campaign's first two years, and ORT use in developing countries increased from less than 1 percent of families to nearly 20 percent.[74] But the targeted nature of GOBI-FFF—the SPHC approach of choosing a package of discrete interventions—was both its strength and its weakness. Its programs had minimal impact on health systems. Without bolstering public health infrastructure, workforce, supply chains, or the provision of primary care services, GOBI-FFF did little to strengthen health systems or improve health indicators other than infant mortality. In other words, the campaign's successes, though significant, were not sustainable.

Further, because UNICEF prioritized oral rehydration therapy and immunizations, the other GOBI-FFF interventions were not as widely deployed; progress on maternal mortality and other health priorities stagnated. In the years after the 1990 conference, UNICEF struggled to maintain momentum on global vaccinations. Immunization rates in a number of countries have since fallen back below 80 percent: by 2010, only half of developing countries had immunized 80 percent of children in 80 percent of their districts for diphtheria, pertussis, and tetanus (DPT). Nearly 53 percent of all developing countries reported no vitamin A distribution to children under the age of five. And even though twenty developing countries eliminated neonatal and maternal tetanus between 2000 and 2011, thirty-eight countries still faced this preventable form of morbidity.[75] UNICEF's inability to sustain its gains after Jim Grant's death in 1995 illustrates the perils of institutionalizing charisma, as Max Weber described: organizations or efforts that depend on a charismatic leader often have difficulty realizing long-term sustainability after that leader's departure (see chapter 2).

At the 2000 World Economic Forum in Davos, Switzerland, the Global Alliance for Vaccines and Immunization (GAVI) was launched with funding from the Bill and Melinda Gates Foundation, in part to reinvigorate the child survival campaign. Working alongside UNICEF and its partners, GAVI targets the millions of children in the developing world who die from vaccine-preventable illnesses every year. This initiative would have been unnecessary had the immunization rates achieved in 1990 been sustained.

UNICEF's *State of the World's Children 2008* report revealed that the effort to combat diarrheal deaths with ORT had also lost steam: diarrhea was still the second leading cause of infant mortality in developing nations, accounting for more than 17 percent of deaths among children under five. At GOBI's inception, UNICEF had hoped to achieve 50 percent ORT use for diarrhea treatment by 1989. By 1990, 61 percent of people worldwide had access to ORT packets through local clinics and pharmacies, but only 32 percent of those individuals actually used the packets to treat diarrhea. Although an estimated 1 million children benefited from ORT use, Grant had sought a better outcome. The *State of the World's Children 2008* report noted that twenty-six thousand children under the age of five died each day in developing countries. "The problem of [infant mortality]," it concluded, "is no less poignant today than it was 25 years ago when the 'child survival revolution' was launched."[76]

So while this "revolution" was touted as a triumph by those who advocated vertical interventions, its gains look more modest in the long term, especially when considering the development of health systems. Oral rehydration packets, for instance, bring short-term benefits but are only a Band-Aid solution to the lack of clean water and modern sanitation in many poor settings. In many ways, the campaign recapitulated the lessons of the disease-specific eradication campaigns earlier in the twentieth century; in 2006, UNICEF itself called GOBI-FFF "a throwback to the mass anti-disease campaigns of the 1950s."[77] Its emphasis on vaccination embodies the vertical approach: technological solutions, not health systems strengthening, were deemed the most prudent investments in international health.

Halfdan Mahler criticized the GOBI campaign for promoting quick fixes rather than building a foundation for international public health. In 1983, he chastised the World Health Assembly for having "little patience for . . . systematic efforts" like those outlined at Alma-Ata; he referred to SPHC initiatives as "the selection by people outside the developing countries of a few isolated elements of primary health care."[78] Mahler's critiques were incisive. Although the GOBI-FFF campaign offered a variety of implementation strategies at the country level, its goals and methods were developed by a UN agency, not the intended beneficiaries. The rhetoric of "community participation" was used to generate support for SPHC among developing nations, but in practice such participation was little reflected in program implementation.[79]

The ascendance of SPHC also reinforced regnant neoliberal ideology. For example, UNICEF's 1987 *Adjustment with a Human Face* offered a groundbreaking critique of the structural adjustment programs of the World Bank and the IMF. Yet the report does not challenge many of the underlying values, rooted in neoliberal economic thinking, that guided the structural adjustment era. For example, it advocated health and education projects to mitigate the harmful social impacts of structural adjustment (as developing countries slashed social-sector spending) without proposing a novel paradigm of health as a human right or health system strengthening as the ultimate end. Furthermore, UNICEF continued to couch international health challenges in terms of cost-containment, embracing cost-effectiveness analyses in its program design. To some extent, SPHC laid the foundations for the World Bank's 1993 *World Development Report,* which enshrined cost-effectiveness as the principal tool for setting priorities in global health.

Above all, SPHC perpetuated a development paradigm that positions health interventions as useful means for achieving economic growth, not as ends per se. According to a UNICEF report, the GOBI-FFF campaign "reversed conventional wisdom. Rates of infant and young child mortality had previously been seen as indicators of a country's development. Now, UNICEF suggested that a direct attack on infant and child mortality might be an instrument of development."[80] But the core assumption that development was the ultimate aim of the program remained unchallenged. Ten years after the World Summit for Children, in the 2000 *Progress of Nations* report, Carol Bellamy—Grant's successor as UNICEF's executive director—wrote that "effective early care for children lies at the very heart of human development. For those most persuaded by economic arguments, investments in services and support for children in the early years have an estimated return as high as 7 to 1."[81] The rhetoric of cost-effectiveness continued to frame debates about child rights and health; the child was seen as a "future agent for economic and social change,"[82] not an individual with inalienable human rights. Arguments about equity, social justice, and health as a human right were not used as levers in health policy debates again until the global AIDS crisis garnered public attention in the late 1990s.

In 2008, the thirtieth anniversary of the Declaration of Alma-Ata, the WHO published *Primary Health Care, Now More Than Ever* as its annual *World Health Report.* In the introduction, WHO Director-General Margaret Chan admits to a "collective failure to deliver in line with the values" of Alma-Ata. "Doing better in the next 30 years," she writes, "means that we need to invest now in our ability to bring actual performance in line with our aspirations."[83] The challenge for the PHC movement now is to articulate clear targets and identify concrete steps that can be taken to strengthen foundational health services in poor countries. As Walsh and Warren noted in 1979, the goals of Alma-Ata are beyond reproach, but they can also be overwhelming when unaccompanied by a clear implementation plan and dedicated financing.[84] Today, armed with lessons from the rise and fall of SPHC, there is new potential to turn the promise of "health for all" into a reality.

A GROWING ROLE FOR THE WORLD BANK IN HEALTH: COST-EFFECTIVENESS AND HEALTH-SECTOR REFORM

The geopolitical and ideological changes of the 1980s had ramifications in global health that went beyond the debate over PHC versus SPHC and the successes of UNICEF's GOBI-FFF campaign. This new ideological climate led to a transformation in the architecture of international health institutions, which had lasting effects on policy and resource allocation worldwide. One of the most important—and lasting—of these transformations was the emergence of the World Bank as an influential actor in global health. This section considers the World Bank's policies and programs in the 1990s; it focuses in particular on the 1993 *World Development Report,* one of the most important global health publications of the decade.

As described earlier, the World Bank promoted structural adjustment lending during the 1980s, advocating cuts in public-sector spending on education and health in many poor countries.[85] A UNICEF report described this agenda of the World Bank and IMF as "exceptionally influential, if not dominant" in developing countries.[86] By 1988, 59 countries had received adjustment loans from the World Bank.[87] In the 1990s, the World Bank adopted a more direct role in global health as a leading policymaker, lender, and funder of health care programs in the developing world. The bank funded HIV prevention, family planning, and nutrition programs as well as microfinance for poverty reduction, even as it also popularized the use of cost-effectiveness as a way to set priorities in the health sector.

As the influence of the World Bank grew, the power of the WHO waned. Still faithful to the "health for all" agenda, the WHO remained influential among ministries of health during the 1980s. But the ministries themselves often faced smaller budgets as a result of structural adjustment. Meanwhile, a restructuring of its own funding base made the WHO less accountable to poor nations. Representation in the World Health Assembly, the governing body of the WHO, is "one country, one vote." However, during the 1980s, rich countries limited their contributions to the WHO to specific initiatives rather than supporting the general operating budget. Although the programs they supported were shielded from generalized funding constraints as a result, this financial structure undermined the accountability of some WHO programs in poor countries as well as the "health for all" agenda.

Facing evidence of deteriorating health systems in low-income countries, the World Bank and the IMF encountered a wave of criticism in the late 1980s, culminating, as noted, in UNICEF's 1987 report *Adjustment with a Human Face*. Although the bank acknowledged that "even a well-designed adjustment program harms some groups,"[88] some mar-

Trade Liberalization and Food

The impacts of neoliberal reforms are complex. Trade liberalization, for example, has led to widespread exportation of cheap food—such as corn meal, corn syrup, and corn oil—from large, subsidized producers in countries like the United States. Small farmers around the world are often unable to compete with the low prices of this imported food; scores have lost their livelihoods—a major "push factor" in global migration and urbanization. Indigenous crops are being displaced by imports or by genetically modified high-yield crops, which require imported inputs such as fertilizer and seed. In addition, traditional diets are giving way to high-salt, high-sugar, high-fat Western diets, contributing to explosive epidemics of heart disease, stroke, and type 2 diabetes in poor countries.[1] On the one hand, access to cheap calories has reduced malnutrition among those earning cash incomes. On the other, dependence on foreign crops has increased the vulnerability of the poor to global market fluctuations. When world food prices skyrocketed in April 2008, Haiti, for example, was hit particularly hard. The crisis should have been less severe, but trade liberalization had transformed Haiti from a net exporter to a net importer of rice, the country's staple grain.[2]

ket advocates held firm that, in the words of Margaret Thatcher, "there is no alternative." The best one could do was mitigate the unintended health effects of structural adjustment by deploying interventions like GOBI-FFF. As a concern of global policymakers, health continued to take a back seat to macroeconomic considerations.

The 1993 World Development Report and Cost-Effectiveness

In the 1990s, the World Bank began to advocate more audibly for greater investment in health. In the *World Development Report 1993: Investing in Health,* the bank outlined a road map for directing health funding toward cost-effective strategies and reforms based on the principles of efficiency and equity.

This *World Development Report* (1993 *WDR*) raised two major issues. First, the bank criticized the high percentage of public funding that went to high-cost tertiary care, typically captured by urban elites, and argued for a reallocation of resources to achieve basic preventive and clinical care for all. While many public-sector health systems provided nominally "free" care, services were concentrated in urban areas and often excluded the rural poor. In Indonesia, for example, in 1990 the richest 10 percent of the population received nearly three times the government subsidy for health as the poorest 10 percent.[89] Similarly, Kenyatta Hospital in Nairobi, Kenya, received more than 50 percent of the government's health budget. Health for all would be attainable, the report argued, only if priority-setting in the health sector was rationalized, and resources were allocated efficiently and equitably.

Second, the 1993 *WDR* proposed cost-effectiveness as the appropriate tool for setting priorities. Using cost-effectiveness analysis, the report posited, planners could achieve the greatest possible improvements in population health, given scarce resources. One obstacle to setting priorities was the absence of a single metric to compare the health benefits of different disease-control efforts. The 1993 *WDR* therefore introduced the Global Burden of Disease project, a collaboration with the WHO, in which the burdens of different diseases and risk factors were calculated using a novel measure: disability-adjusted life years, or DALYs. DALYs combine years lost to premature death and years lived with a disability in a single metric to estimate the burden of a particular disease in a specific population. DALYs enable policymakers to compare the burden of various diseases and the cost-effectiveness of different interventions. (Chapter 8 explains this metric and its use in more detail.)

The 1993 *WDR* calculated that governments in low-income countries that invested in a package of basic public health programs and essential clinical services could reduce their burden of disease by one-third at a cost of $12 per capita per year.[90] This package included these components:

Immunizations

Deworming drugs and micronutrients at schools

Information campaigns on family planning, nutrition, and household hygiene

Programs to reduce alcohol and tobacco use

HIV-prevention programs

Clinical services such as family planning and maternal care, treatment of tuberculosis, control of sexually transmitted diseases, and care for common childhood illnesses such as malaria, respiratory infections, and diarrheal disease[91]

The report observed that reallocating resources to cost-effective treatments implied excluding such interventions as heart surgery, antiretroviral treatment for HIV/AIDS, and intensive care for premature babies from the basic publicly financed package.[92] Noting that some governments spent as little as $6 per capita per year on health, the bank argued for a substantial increase in funding from governments and donors and for cost-sharing by individuals, households, and communities. In a notable departure from past policy, the bank advocated, among other things, that low-income governments increase spending on health to provide the basic package of essential services. The bank also expressed a more nuanced view of the balance between health needs and its vision for long-term growth through structural adjustment: "Such adjustment is clearly needed for long-run health gains. But during the transitional period, and especially in the earliest adjustment programs, recession and cuts in public spending slowed improvements in health."[93]

The 1993 *World Development Report* signaled the World Bank's increasing influence as a funder and standard-setter in global health. Lending by the bank's Health, Nutrition, and Population Division increased from under $100 million in 1978 to over $1 billion by the mid-1990s (see figure 4.9). The report once again manifested the growing importance of economics in global health policymaking and pro-

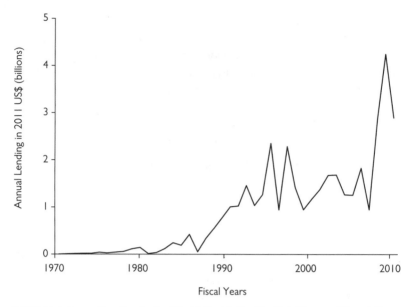

FIGURE 4.9. Annual lending by the World Bank's Health, Nutrition, and Population Division, 1970–2011. Data courtesy of the World Bank's Health, Nutrition, and Population Division; graph adapted from Joy A. de Beyer, Alexander S. Preker, and Richard G. A. Feachem, "The Role of the World Bank in International Health: Renewed Commitment and Partnership," *Social Science and Medicine* 50, no. 2 (2000): 169–176.

gram design. Arguments for using cost-effectiveness to set priorities rested on the assumption that resources for health were scarce. Over the next two decades, however, the validity of this assumption would be challenged (and shaken), as the next chapter describes.

CONCLUSION

The two decades examined in this chapter—the mid-1970s to the mid-1990s—witnessed a dramatic shift in global health policy and practice. The coalescence of political will at Alma-Ata proved fragile in the wake of the debt crisis in the developing world and the political changes in the United States and the United Kingdom. With the ascendance of neoliberalism, support for building (or strengthening) primary health care delivery systems dried up; instead, advocates of targeted and limited health interventions—selective primary health care—found political traction.

International financial institutions gained increasing influence during the latter decade, prompting changes in resource allocation and the vocabularies used to formulate global health policy. Market-based strategies and cost-effectiveness analysis became standard practice for many health reformers and policymakers. Some of these trends led to great feats in promoting health equity: UNICEF's child survival revolution hugely expanded access to lifesaving vaccines; cost-effectiveness analysis guided a number of developing countries away from overemphasis on tertiary care in urban centers.

But the vision that began this period—primary health care for all—was shelved and in some ways reversed. Declining public investment in health programs (triggered by the debt crisis and structural adjustment) and widespread adoption of user fees undermined already limited access to health services among the world's poorest. The drafters of the Alma-Ata Declaration failed to design and implement a road map and financing strategy for their vision. But "health for all" has not been abandoned entirely. Today, advocates of global health equity often hark back to the principles enshrined at Alma-Ata in 1978. The next chapter considers how an unlikely coalition of health professionals, scientists, activists, and policymakers around the world managed to increase U.S. government funding for global AIDS tenfold in the space of a few years—one of the most significant steps toward "health for all" in history.

SUGGESTED READING

Acemoglu, Daron, and James Robinson. *Why Nations Fail: The Origins of Power, Prosperity, and Poverty.* New York: Crown Press, 2012.

Adamson, Peter. "The Mad American." In *Jim Grant: UNICEF Visionary,* edited by Richard Jolly, 19–38. Florence, Italy: UNICEF, 2001.

Brown, Theodore M., Marcos Cueto, and Elizabeth Fee. "The World Health Organization and the Transition from 'International' to 'Global' Public Health." *American Journal of Public Health* 96, no. 1 (2006): 62–72.

Cornia, Giovanni Andrea, Richard Jolly, and Frances Stewart, eds. *Adjustment with a Human Face: Protecting the Vulnerable and Promoting Growth—A Study by UNICEF.* Oxford: Clarendon Press, 1987.

Cueto, Marcos. "The Origins of Primary Health Care and Selective Primary Health Care." *American Journal of Public Health* 94, no. 11 (2004): 1864–1874.

de Beyer, Joy A., Alexander S. Preker, and Richard G. A. Feachem. "The Role of the World Bank in International Health: Renewed Commitment and Partnership." *Social Science and Medicine* 50, no. 2 (2000): 169–176.

de Quadros, Ciro A. "The Whole Is Greater: How Polio Was Eradicated from the Western Hemisphere." In *The Practice of International Health: A Case-*

Based Orientation, edited by Daniel Perlman and Ananya Roy, 54–70. London: Oxford University Press, 2009.

Easterly, William. *The Elusive Quest for Growth: Economists' Adventures and Misadventures in the Tropics.* Cambridge, Mass.: MIT Press, 2001.

Ferguson, James. *Global Shadows: Africa in the Neoliberal World Order.* Durham, N.C.: Duke University Press, 2006.

Kim, Jim Yong, Joyce V. Millen, Alec Irwin, and John Gershman, eds. *Dying for Growth: Global Inequality and the Health of the Poor.* Monroe, Maine: Common Courage Press, 2000.

Litsios, Socrates. "The Long and Difficult Road to Alma-Ata: A Personal Reflection." *International Journal of Health Services* 32, no. 4 (2002): 709–732.

Morgan, Lynn M. "The Primary Health Care Movement and the Political Ideology of Participation in Health." In *Community Participation in Health: The Politics of Primary Care in Costa Rica,* by Lynn M. Morgan, 62–82. Cambridge: Cambridge University Press, 1993.

Paluzzi, Joan. "Primary Health Care since Alma Ata: Lost in the Bretton Woods?" In *Unhealthy Health Policy: A Critical Anthropological Examination,* edited by Arachu Castro and Merrill Singer. Walnut Creek, Calif.: Altamira Press, 2004.

Pavignani, Enrico. "Can the World Bank Be an Effective Leader in International Health?" *Social Science and Medicine* 50, no. 2 (2000): 181–182.

Rodrik, Dani. "Goodbye Washington Consensus, Hello Washington Confusion? A Review of the World Bank's Economic Growth in the 1990s: Learning from a Decade of Reform." *Journal of Economic Literature* 44, no. 4 (December 2006): 973–987.

Rowden, Rick. *The Deadly Ideas of Neoliberalism: How the IMF Has Undermined Public Health and the Fight against AIDS.* London: Zed Books, 2009.

Sachs, Jeffrey. *The End of Poverty: Economic Possibilities for Our Time.* New York: Penguin Press, 2005.

Stein, Howard. *Beyond the World Bank Agenda: An Institutional Approach to Development.* Chicago: University of Chicago Press, 2008.

Stiglitz, Joseph E. *Globalization and Its Discontents.* New York: Norton, 2002.

Stuckler, David, and Karen Siegel, eds. *Sick Societies: Responding to the Global Challenge of Chronic Disease.* New York: Oxford University Press, 2011.

Walsh, Julia A., and Kenneth S. Warren. "Selective Primary Health Care: An Interim Strategy for Disease Control in Developing Countries." *New England Journal of Medicine* 301, no. 18 (1979): 967–974.

Williamson, John. "What Washington Means by Policy Reform." In *Latin American Adjustment: How Much Has Happened?* edited by John Williamson, 7–39. Washington, D.C.: Institute for International Economics, 1990.

Redefining the Possible

The Global AIDS Response

LUKE MESSAC, KRISHNA PRABHU

THE GOLDEN AGE OF GLOBAL HEALTH

No past effort to combat disease captures the promise of medicine and global health like the worldwide response to AIDS. Medicine has been termed the "youngest science": the great tools of medicine—diagnostics, preventatives, therapeutics—were late twentieth-century innovations. Then came AIDS, and in the space of thirty years scientists identified the pathogen and developed the necessary tools to turn what had been a death sentence into a manageable chronic disease. This is modern medicine at its best. What's more, there was an equity plan: led by the U.S. President's Emergency Plan for AIDS Relief (PEPFAR), the Global Fund to Fight AIDS, Tuberculosis and Malaria, and the Bill and Melinda Gates Foundation, great strides have been made to ensure that the world's poor have access to these fruits of modern medicine. In November 2011, U.S. Secretary of State Hillary Clinton even spoke of an "AIDS-free generation."[1] Will this audacious vision come to pass in the next decade? How might global health practitioners and policymakers sustain and strengthen the progress made in the first decade of the twenty-first century? In addressing these and other similar questions, this chapter explores some of the major forces underpinning the golden age of global health.

The first years of this century saw an unprecedented rise in both public attention and funding directed to global health. Health researcher

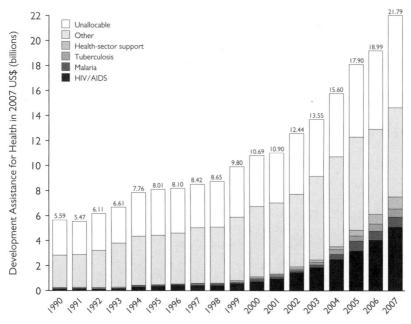

FIGURE 5.1. Development assistance for health, from public and private institutions, 1990–2007, by disease. Source: Nirmala Ravishankar, Paul Gubbins, Rebecca J. Cooley, Katherine Leach-Kemon, Catherine M. Michaud, Dean T. Jamison, and Christopher J. L. Murray, "Financing of Global Health: Tracking Development Assistance for Health from 1990 to 2007," *Lancet* 373, no. 9681 (2009): 2113–2124.

Nirmala Ravishankar and colleagues estimate that development assistance for health from public and private institutions rose from $8.65 billion in 1998 to $21.79 billion in 2007 (see figure 5.1).[2] Between fiscal years 2000 and 2006, the U.S. government increased funding for international AIDS prevention and treatment more than tenfold.[3] Private philanthropists also devoted greater sums to research and service programs. Burgeoning public activism around global health was evidence of the growing recognition that epidemic scourges such as HIV and malaria are treatable diseases. International institutions began new initiatives to galvanize and coordinate state and nonstate actors. The new funding, transnational activism, and refashioned institutional architecture of health care delivery around the world triggered some of the greatest advances toward global health equity in history.

At the turn of the twenty-first century, the U.S. government seemed an unlikely champion of people living with AIDS in developing countries. A number of congressional leaders and the newly inaugurated president, George W. Bush, had a record of coolness toward foreign aid.[4] In the years following the 1994 "Republican revolution," when Republicans gained majorities in both houses of Congress, some conservatives decried foreign aid as wasteful. Senator Jesse Helms (R-N.C.), chair of the Senate Committee on Foreign Relations from 1995 until 2001, boasted that he had "never voted for a foreign aid giveaway."[5] The prospects of global AIDS funding in particular appeared especially dim, as influential Christian conservative leaders had a history of opposing federal funding for AIDS treatment and research even in the United States during the 1980s and 1990s: "AIDS is God's punishment" for homosexuality and promiscuity, proclaimed Reverend Jerry Falwell in 1983.[6] Given the skepticism about foreign aid in the Republican Party, and the stigma and rhetoric of blame associated with AIDS, few would have predicted that the U.S. government would launch one of the largest and most successful global health programs in history—the U.S. President's Emergency Plan for AIDS Relief—dedicating billions of dollars to combating AIDS around the world.

Nonetheless, it was during an era of Republican control over the U.S. executive and legislative branches that federal appropriations for international AIDS prevention, care, and treatment programs increased from approximately $300 million in fiscal year 2000 to more than $3.4 billion by fiscal year 2006.[7] This influx of funds dramatically increased access to services in many developing countries affected by the pandemic. In 2000, the United States funded lifesaving antiretroviral therapy (ART) for no more than a few hundred patients around the world; by late September 2009, the U.S. State Department claimed that PEPFAR supported (in whole or in part) treatment for some 2.5 million people in twenty-four foreign nations[8] and interventions for 509,800 HIV-positive pregnant women that allowed them to avert mother-to-child HIV transmission.[9] It is no exaggeration to credit PEPFAR with preventing millions of deaths.[10]

Private foundations also helped to transform common conceptions of the possible. Established in 1994, the Bill and Melinda Gates Foundation has become the largest private funder of global health research and implementation. By 2009, the Gates Foundation—its assets nearly doubled by investor Warren Buffett—had disbursed over $10 billion for global health.[11] Funding priorities of the foundation's Global Health Program focus on discovery, delivery, and policy advocacy to fight and prevent major global health problems, including enteric and diarrheal diseases; HIV/AIDS; malaria; pneumonia; tuberculosis; neglected diseases; family planning; nutrition; maternal, neonatal, and child health; tobacco control; and vaccine-preventable diseases.

In addition, international institutions have played a critical role. The Global Fund to Fight AIDS, Tuberculosis and Malaria—an independent, multilateral organization established in 2002—receives public and private donations, which it allocates to countries with coordinated strategies for combating the three leading infectious killers on the planet. As of December 2011, the Global Fund had approved US$22.6 billion for more than a thousand grants in 150 countries.[12] Beginning in 1996, the World Bank and the International Monetary Fund began offering debt relief to heavily indebted poor countries, writing off more than $76 billion in debt by 2011 and thereby increasing the resources available for public health in the government budgets of poor countries.[13]

New international health policy initiatives have also served as catalysts for this unprecedented increase in funding for HIV/AIDS treatment in developing countries. One such effort, the "3 by 5" initiative launched by the World Health Organization (WHO) and the Joint United Nations Programme on HIV/AIDS (UNAIDS) in 2003, set a goal of extending antiretroviral treatment to 3 million people living with AIDS in low- and middle-income countries by the end of 2005. By setting an ambitious treatment target, the WHO leveraged its unique position as the principal standard-setting body in global health to reimagine worldwide access to antiretroviral treatment. This initiative was not without its detractors. Many remained unconvinced that ART could be delivered effectively and at large scale in developing countries; at the end of 2003, only one hundred thousand people— 2 percent of those in need—were receiving treatment in sub-Saharan Africa.[14] Nonetheless, this clear target helped to coalesce a diverse set of actors—multilateral and bilateral donors, health practitioners, international policymakers, governments of AIDS-afflicted countries, AIDS patients and their advocates throughout the world—around further ART scale-up initiatives. By measuring success according to the number of people being treated rather than the amount of money donated, the 3 by 5 campaign also encouraged accountability among donors. By the end of 2005, the number of people receiving antiretroviral therapy in sub-Saharan Africa had increased eightfold, covering 17 percent of those in need.[15] Although the treatment target was reached in 2007, not 2005, the 3 by 5 initiative helped galvanize the global AIDS effort.

The WHO's early leadership set an example that would give direction to many subsequent initiatives. By the end of 2011, UNAIDS estimated that nearly 6.6 million people were receiving antiretroviral therapy.[16]

As Ravishankar and colleagues noted in *The Lancet* in June 2009, the increase in development assistance for health during the 1990s—from $5.6 billion in 1990 to $9.8 billion in 1999—pales in comparison to the rise during the 2000s: $21.8 billion was disbursed for global health programs in 2007.[17] What factors led to this surge in available resources? Why did AIDS—a chronic disease that demands a more expensive and complex treatment regimen than that for many leading causes of death and disability around the world—spark this surge, at least in part? Accounting for the golden age of global health demands biosocial analysis that is geographically deep and historically broad.

How did this bold vision of global health equity enter the public imagination? How did the conception of the possible shift so dramatically in the space of a decade? One way to answer this question draws on the concept of institutionalization, as explained by sociologists Peter Berger and Thomas Luckmann (see chapter 2). Before the 2000s, low expectations (and paltry resources) for international health were the norm. Over time, policymakers, donors, and health professionals had all become socialized for scarcity: they focused on optimizing use of a tiny resource pie instead of also reimagining and seeking to expand the size of that pie. Health providers in poor countries became accustomed to targeting the "low-hanging fruit" of public health—vaccines, handwashing, bed nets, condoms, the GOBI interventions (discussed in chapter 4), to name a few examples—just as donors became accustomed to disbursing modest sums for global health programs. The high prices of lifesaving interventions, including antiretroviral therapy and second-line TB treatment, were accepted as fixed. In other words, constraint was *institutionalized* as the status quo in global health.

This had far-reaching effects on what the "stakeholders" in global health, including poor people in need of basic medical care, considered possible. "Habitualization carries with it the important psychological gain that choices are narrowed," write Berger and Luckmann.[18] For many years, the only approach deemed possible in global health was harvesting the low-hanging fruit. But high drug costs, paltry funding, and low expectations were constructs—institutionalized habits—vulnerable to large-scale social change. In the next decade, the bar would be raised.

FROM DEATH SENTENCE TO CHRONIC CONDITION:
AIDS IN THE TIME OF ANTIRETROVIRAL THERAPY

During the 1980s and into the early 1990s, an HIV diagnosis was a guarantee of early death. In the first years of the pandemic, physicians in both rich and poor settings lacked therapeutic tools capable of suppressing the virus and preventing the onset of clinical symptoms. The best they could do was treat opportunistic infections associated with HIV, such as pneumonia and herpes. Azidothymidine (AZT), the first drug found to safely and effectively slow replication of HIV in the body, won approval from the U.S. Food and Drug Administration (FDA) for use against AIDS in 1987.[19] Until the introduction of didanosine in 1991, AZT monotherapy was the only treatment option—and it was accessible only to patients who could afford its $8,000 annual cost.[20] Although AZT suppressed the virus for a time, HIV replication remained high enough that AZT-resistant strains soon emerged.[21] Without therapy capable of stopping the progression from HIV infection to full-blown AIDS, mortality rates from the disease increased steadily in the United States between 1987 and 1995.[22]

Meanwhile, AIDS was taking an even greater toll in the developing world. But addressing AIDS on a global scale did not figure high on the agenda of most policymakers and activists in rich countries. In *The Invisible People,* a chronicle of the history of the AIDS pandemic from the 1980s to the early 2000s, Greg Behrman notes that few AIDS activists in the United States understood the magnitude of the international pandemic; even fewer were willing to expand their campaigns beyond U.S. borders.[23] While thousands formed human blockades in New York City and protested outside federal buildings in Washington, D.C., calling for increased access to AZT monotherapy, greater appropriations for research, more rapid FDA approval of new therapies, nondiscrimination in the workplace, subsidized housing, condom distribution, and other measures in care, prevention, and treatment, only a few concurrently demanded similar interventions for at-risk populations and people living with AIDS in developing countries.[24] According to Eric Sawyer, co-founder of the activist group AIDS Coalition to Unleash Power (ACT UP), as late as the mid-1990s only 10 percent of the domestic activist community paid attention to the global pandemic.[25]

The year 1996 marked a turning point in the search for effective therapeutics against AIDS. In 1995, the FDA had approved saquina-

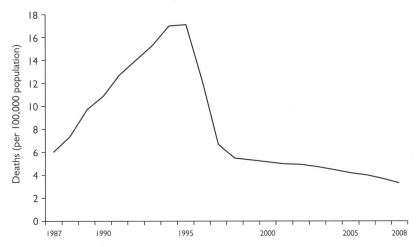

FIGURE 5.2. Deaths from HIV/AIDS in the United States, 1987–2008. (Estimates based on the age distribution of the U.S. population in 2000.) Source: Centers for Disease Control and Prevention, *HIV Mortality: Trends (1987–2008)*, "Slide 5: Trends in Annual Age-Adjusted Rate of Death Due to HIV Disease: United States, 1987–2008," www.cdc.gov/hiv/pdf/statistics_surveillance_statistics_slides_HIV_mortality.pdf. Courtesy Centers for Disease Control and Prevention.

vir, the first in a new class of antiretrovirals called protease inhibitors. In 1996, nevirapine, the first in another class of antiretrovirals known as non-nucleoside reverse transcriptase inhibitors (NNRTIs), received FDA approval. Later that year, the Eleventh International Conference on AIDS affirmed the promise of these new therapeutics. At that meeting, held in Vancouver, David Ho, scientific director and CEO of the Aaron Diamond AIDS Research Center in New York, announced study results demonstrating that regimens containing three antiretroviral drugs from at least two different classes of antiretrovirals—regimens that came to be known as Highly Active Antiretroviral Therapy, or HAART—suppressed the virus and restored patients' immune systems for sustained periods.[26]

Evidence of the effectiveness of HAART continued to mount in scientific studies published in the subsequent months.[27] For those who could access the drugs, it began to seem possible that AIDS would become a manageable chronic disease rather than a certain killer. According to the U.S. Centers for Disease Control and Prevention (CDC), age-adjusted mortality from AIDS-related causes in the United States declined 28 percent between 1995 and 1996, 46 percent between 1996 and 1997, and 18 percent between 1997 and 1998.[28] By 1998, fewer people in the United States were dying of AIDS-related causes than had been the case in 1991 (see figure 5.2).

ONE WORLD, ONE HOPE? DIFFERENT INCOMES, DIFFERENT OUTCOMES

The theme of the Vancouver Conference was "One World, One Hope." Yet even with the reported promise of HAART, not all attendees were flush with optimism. Initially, pharmaceutical companies set prices for antiretroviral treatment with a three-drug cocktail at $10,000 to $15,000 per patient per year—far out of reach for most people living with AIDS in developing countries. Speaking at the Vancouver Conference, Eric Sawyer argued that "drug companies should consider developing a two-tier pricing system. . . . AIDS treatments must also be made available to the poor everywhere, at cost or at very minimal levels of profit."[29]

The discovery of effective drug therapy inspired some American AIDS activists to join with advocacy groups in the developing world.[30] But as therapeutic advances and improved public services for affected individuals made HIV infection less of a mortal crisis for many erstwhile advocates, the activist movement in the developed world dwindled in numbers and militancy. At its peak in 1992, ACT UP had thousands of active members spread across seventy chapters in the United States and Europe. But by the late 1990s, many of these chapters had folded, and even the largest surviving chapters—New York City, Philadelphia, San Francisco, and Washington, D.C.—counted far fewer members at weekly meetings.[31]

Meanwhile, prominent voices in international public health and development circles were arguing against treating AIDS in poor countries. In 2002, two articles in *The Lancet,* a highly regarded medical journal, posited that HAART was not cost-effective in poor countries. Elliot Marseille and colleagues concluded that "data on the cost-effectiveness of HIV prevention in sub-Saharan Africa and on highly active antiretroviral therapy indicate that prevention is at least 28 times more cost effective than HAART."[32] Andrew Creese and colleagues reached a similar conclusion: "The most cost-effective interventions are for prevention of HIV/AIDS and treatment of tuberculosis, while HAART for adults, and home based care organized from health facilities, are the least cost-effective."[33] In both articles, prevention and treatment were deemed mutually exclusive activities; assuming scarce resources for health care delivery in poor countries, investing in AIDS treatment instead of prevention would, by these accounts, cost lives. Such claims were echoed among foreign aid officials. "If we used antiviral drugs in treatment regimens similar to those used in the U.S.," argued the chief of the HIV/AIDS division in the U.S. Agency for International Development (USAID) in 1998, "it would cost approximately $35 billion per year to treat those infected in the developing world. We are talking about medical regimens that cost $5,000 to $10,000 a year and require sophisticated health provider and laboratory infrastructure. . . . How can we get involved in care in the face of such staggering statistics?"[34]

Others argued that HAART was too complex to deliver in resource-poor settings. In testimony before the House of Representatives Committee on International Relations in June 2001, Andrew Natsios, head of USAID, said, in reference to UN Secretary-General Kofi Annan's proposed budget for a possible global fund:

> The biggest problem, if you look at Kofi Annan's budget, half the budget is for antiretrovirals. If we had them today, we could not distribute them. We could not administer the program because we do not have the doctors, we do not have the roads, we do not have the cold chain. This sounds small and some people, if you have traveled to rural Africa you know this, this is not a criticism, just a different world. People do not know what watches and clocks are. They do not use Western means for telling time.[35]

Natsios's claim about watches and "Western means for telling time" cast aspersions on Africans' ability to adhere to treatment regimens. Antiretroviral therapy demands strict, lifelong adherence; missing even a few doses per month increases the risk that resistant strains will develop, rendering first-line treatment ineffective. Second- and third-line regimens for resistant strains are expensive. Confident that such treatments could not be effectively delivered, Natsios argued against the comprehensive and recalibrated response to the pandemic advocated by Kofi Annan and others. Natsios and many public health "experts" instead promoted prevention and palliation, even as the fatality rates of these diseases dropped in affluent parts of the world. Lack of access to treatment in the face of explosive epidemics remained the norm across the developing world.[36]

As such immodest claims—reflecting a restrictive conception of the possible—were aired in policy circles and the media, evidence was mounting about the feasibility (and effectiveness) of treating AIDS in resource-poor settings. In 2001, the *Bulletin of the World Health*

Organization published the results of a Partners In Health study that followed 150 patients receiving HAART in Haiti's rural Central Plateau. While Natsios had argued that patients in such settings would not adhere to therapy, this study found adherence rates *above* those documented in many parts of the United States.[37] Another study that followed 288 adults receiving HAART beginning in 2001 in a community-based program operated by Médecins Sans Frontières (Doctors Without Borders) in Khayelitsha township—a poor urban neighborhood outside Cape Town, South Africa—found immune restoration, viral load suppression, and high adherence rates in the vast majority of the patient cohort.[38] Furthermore, these studies challenged the presumed dichotomy between prevention and treatment. When HAART became available, more people began seeking voluntary counseling and testing—a pillar of HIV prevention. In other words, the possibility of receiving treatment functioned as an incentive for people to learn their status. The findings of these studies contradicted immodest claims about adherence and about the supposed conflict between treatment and prevention.

Armed with examples of successful HAART delivery in impoverished settings, a small coalition of health providers, policymakers, activists, and academics in rich and poor countries decried the lack of access to HAART globally. In 2001, 133 Harvard University faculty members signed a "Consensus Statement on Antiretroviral Treatment for AIDS in Poor Countries," declaring that "the objections to HIV treatment in low-income countries are not persuasive and . . . there are compelling arguments in favor of a widespread treatment effort."[39] This statement helped policymakers reimagine the possible in global health: if delivering HAART—chronic care for a chronic disease—was feasible in Haiti and South Africa, why not scale it up around the world? Why not use HAART to usher in a more ambitious agenda of health system strengthening globally?

The Harvard consensus statement noted two principal barriers to expanding access to HAART: the high price of antiretrovirals and insufficient funding for implementation. These hurdles were well known to AIDS activists. U.S. AIDS advocacy organizations such as ACT UP Philadelphia were, by the early 2000s, made up mostly of low-income, HIV-positive African American individuals who had personal experience with a health system that divided patients according to their ability to pay for lifesaving medications—what they termed "medical apartheid."[40] These groups had led struggles to expand access to anti-

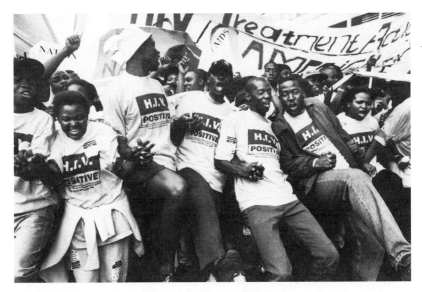

FIGURE 5.3. A demonstration organized by the Treatment Action Campaign at the 2000 International AIDS Conference in Durban, South Africa. Courtesy Gideon Mendel/CORBIS.

retroviral drugs, including a successful campaign to get Pennsylvania Medicaid—government insurance for the poor—to cover antiretroviral drug costs. Realizing the links between their own campaigns for access and the growing treatment gap between the rich and poor worlds, these groups established transnational alliances with AIDS activists in developing countries.[41] For example, the Health Global Action Project (Health GAP) and ACT UP joined forces with a South African civil society group, made up largely of poor people living with HIV/AIDS, called the Treatment Action Campaign (see figure 5.3). Together, these organizations led a worldwide campaign to lower the costs of antiretroviral drugs in poor countries.

UNPACKING THE "COST" OF AIDS TREATMENT: INTELLECTUAL PROPERTY AND CIVIL SOCIETY

Intellectual property rights lay at the heart of the first transnational battle for expanded access to antiretrovirals. In the mid-1990s, public laboratories and privately owned companies in Brazil began producing generic versions of patented ARV (antiretroviral) medications; Brazil also imported generic antiretrovirals from suppliers in India.

These actions precipitated a 70 percent drop in Brazil's domestic price of HAART by 2001.[42] Some countries attempted to emulate Brazil's strategy by passing legislation that permitted generic production of certain patented drug formulations.[43] In late 1997, South Africa's parliament approved the Medicines Act, which stipulated that in the case of a national health emergency, the government could allow both compulsory licensing (generic production of patented antiretroviral medicines without the permission of the patent holder, who would, however, be paid an appropriate royalty) and parallel importation (importation of these drugs from countries where they are sold at lower prices). These measures aimed to lower prices for antiretroviral therapy in South Africa, where, in 2000, only an estimated 1 percent of the half million South Africans in need of antiretrovirals received them.[44]

Thirty-nine pharmaceutical companies, alarmed by the prospect of losing the exclusive rights guaranteed by their patents, filed suit in South African courts in 1998 to overturn the Medicines Act. These companies argued that the legislation undermined the notion of intellectual property, thereby weakening incentives for innovation and decreasing funds for pharmaceutical research and development. Advocates of the law, including AIDS activists in the United States and South Africa, pointed out that brand-name pharmaceutical companies in the United States derived only 5 to 7 percent of their profits from low- and middle-income countries.[45] They argued further that branded antiretroviral prices far exceeded outlays for production, research, and development, contending that companies set ARV prices high to increase profits at the margins.

Initially, the Clinton administration sided with the pharmaceutical companies. Vice President Al Gore, who served with Deputy Prime Minister Thabo Mbeki of South Africa as co-chairs of a bilateral commission to promote democracy in South Africa, used the forum to express the U.S. government's opposition to the Medicines Act. When President Nelson Mandela and the South African legislature remained unmoved, Charlene Barshefsky, President Clinton's U.S. trade representative, placed South Africa on a "priority watch list"—a diplomatic precursor to trade sanctions—in March 1999, citing the Medicines Act as South Africa's major transgression. In Barshefsky's words, the passage of the Medicines Act merited this response because it could "abrogate patent rights."[46]

American AIDS activists and members of the Congressional Black Caucus called on the Clinton administration to stop pressuring South

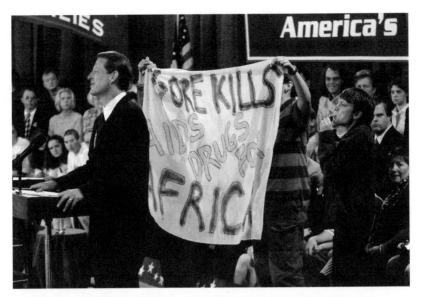

FIGURE 5.4. Activists interrupted the first three events of Vice President Al Gore's presidential campaign in 1999, before the 2000 election. Within a year, President Bill Clinton issued an executive order meeting the activists' demands that the United States not interfere with South Africa's generic licensing policies for lifesaving medications. Courtesy Luke Frazza/AFP/Getty Images.

Africa to repeal the Medicines Act. Members of what would become Health GAP targeted Gore's presidential campaign rallies (see figure 5.4). As he announced his candidacy on June 16, 1999, in a carefully choreographed event in Carthage, Tennessee, activists interrupted his speech with whistles, banners, and chants of "Gore's greed kills! AIDS drugs for Africa!"[47] In the ensuing days, similarly disruptive protests took place at other campaign events, lending the bilateral dispute prominence in the U.S. press.

Soon after these protests, the political winds shifted decidedly against the pharmaceutical lobby. In September 1999, just three months after the Carthage demonstration, Barshefsky announced the Clinton administration's support for the Medicines Act. In December, Clinton announced that the United States would not pressure any sub-Saharan African country into purchasing brand-name AIDS drugs and would support parallel importation or generic production as a means to lower prices.[48]

By April 2001, all thirty-nine pharmaceutical companies had withdrawn their lawsuits.[49] Later that year, the Doha Declaration, adopted

University Students and Access to Medicines: Yale and d4t

Although deprived of political support after President Clinton publicly backed South Africa's Medicines Act in 1999, the thirty-nine pharmaceutical companies continued to sue the South African government in an effort to overturn the Medicines Act and retain their exclusive patents. In opposition, Amy Kapczynski, a first-year Yale University law student who had recently returned from the Durban International AIDS Conference, helped launch a campaign to improve treatment access by leveraging Yale's intellectual property rights.[1]

In the mid-1980s, a team of researchers led by Yale's William Prusoff had detected the potency of d4t, an antiretroviral also known as stavudine, against HIV; and Yale secured a patent for the discovery. In 1988, Yale issued an exclusive license to Bristol-Meyers Squibb (BMS) to produce and sell d4t. By 1999, this license alone accounted for approximately $40 million of the $46.12 million that the university collected in royalties. As it became a mainstay in first-line HAART regimens, d4t garnered $578 million in sales for BMS in 2000. In 2001, d4t (sold by BMS under the brand name Zerit) cost nearly $1,600 per patient per year in South Africa, a nation with a per capita GDP of approximately $3,000. BMS, one of the parties to the suit challenging South Africa's Medicines Act, was strongly opposed to generic production or importation of d4t in South Africa.[2]

In 2001, Amy Kapczynski and her classmates, working alongside Médecins Sans Frontières (MSF), demanded that Yale renegotiate its license for d4t with BMS and that the university "issue a voluntary license to allow the importation and use of generic stavudine in South Africa."[3] Yale initially denied this request, explaining that it had granted exclusive rights to the company and that only BMS could renegotiate the license.[4] MSF responded that Yale should breach its contract to ensure that d4t could reach poor patients unable to afford Zerit's high price. The students protested and gathered petition signatures (drawing media attention in the process) and convinced Prusoff to pen a *New York Times* op-ed arguing that "d4t should be either cheap or free in sub-Saharan Africa."[5] Within one month of MSF's original request, Yale and BMS announced that they would permit the sale of generic d4t in South Africa.[6] In June 2001, BMS signed an "agreement not to sue" with Aspen Pharmacare, a generic manufacturer in South Africa. The price of d4t in South Africa subsequently dropped by 96 percent.[7]

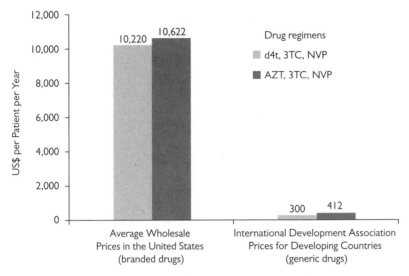

FIGURE 5.5. Prices of first-line HIV/AIDS drug regimens, branded versus generic, 2002. Sources: Internal Partners In Health data and Médecins Sans Frontières.

at a ministerial meeting of the World Trade Organization (WTO), reaffirmed that the 1995 international agreement on intellectual property protections, known as TRIPs, "does not and should not prevent Members from taking measures to protect public health." The agreement recognized the right of each WTO member "to grant compulsory licenses and the freedom to determine the grounds upon which such licenses are granted."[50] In other words, the world's most powerful states had agreed, for the moment at least, that access to medicines could, in certain instances, trump patent protections.

This nascent international political and legal consensus opened the door to generic production of patented HIV drugs for poor countries. Realizing this opportunity, the William J. Clinton Foundation—established in 2001 after President Clinton left the White House—and other institutions sought rapid reductions in treatment costs. Beginning in 2002, the Clinton Foundation's HIV/AIDS Initiative worked to generate demand, securing agreements from the governments of developing countries to place large orders of generic antiretrovirals at specified prices. Generic producers in India and South Africa, in turn, agreed to alter their business models, producing higher volumes and improving production processes to lower unit costs, while seeking smaller margins per pill sold. By harnessing newfound economies of scale, generic producers of antiretrovirals realized higher profits (after suffering some anticipated losses in the short term), while purchasers secured substantial price reductions.[51] The lowest available annual per-patient price of the most common first-line HAART regimen in the developing world fell from $10,000–$15,000 in the late 1990s to $300 in 2002 and to $87 in 2007. Figure 5.5 contrasts the 2002 costs of branded drugs in the United States with the costs of generic drugs in developing countries.[52]

This precipitous decrease in drug prices created new opportunities to scale up AIDS treatment programs globally. Yet another hurdle remained—the lack of dedicated funding for implementation in poor countries.

STRANGE BEDFELLOWS IN THE FIGHT FOR FUNDING

With growing consensus that antiretroviral therapy could be delivered effectively and affordably in resource-poor settings, advocates continued calling for increased funding for global AIDS treatment programs. The World Health Organization's Commission on Macroeconomics and Health, chaired by economist Jeffrey Sachs, published a report in 2001 providing evidence that improved health outcomes could boost economic growth. (The economic effects of health programs are difficult to capture in metrics used to formulate development policy.) The report also suggested that donor dollars had an important role to play in fostering the virtuous cycle of growth and health improvements in poor countries.[53]

Earlier that year, Sachs and Harvard colleague Amir Attaran had published an article in *The Lancet* proposing a practical application of these findings: a new funding stream dedicated to controlling the world's greatest infectious killers. Funded by increased foreign aid commitments from rich nations, this new body would use a competitive and transparent process to distribute grants, rather than loans, to health projects in developing countries. Grants would be "directed toward funding projects which are proposed and desired by the affected countries themselves, and which are judged as having epidemiological merit against the pandemic by a panel of independent scientific experts."[54] UN Secretary-General Kofi Annan vocally endorsed the plan, and leaders of the developed world launched the Global Fund to Fight AIDS, Tuberculosis and Malaria at the G8 Summit in Genoa, Italy, in 2001. In 2002, the fund made its first disbursements.[55]

In rich countries, the political capital of global health increased rapidly in the early 2000s. In 2001, students at Harvard's undergraduate campus and the Kennedy School of Government jointly founded the Student Global AIDS Campaign, an advocacy group that by 2004 boasted more than eighty chapters at colleges and universities across the country.[56] A number of global AIDS advocacy organizations soon established a presence in Washington, including the Health Global Access Project (June 1999), the Global AIDS Alliance (March 2001), Prescription for Hope (2002), and DATA (Debt, AIDS, Trade, Africa) (2002). Once established, the AIDS lobby—made up of conservative evangelical Christians, college students, gay rights activists, African Americans, and people living with AIDS—began exerting significant pressure on the federal appropriations process.

The AIDS movement also drew considerable support from opinion leaders and celebrities. Franklin Graham, founder of the Christian charity Samaritan's Purse and son of the renowned evangelist Billy Graham, helped convince Senator Jesse Helms that AIDS afflicted the "blameless" just as often as it afflicted homosexuals, whom Helms judged to be immoral.[57] Helms, chair of the Senate Committee on Foreign Relations, noted that Graham was the first to explain to him the toll taken on "innocent victims of this sexually transmitted disease"— the millions of children who had either contracted the infection from their mothers or been orphaned by the death of a parent.[58] Bono, lead singer of the Irish rock band U2, who had already played a key role in the Jubilee 2000 campaign advocating debt forgiveness for poor countries, emerged as a champion of worldwide AIDS efforts. In a meeting with Helms, he pointed out that the Bible mentions poverty in 2,103 verses, while it mentions sexual behavior in only a few.[59] Helms would repeat this observation in a press conference, and soon thereafter he would publicly apologize for not supporting AIDS care and treatment efforts in the past.[60] In late 2001, Helms joined his colleague William Frist (R-Tenn.) in sponsoring a $500 million initiative—which came to be known as the Helms Legacy Amendment—to prevent mother-to-child transmission of HIV in poor countries.

The most important convert was, in some ways, the least likely: President George W. Bush. During Bush's tenure as governor of Texas, his senior health advisor had observed that "the one thing Bush is really uncomfortable dealing with is AIDS" because of supposed links (much-discussed in conservative media) between the disease, homosexuality, and promiscuity.[61] During his 2000 presidential campaign, Bush told

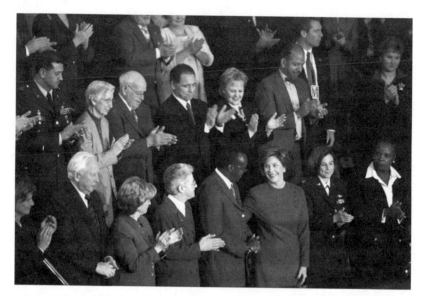

FIGURE 5.6. Ugandan physician and AIDS expert Peter Mugyenyi attends President George W. Bush's 2003 State of the Union address as a special guest of First Lady Laura Bush. Dr. Mugyenyi's efforts to provide AIDS treatment and prevention services at the Joint Clinical Research Centre in Uganda helped convince President Bush to launch PEPFAR. Courtesy George W. Bush Presidential Library.

journalist Jim Lehrer that Africa "doesn't fit into the national strategic interests" of the United States and would therefore not figure prominently in his foreign policy agenda.[62]

But in January 2003, Bush reinvented himself as one of the great champions of global AIDS relief. During his State of the Union Address that year (see figure 5.6), he proposed a sweeping new international AIDS initiative:

> AIDS can be prevented. Antiretroviral drugs can extend life for many years. . . . Seldom has history offered a greater opportunity to do so much for so many. . . . To meet a severe and urgent crisis abroad, tonight I propose the Emergency Plan for AIDS Relief—a work of mercy beyond all current international efforts to help the people of Africa. . . . I ask the Congress to commit $15 billion over the next five years, including nearly $10 billion in new money, to turn the tide against AIDS in the most afflicted nations of Africa and the Caribbean.[63]

No one in Congress—Democrat or Republican—had formally proposed $3 billion in annual spending on global AIDS programs. Prodded by Bush's powerful proposal, both houses of Congress passed legislation in May 2003 authorizing the five-year $15 billion U.S. President's Emergency Plan for AIDS Relief.[64]

Spurred by the same forces—lower drug prices, growing evidence of treatment efficacy in resource-poor settings, grassroots activism, and advocacy by elites—other rich nations also increased their allocations to global AIDS programs. At the G8 summit in Gleneagles, Scotland, in 2005, leaders of rich countries pledged to double aid to Africa and to ensure "as close as possible to universal access to treatment for AIDS" by 2010.[65] UNAIDS reported that disbursements by the G8 and the

---

The Politics of Global AIDS Funding in the American Heartland

The nascent global AIDS lobby proved its clout in 2004, convincing a congressional committee chair to reverse a budgetary decision that could have decreased U.S. AIDS appropriations. In April 2004, as the House considered the fiscal year 2005 budget resolution, Representative Jim Nussle (R-Ind.), then chair of the House Budget Committee, proposed $3.6 billion less for the international affairs account than had been proposed by either the Senate Budget Committee or the president's budget.[1] Because the majority of global AIDS spending came from that account, AIDS activists worried that Nussle's proposal would lower the U.S. contribution to treatment and prevention programs abroad. In response, Student Global AIDS Campaign members at Luther College—Nussle's alma mater—petitioned the college president to revoke Nussle's forthcoming public service award and staged a protest at one of his town hall events. Meanwhile, advocacy groups such as DATA and the Global AIDS Alliance convinced sympathetic religious leaders in Nussle's district to express public disapproval of this funding shortfall. Lutheran bishop Phillip Hougen, one such leader, emphasized his congregation's ties to Tanzania, telling a reporter from *Roll Call:* "Iowans are somewhat more globally aware than people give them credit for."[2]

Faced with a surge of political pressure during an election year, Nussle relented.[3] In late May, he announced that he would request an additional $2.8 billion for the international affairs account when the budget resolution was negotiated in conference committee. Nussle spokesperson Sean Spicer acknowledged the influence of constituent activists: "He wanted to make sure they understood that he truly was supportive" of AIDS funding.[4] Global AIDS once again proved to be a political issue that could unite people across the ideological spectrum.

European Community for HIV/AIDS prevention, care, and treatment programs in the developing world rose from $1.2 billion in 2002 to $7.6 billion in 2009, though this figure fell to $6.9 billion in 2010. Leading public donors to global AIDS programs in 2010 were the United States ($3.7 billion), the United Kingdom ($0.9 billion), and the Netherlands, Germany, and France (each about $0.4 billion).[66]

In some cases, AIDS funding increases proved to be a beachhead for new resources for other global health priorities. For instance, the WHO estimates that international funding disbursements for malaria increased from $249 million in 2004 to $1.25 billion in 2008.[67] The second five-year iteration of PEPFAR, authorized by the U.S. government in mid-2008, established new goals to strengthen health infrastructure—recruiting and training (and retaining) 140,000 health care professionals and paraprofessionals in partner countries by 2013, for example—in addition to expanding AIDS treatment and prevention services.[68]

AFTER THE GOLDEN AGE

The first decade of the twenty-first century raised the bar in global health. The failures of imagination that had long been the status quo fell prey to evidence of effective health care delivery in resource-poor settings matched with bold visions of global health equity. Although some public health "experts" had declared lifesaving interventions such as antiretroviral treatment too complex or too expensive for resource-poor settings, pioneering programs proved otherwise. The costs of numerous preventatives, therapeutics, and diagnostics decreased significantly after transnational activism and innovative market coordination opened the door to generic production as well as new strategies for financing and procurement. Funding for global health increased to unprecedented levels; long socialized for scarcity, health practitioners and policymakers around the world were able to reimagine global health equity. By 2010, drug prices were lower and international funding levels were higher than almost anyone had thought possible a decade earlier.

Yet it is still a long road to "health for all." Although getting 6.6 million people on antiretroviral treatment is a feat that affirms the promise of global health and modern medicine, such progress must be sustained and expanded. Millions more are in need of antiretroviral treatment around the world. In the wake of the worldwide economic downturn in 2008, many countries, including the United States, faltered on their foreign aid pledges.[69] Across the developing world, hospitals and clinics have had to turn away new AIDS patients.

This slowdown was especially poignant because it came on the heels of breakthrough evidence about AIDS treatment and prevention. In May 2011, a study funded by the National Institutes of Health found that antiretroviral treatment reduces the rate of transmission by 96 percent.[70] Put another way, treatment *is* prevention. For the first time in three decades, it became possible to imagine the "end of AIDS." Redoubled commitment to HIV-control initiatives around the world could slow (or even stop) the pandemic. Such an effort would demand not only increased funding but also better use of the dollars available. Much of PEPFAR's funding is distributed to contractors, including universities and NGOs, which are tasked with implementing PEPFAR programs. In 2008, journalist Laurie Garrett reported that although PEPFAR did not provide details on contractor "overhead" rates—that is, the percentage of funding going toward expenses such as NGO salaries and office expenses rather than treatment, prevention, and education—reports indicated that rates of 30 to 60 percent were the norm.[71] If fewer dollars were siphoned off en route to poor patients, many more would have access to life-saving treatment.

Beyond AIDS, the golden age of global health ushered in significant advances against other leading causes of suffering and premature death around the world. Some health providers learned to use "vertical" AIDS programs to simultaneously provide "horizontal" primary health care services and strengthen health systems. Delivering services for complex chronic conditions like AIDS requires a full-time salaried staff; modern facilities; trained community health workers, supported by stipends; and a robust referral network. It can therefore have powerful spillover effects on other health priorities. Health practitioners, including community health workers, who are focusing on HIV control can be trained to simultaneously address other pathologies of poverty: HIV patients infected with tuberculosis, children with pneumonia or diarrheal disease, families without sufficient food or access to clean water. In other words, AIDS treatment can be used as a wedge to strengthen health systems.[72] The next chapter explores one model of care based on this approach.

SUGGESTED READING AND OTHER MEDIA

Behrman, Greg. *The Invisible People: How the U.S. Has Slept through the Global AIDS Pandemic, the Greatest Humanitarian Catastrophe of Our Time.* New York: Free Press, 2004.

"Consensus Statement on Antiretroviral Treatment for AIDS in Poor Countries, by Individual Members of the Faculty of Harvard University." March 2001. www.cid.harvard.edu/cidinthenews/pr/consensus_aids_therapy.pdf.

d'Adesky, Anne-Christine. *Moving Mountains: The Race to Treat Global AIDS.* London: Verso, 2004.

Epstein, Steven. *Impure Science: AIDS, Activism, and the Politics of Knowledge.* Berkeley: University of California Press, 1996.

Farmer, Paul, Fernet Léandre, Joia Mukherjee, Rajesh Gupta, Laura Tarter, and Jim Yong Kim. "Community-Based Treatment of Advanced HIV Disease: Introducing DOT-HAART (Directly Observed Therapy with Highly Active Antiretroviral Therapy)." *Bulletin of the World Health Organization* 79, no. 12 (2001): 1145–1151.

Gupta, Rajesh, Jim Y. Kim, Marcos A. Espinal, Jean-Michel Caudron, Bernard Pecoul, Paul E. Farmer, and Mario C. Raviglione. "Responding to Market Failures in Tuberculosis Control." *Science* 293, no. 5532 (2001): 1049–1051.

Kapczynski, Amy, Samantha Chaifetz, Zachary Katz, and Yochai Benkler. "Addressing Global Health Inequities: An Open Licensing Approach for University Innovations." *Berkeley Technology Law Journal* 20, no. 2 (2005): 1031–1114.

PBS. *The Age of AIDS.* Frontline documentary series directed by William Cran and Greg Barker. 2006. www.pbs.org/wgbh/pages/frontline/aids/.

Public Square Films. *How to Survive a Plague.* Documentary directed by David France. 2012.

Siplon, Patricia D. *AIDS and the Policy Struggle in the United States.* Washington, D.C.: Georgetown University Press, 2002.

Smith, Raymond A., and Patricia D. Siplon. *Drugs into Bodies: Global AIDS Treatment Activism.* London: Praeger, 2006.

6

Building an Effective Rural Health Delivery Model in Haiti and Rwanda

PETER DROBAC, MATTHEW BASILICO, LUKE MESSAC, DAVID WALTON, PAUL FARMER

Thus far, this book has focused on theories we have found useful in understanding global health and on the history of the term and its predecessor paradigms. Underpinning much of these reflections is an awareness that poverty and social disparities of all sorts determine the fate of millions. But what do large-scale social forces such as poverty or political violence mean at the point of care for people living in such conditions? How might social theory and history inform efforts to improve the *delivery* of health services? This chapter explores the experiences of Partners In Health, an institution that seeks to strengthen health systems in the rural reaches of some of the most underserved parts of the developing world. PIH's approach links delivery of high-quality care for individual patients to efforts to redress some of the structural barriers to good health, such as unemployment, insufficient access to food and clean water, shoddy (or absent) health infrastructure, high transport costs, and poor housing, to name just a few. We focus on PIH because we know its work well; other organizations have met similar goals using comparable approaches, which seek to deliver care to the poor while bolstering public capacity to do so. All have relied on efforts to learn how to improve care delivery by studying the process and training others to do so. Many, including GHESKIO in Haitia, AMPATH in Kenya, CIDRZ in Zambia, and Health Alliance International in several countries, are linked to universities, as is PIH.[1]

An exploration of PIH's work starts with its roots in rural Haiti in the 1980s. As this chapter documents, an understanding of the local context—drawing on an understanding of burden of disease but also on history, political economy, and ethnography—enabled PIH and its sister organizations to design (and redesign) an effective health system capable of delivering care in settings of poverty and disruption. But this success was not the result of a tidy application of theory to a particular setting with enormous and unmet needs; nor did the work proceed smoothly. PIH's first years were grounded in trial and error and slow correction of course. But these tumultuous years taught us the importance of learning from those we sought to serve and of studying delivery. The successes and failures of these years also help to explain our conviction that partnership itself is a way forward; that health equity is a worthy aspiration; and that training and research are necessary, from the outset, to improve services and, at times, to reset course entirely.

Some of that course was set by PIH's first partners, a group of displaced peasant farmers in central Haiti. This chapter thus begins with a brief overview of the region before turning to an exploration of PIH's health delivery model in rural Haiti. The second part of the chapter discusses the expansion of PIH's work in rural Rwanda. As we note, these two countries have much in common—violent (and contested) histories, populations of about 10 million, largely agrarian economies, low average income, and limited access to health services—and therefore have much to learn from each other, as we have much to learn from them.

The last part of this chapter addresses an event that has posed a grave threat to health in Haiti and to the progress made in the previous decades: the 2010 earthquake. No one—including public health experts, medical practitioners, disaster-preparedness experts, and humanitarians—could have been ready for the massive earthquake that leveled much of Port-au-Prince on January 12 of that year. The quake struck the nerve center of the country—and its frail health system—claiming hundreds of thousands of lives and causing untold disability. The country's biggest hospitals were damaged or destroyed; the state nursing school collapsed altogether. Understanding the lessons of January 2010 is important if we are to "reimagine global health" because responses to such events, whether termed natural or unnatural disasters, lead to consequences intended and unintended. They shape an emerging field as do colonial practices and subsequent paradigms.

HAITI

History in Brief

The history of poor health in Haiti's Central Plateau begins well before the 1919 founding of the Ministry of Public Health and Population, the government agency charged with providing health services. Haiti's history is characterized by tumult and frequent incursions from beyond its borders. The indigenous inhabitants of Haiti—the Taíno Amerindians, numbering in the hundreds of thousands or even millions in the fifteenth century—had all but perished, as a result of conquest and infectious disease, a mere century after Christopher Columbus reached the island of Hispaniola in 1492. The dwindling Taíno population proved insufficient as slave labor on lucrative sugar and coffee plantations, so the Spanish colonists began importing African slaves. The western third of the island, ceded to the French in 1697, was transformed into one of the most profitable European colonial possessions in the New World, becoming the world's largest supplier of sugar and coffee in the late eighteenth century. By 1791, on the eve of revolution, slaves outnumbered Europeans nine to one.[2]

This brutal labor system gave way to the largest slave revolt in history: even though Napoleon sent his brother-in-law at the head of the largest armada ever to set forth from Europe to the Americas, to retake Haiti, the French were defeated and ousted. The second republic in the Western Hemisphere—the first black republic in the world—was born in 1804.

But independence did not mean protection from foreign intruders and predatory local elites. The spirit of resistance and the rejection of forced labor that led to revolution also stymied efforts by early rulers to re-create a system of export-led plantation agriculture, which depended on large reserves of cheap labor to do such backbreaking work as cutting sugarcane. Many former slaves did work on others' land, but by the late nineteenth century there were more small landowners in Haiti than in other countries in the region. Most Haitians instead opted for independent farming—what one historian calls a "counter-plantation system"[3]—even if it meant relocating to remote regions such as the mountainous Central Plateau. Anthropologist Michel-Rolph Trouillot describes the situation: "The peasantry, conscious of its new-found liberty and stubbornly holding onto its rights, was not responsive to the lure of money. When it had to choose between a higher income and direct control of the labor process, it chose control."[4]

With reorganization into estate farming ruled out as a viable option, many rural landowners gradually lost their political and economic influence through dwindling parcel size and diminishing productivity; some liquidated their holdings to join the more prosperous merchant class. By the turn of the twentieth century, members of Haiti's small elite, who controlled the state and almost all foreign trade, were densely clustered in Port-au-Prince and a couple of smaller coastal cities. In 1881, trade duties made up more than 98 percent of state income.[5] The majority of the population, however, remained rural smallholder farmers, increasingly excluded from the power structure of the capital, and continued to be the chief producers of the country.

International pressure and local misrule paralyzed rural economic development. The United States and most of Europe refused to recognize Haiti until the late nineteenth century and often practiced gunboat diplomacy to get their way.[6] In 1825, a French naval delegation demanded an indemnity of 150 million francs from Haiti for the "losses"—land, capital, and the bodies of slaves themselves—endured by the French plantation owners during the revolution. Haiti continued to pay off this odious debt ($21 billion in today's dollars) until 1922.[7] Foreign meddling was far from over in the twentieth century. Seeking influence in the Caribbean and control of the Haitian customs houses, the U.S. Marine Corps invaded Haiti in 1915 and occupied the country militarily until 1934, cementing a relationship of dependence between the two oldest republics in the hemisphere. U.S. leaders rewrote the Haitian constitution to allow foreign ownership of land and to open more markets to U.S. investors, which seemed to further concentrate power in Port-au-Prince. The modern Haitian army was also established by an act of the U.S. Congress during this period.

These years saw little in the way of new resources for development or social services for the poor, which ruling elites showed little inclination to provide in the first place. They continued trying, with scant success, to resuscitate the one economic activity that had a proven record of generating revenues on the island: export agriculture. Once again, public revenues—meager as they were—came largely from rural peasantry, who toiled on but remained cut off from most services and profits.[8] These uses and abuses of Haiti left the beleaguered country with neither capacity nor resources for rural development, to say nothing of education or health care.

The post–World War II era of decolonization and "big push" development schemes (which called for a surge of investment to jumpstart growth in poor countries) might have been a turning point for Haiti.[9] But it was not to be. The infrastructure gap was not breached any more than failures to invest in human capital were addressed. From 1804 to the mid-twentieth century, few high schools or hospitals or roads had been completed, except for those built during the occupation; and Haiti remained largely without electricity in spite of the 1956 construction of the Péligre Dam. The knockout blow arrived with the ascension of François "Papa Doc" Duvalier in 1957. With the help of his paramilitary force, the *tonton macoutes,* Duvalier ensured political control by silencing opposition—including some thirty thousand politically driven murders—until his death in 1971.[10] His reign further intensified the centralization of wealth and power in the nation's capital: by the end of it, 80 percent of the government budget was consumed in Port-au-Prince, which housed less than 20 percent of the Haiti's population.[11] Like electricity, health care and higher education were also heavily concentrated in what Haitians call "The City."

Duvalierism, which was focused less on ideology and more on iron rule, widened the divide between the state and the poor and further undermined the capacity (and will) of the government to provide services for its citizens. Duvalier turned the civil service, long weak and ineffective, even further away from official mandates and, with liberal use of brutality and outright terror, built a political machine that ran on graft and cronyism.[12] Across Haiti, what scant health and education infrastructure existed withered away; concrete carcasses of half-finished, half-hearted investments dotted the urban landscape but provided little in the way of services. Papa Doc's son, Jean-Claude Duvalier (both are pictured in figure 6.1), maintained this status quo until he fled the country in 1986.[13] Despite the brutality of the Duvaliers, some nations, especially the United States, perceived the family dictatorship as a "bulwark against communism" and so propped up the regime with a steady stream of resources—a stream that grew more substantial toward the end of the Cold War. Such assistance contributed substantially, if indirectly, to the rulers' personal wealth and to a system of state-sponsored terrorism.[14]

Haiti, facing a growing ecological crisis—deforestation had triggered erosion and decreased crop yields—was further pushed into hunger by the unfair trade practices that wiped out Haiti's rice production and left it a net importer of sugar. In the embrace of U.S. and international trade regimes, Haiti could do little to protect its own agriculture. During the last half of the twentieth century, heavily subsidized

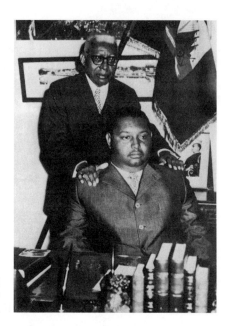

FIGURE 6.1. François and
Jean-Claude Duvalier. Courtesy
Keystone-France/Getty Images.

U.S. products flooded its markets.[15] Hunger riots erupted in 1985, and within months, Baby Doc fled, leaving the reins of government in the hands of the Haitian army. Established during the U.S. occupation, the modern army had never known a non-Haitian enemy.

After years of coups and instability, 1990 brought hope to Haiti. The first free and fair elections in Haitian history led to the presidency of Jean-Bertrand Aristide, a liberation theologian with far-reaching support among the peasantry and urban poor.[16] But these hopes were soon dashed: a military coup forced Aristide from office only nine months later. After several years of international negotiations, Aristide was reinstated with the help of the United States and the United Nations; but the deal came with conditions, including further "reforms" of the Haitian economy that followed structural adjustment policies.[17] As chapter 4 discusses, such stipulations capped social-sector spending. The public health and education systems remained starved of resources. And despite promises to the contrary, foreign aid for public-sector services remained paltry during the remainder of Aristide's term and that of his successor, René Préval.[18] Elections returned Aristide to the presidency in 2001, and Préval became the first democratically elected president in the republic's two-hundred-year history to hand over power after a full term in office. Not coincidentally, the Aristide administration had demobilized the Haitian army and began integrating, by gender, the police force.

Aristide may have won the popular vote handily. But he was not universally supported by those recently put in charge of U.S. foreign policy toward Haiti, Cuba, and Venezuela at the time. Although the United States had funneled a great deal of aid to and through the Duvalier dictatorships, Washington's leaders, in concert with France and Canada, quietly implemented an aid embargo on the Haitian government over alleged discrepancies involving six minor district-level seats in the 2001 elections.[19] This diplomatic action signaled displeasure with Aristide's policies, which included democratizing political and economic institutions in Haiti and providing services designed to benefit the poor majority. This was met by open hostility from some sectors of the Haitian elite and by attacks by former soldiers and Army officers, who had formed bases in the neighboring Dominican Republic. In 2004, Aristide was once again forced from office and into exile by a coup—the origins and financing of which continue to be debated— leaving Haiti involuntarily on a U.S. plane. [20]

The governments that followed, whether cobbled together or elected, have had an uphill challenge to find firm footing. Buffeted by political instability and international economic forces, not to mention a series of devastating hurricanes, the country struggled, and the social conditions of the poor in Haiti remained dire.

This relatively recent period of Haiti's history, from the mid-1980s into the first decade of the new millennium, formed the immediate backdrop against which the team of Partners In Health and Zanmi Lasante carried out its work and began to develop a model of health care delivery, as described in the following sections. But as the organization's workers learned, they were never far from the deep roots of Haiti's colonial past.

Health Care in Haiti

It comes as no surprise that after centuries of misrule and foreign interference, Haiti has long had some of the worst health indices in the Western Hemisphere.[21] Despite the importance of colonial Haiti to the French economy, France's investments in health care infrastructure were negligible. On the eve of the revolution that began on the island in 1791, only a few military hospitals were in operation. Ill members of the white minority were treated at home. Members of the black majority, if treated at all, received such care as was available in plantation sickbays. One plantation's records show that a third of the newly acquired slaves were dead within "a year or two."[22]

A decade later, after the war for independence, the situation had not improved. According to Ary Bordes, one chronicler of public health in Haiti, all of the island's doctors and surgeons had fled. The majority of hospitals and other institutions had been destroyed; only the military hospitals in Port-au-Prince and Cap-Haïtien remained. The towns were in shambles, without sewers or latrines. What little care could be delivered was offered by orderlies who had worked in hospitals or by midwives, herbalists, and bonesetters. Bordes writes of a "host of technically unprepared health workers in the presence of a population newly liberated from slavery, living for the most part in primitive huts, without water or latrines, and undermined and decimated by the infectious diseases against which they were so poorly protected. [This was the] oppressive legacy from our former masters, thirsty for profits, and little interested in the living conditions and health of the indigenous population."[23]

This oppressive legacy is very much alive in rural Haiti. With a rural per capita income under $300 per year, Haiti has long teetered on the edge of famine, and its people are faced with a long list of health problems worsened by chronic undernutrition. Adequate housing and sanitation systems remain rare. In 2009—just before the earthquake—World Bank estimates suggested that, for rural Haitians, only 51 percent had access to an improved water source and only 10 percent had access to improved sanitation facilities.[24] More than half of Haitians lived on less than $1.25 per day, with 58 percent of children undernourished. More than half of all school-age children were not in school.[25]

On the eve of the January 2010 earthquake, healthy life expectancy stood at sixty-one years, while mortality rates for children under five were estimated to be close to 72 per 1,000.[26] Diarrheal disease exacts a toll on children of all ages. It is the leading cause of death among poorly nourished preschoolers and the chief cause of missed school among those fortunate enough to attend.[27] Malaria, eradicated in the surrounding islands, continues to take lives in Haiti. In 2006, the physician-to-population ratio stood at 25 per 100,000.[28] (In the United States, the figure is 256 per 100,000.)[29]

On top of these challenges was a disease caused by a new pathogen, likely introduced to Haiti by tourists in the 1970s.[30] The disease was eventually called AIDS and in 1983 shown to be caused by HIV. Urban Haiti was one of the epicenters of the American epidemic and also, thanks to GHESKIO, one of the settings in which some of the early knowledge of the epidemic was generated and shared, locally and internationally. By the mid-1990s, the virus had taken hold among marginalized populations in the slums of Port-au-Prince and had begun making its way into rural communities; prevalence increased to 5.6 percent nationally.[31] This chapter recounts efforts to confront AIDS in rural Haiti by seeking to adhere to PIH's mission statement—to "draw on the resources of the world's leading medical and academic institutions and on the lived experience of the world's poorest and sickest communities."[32] It also asserts that efforts to integrate prevention and care helped to turn the AIDS epidemic around in Haiti and elsewhere.

Cange

Partners In Health and its sister organization, Zanmi Lasante, were launched in the mid-1980s in Haiti's Central Plateau (see map 6.1), with the founding of a small clinic in Cange. Pictured in figure 6.2, Cange was a squatter settlement of displaced peasant farmers who had lost their land, their homes, and their livelihoods when the construction of a giant dam and reservoir flooded their fertile valley. In 1956, when the Péligre Dam (shown in figure 6.3) was completed, it was the tallest buttress dam in the Western Hemisphere. Designed and built during the height of "big push" development enthusiasm and constructed by the U.S. company Brown and Root (later acquired by Halliburton), the dam provided electricity to far-off Port-au-Prince, skipping rural towns along the way—and also skipping poor residents of the capital. (Some forty-seven years later, President Aristide saw that Cange got electricity, too.)[33]

Official documents claim that those who built the dam had warned local denizens of the impending flood. But interviews with many of the displaced suggested that some area inhabitants were unaware of the dam's completion until waters started rising, swallowing their houses and farmland. These "water refugees," at least the ones in Cange, complained that most had not received any compensation from the government or the companies involved.[34]

That the lives of those who inhabited the low-lying lands behind the dam were disrupted by large-scale social forces far beyond their control is not a difficult argument to make. We can point to grow-

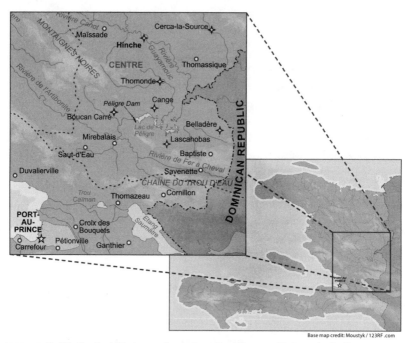

MAP 6.1. Haiti's Central Plateau, situated north of Port-au-Prince, including the locations of Zanmi Lasante/Partners In Health facilities such as Cange, Lascahobas, and Mirebalais. Source: Thomas McIntyre, Christopher D. Hughes, Thierry Pauyo, Stephen R. Sullivan, Selwyn O. Rogers, Maxi Raymonville, and John G. Meara, "Emergency Surgical Care Delivery in Post-Earthquake Haiti: Partners In Health and Zanmi Lasante Experience," *World Journal of Surgery* 35, no. 4 (2011): 745–750.

ing government enthusiasm for big infrastructure projects, or to the creation of development agencies that pushed such projects, or to the rise of authoritarian governments that followed the U.S. military occupation and preceded the Duvalier dictatorships as the immediate precursors of their displacement. We can also reach back to Haiti's history as a slave colony, and to the lack of education and fair land-titling practices in rural Haiti, to understand the roots of their vulnerability. In either case, it is clear that many of that region's small farmers were buffeted by economic and political developments that washed over them much as the impounded waters of the Artibonite River washed over their small plots of land. What did these developments mean for families and individuals trying to make a living in this troubled squatter settlement? How are the history and political economy of Haiti manifested, as sickness, in the bodies of the

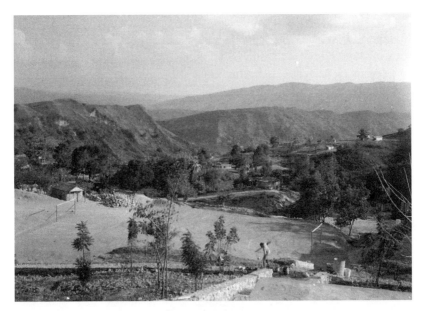

FIGURE 6.2. A view of Cange, circa 1985. Courtesy Partners In Health.

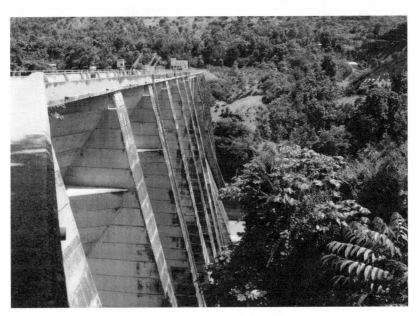

FIGURE 6.3. The Péligre Dam, built in 1956. Courtesy Arjun Suri.

"water refugees" and their descendants? Do such forces need to be understood by those seeking to deliver health care? If so, how do they matter? How might such understandings be "built into" efforts to prevent or alleviate suffering caused by poverty and disease? To answer these questions, we will look at both the experience of AIDS and tuberculosis in a squatter settlement in central Haiti and also at attempts to address illness, and especially chronic disease, with a health system that can deliver care to patients who struggle against both poverty and disease.

Acéphie's Story

Acéphie Joseph was the daughter of a couple who had lost their home and land when the water rose. She and her twin brother attended primary school in a banana bark–thatched open shelter in which children and young adults received the rudiments of literacy. "She was the nicest of the Joseph sisters," recalled one of her classmates. "And she was as pretty as she was nice."

Acéphie's beauty—she was tall and fine-featured, with enormous dark eyes—and her vulnerability may have sealed her fate as early as 1984. Though still in primary school then, she was already nineteen years old; it was time for her to help generate income for her family, which was sinking deeper and deeper into poverty. Acéphie began to help by carrying produce to a local market on Friday mornings. On foot or with a donkey, it took over an hour and a half to reach the market, and the road led right through Péligre, site of the dam and a military barracks. The soldiers liked to watch the parade of women on Friday mornings. Sometimes they taxed them, literally, with haphazardly imposed fines; sometimes they levied a toll of flirtatious banter.

Such flirtation is seldom rejected, at least openly. In rural Haiti, entrenched poverty made the soldiers—then the region's only salaried men—more attractive. Hunger was a near-daily reality for the Joseph family; by 1985, the times were as bad as those right after the flooding of the valley. So when Acéphie's good looks caught the eye of Captain Jacques Honorat, a native of Belladère, formerly stationed in Port-au-Prince, she returned his gaze. Acéphie knew, as did everyone in the area, that Honorat had a wife and children. He was known, in fact, to have more than one regular partner. But Acéphie was taken in by his persistence, and when he went to speak to her parents, a long-term liaison was, from the outset, a serious possibility:

What would you have me do? I could tell that the old people were uncomfortable, worried; but they didn't say no. They didn't tell me to stay away from him. I wish they had, but how could they have known? . . . I knew it was a bad idea then, but I just didn't know why. I never dreamed he would give me a bad illness, never! I looked around and saw how poor we all were, how the old people were finished . . .

What would you have me do? It was a way out, that's how I saw it.

Acéphie and Honorat were sexual partners only briefly—for less than a month, according to Acéphie. Shortly thereafter, Honorat fell ill with unexplained fevers and kept to the company of his wife in Péligre. As Acéphie was looking for a *moun prensipal*—a "main man"—she tried to forget about the soldier. Still, it was shocking to hear, a few months after they parted, that he was dead.

Acéphie was at a crucial juncture in her life. Returning to school was out of the question. After some casting about, she went to Mirebalais, the nearest town, and began a course in what she euphemistically termed a "cooking school." The school—really just an ambitious woman's courtyard—prepared poor girls like Acéphie for their inevitable turn as servants in the city. Indeed, becoming a maid was fast developing into one of the rare growth industries in Haiti; and, as much as Acéphie's proud mother hated to think of her daughter reduced to servitude, she could offer no viable alternative.

And so Acéphie, twenty-two years old, went off to Port-au-Prince, where she found a job as a housekeeper for a middle-class Haitian woman who worked for the U.S. embassy. Acéphie's looks and manners kept her out of the backyard, the traditional milieu of Haitian servants. In addition to cleaning, she answered the door and the phone. Although Acéphie was not paid well—she received thirty dollars each month—she recalled the gnawing hunger in her home village and managed to save a bit of money for her parents and siblings, especially her brother, who had never been able to find a paying job.

Still looking for a *moun prensipal*, Acéphie began seeing Blanco Nerette, a young man with origins similar to her own: Blanco's parents were also "water refugees," and Acéphie had known him when they were both attending the parochial school in Cange. Blanco had done well for himself, by local standards: he chauffeured a small bus between the Central Plateau and the capital. In a setting in which the unemployment rate was greater than 60 percent, he could command considerable respect. He turned his attentions to Acéphie. They planned to marry, she later recalled, and started pooling their resources.

Acéphie remained at the "embassy woman's" house for more than three years, staying until she discovered that she was pregnant. She told Blanco, who immediately became nervous. Nor was her employer pleased: it is considered unsightly to have a pregnant servant. And so Acéphie returned to Cange, where she had a difficult pregnancy. Blanco came to see her once or twice. They had a disagreement, and then she heard nothing more from him. Following the birth of her daughter, Acéphie was sapped by repeated opportunistic infections. A regular visitor to the clinic, she was soon diagnosed with AIDS.

Within months of her daughter's birth, Acéphie's life was consumed with managing her own drenching night sweats and debilitating diarrhea while attempting to care for the child. "We both need diapers now," she remarked bitterly, toward the end of her life. As political violence hampered her doctors' ability to open the clinic, Acéphie was faced each day not only with diarrhea but also with a persistent lassitude. As she became more and more gaunt, some villagers suggested that Acéphie was the victim of sorcery. The clinic doctors diagnosed disseminated tuberculosis. Others recalled her liaison with the soldier and her work as a servant in the city, by then widely considered (among care providers) to be risk factors for AIDS and tuberculosis, the most opportunistic infection seen in Haiti. Acéphie herself knew that she had AIDS, although she was more apt to refer to herself as suffering from a disorder brought on by her work as a servant: "All that ironing, and then opening a refrigerator." She died far from refrigerators or other amenities as her family and caregivers stood by helplessly.

But this is not simply the story of Acéphie and her daughter, also infected with the virus. There is also Jacques Honorat's first wife, who each year grew thinner. After Honorat's death, she found herself desperate, with no means of feeding her five hungry children, two of whom were also ill. The widow's subsequent union was again with a soldier. Honorat had at least two other partners, both of them poor peasant women, in the Central Plateau. One was HIV-positive and the mother of two sickly children. And there was Blanco, apparently in good health, plying the roads from Mirebalais to Port-au-Prince. Who knew if he carried the virus? As a chauffeur, he had several girlfriends.

Nor is this simply the story of those infected with HIV. The pain felt by Acéphie's mother and twin brother was manifestly intense. But few understood her father's anguish. Shortly after Acéphie's death, he hanged himself with a length of rope.[35]

. . .

Living in Cange, among the "water refugees" whose lives had been upended by decisions made elsewhere, provided as good a setting as any to learn that regnant models of health care financing and delivery would not lead to good outcomes among the landless poor. (Such models were increasingly based on crude notions of cost-effectiveness and selective primary health care.) The water refugees and their descendents called for equity and redress; they became the teachers of PIH. Few others could have explained how poverty and landlessness—forces termed "structural" in this volume and elsewhere[36]—constrain agency and fuel migration to urban slums. Starting in a squatter settlement in rural Haiti taught us, in short, how to design medical and educational services not on the basis of cost-effectiveness but rather as fundamentally reparative efforts to promote basic social and economic rights.

Working in Cange also taught PIH how to design interventions seeking to counter the effects of structural violence: programs to diagnose and treat patients with tuberculosis and without sufficient food, for example, or AIDS prevention efforts targeting women whose choices had been sharply circumscribed by poverty and gender inequality.[37] These lessons were learned in part through a series of studies, including community health assessments conducted in Cange and surrounding villages; others involved qualitative methods, including ethnography and semi-structured interviews. Most lessons were learned in a more painful way: by making mistakes and then seeking to correct them.

The life experiences of Acéphie and other Haitians living in poverty—in addition to knowledge of Haiti's history and political economy and of the ranking health problems facing the population—began to inform the early decisions made by PIH and its Haitian sister organization Zanmi Lasante. Taking a hard look at the poor outcomes of tuberculosis care was especially instructive. In fact, this small program taught us all hard lessons about the importance of designing programs to meet the needs of patients facing both poverty and chronic illness. Since it shaped not only our thinking but also subsequent efforts to respond to AIDS and other health problems, we examine it in some detail.

Tuberculosis in Haiti

The experience of tuberculosis in rural Haiti is strongly conditioned by historical contingencies and material constraints.[38] Most available documentation suggests that the slave forebears of contemporary Haitians were ill indeed, as the anthropologist Jean Weise noted: "The slaves brought from Africa to Haiti carried with them the remnants of their cultural systems, yellow fever, yaws and malaria. The Spanish gave them sugar cane, vicious slavery, a form of Catholicism, smallpox, measles, typhoid and tuberculosis. The French, in their turn, gave the Haitians a language, traces of French culture and continued vicious servitude."[39] The introduction of tuberculosis, whenever it took place, would prove to be of enduring significance. By 1738, the disorder was widespread enough to alarm French doctors visiting the island.[40] One historian noted that the rainy season was particularly hard on the colony's *poitrinaires,* a term still commonly used in reference to tuberculosis in rural Haiti.[41] A later observer estimated that *les tubercules* were, after dysentery, the most common chronic illness.[42]

Tuberculosis remained a ranking threat two centuries later. "Of all the health problems cited," observed Jean Wiese in 1971, "one stands out from the others by virtue of its insidious onset, its tenacity, and its prevalence—pulmonary tuberculosis."[43] The prevalence of tuberculosis in Haiti is estimated to be the highest in the hemisphere. Little is known of the disease during the nineteenth century, but in 1941 one scholar wrote that, in a series of seven hundred autopsies performed in the Port-au-Prince General Hospital, 26 percent of deaths were deemed due to tuberculosis.[44] The United Nations reported that in 1944 "tuberculosis was the most important cause of death among hospitalized patients" in Haiti. Linking the high incidence of the disorder to poor sanitation and poverty, the UN predicted that "for many years to come tuberculosis will, it is feared, continue to take a heavy toll of human lives in Haiti."[45]

This prediction came true. The Pan American Health Organization estimated the prevalence of tuberculosis in 1965 at 3,862 cases per 100,000 inhabitants.[46] Available data indicate that tuberculosis remained the leading cause of death among individuals between the ages of fifteen and forty-nine until the turn of the millennium (when it was supplanted by AIDS). Studies from the Hôpital Albert Schweitzer in the 1980s suggested that, in this age group, tuberculosis caused two to three times as many deaths as the next most common diagnosis.[47]

By the 1990s, the situation had worsened. The high prevalence of tuberculosis was complicated by the advent of HIV. In sanatoriums in urban Haiti, some 45 percent of all tuberculosis patients reportedly were co-infected with HIV. In a survey of over 7,300 ostensibly healthy adults living in a densely populated slum, 70 percent of those screened were deemed infected with latent strains of *Mycobacterium tuberculosis* and more than 15 percent were HIV-positive. More alarming, community-based screening detected a prevalence of 2,281 *active* pulmonary tuberculosis cases per 100,000 adults.[48] One study conducted at about this time in rural regions found that 15 percent of patients diagnosed with tuberculosis disease were also infected with HIV. In another rural setting, at the Hôpital Albert Schweitzer, 24 percent of all patients with tuberculosis were co-infected with HIV.[49]

Adding to this noxious synergy was the emergence of resistance to first-line antituberculous drugs. There are few published studies of drug resistance in Haiti, in large part because it is difficult to culture *Mycobacterium tuberculosis* in settings with no reliable source of electricity and little in the way of modern laboratories. One of the only large series including culture data revealed that 22 percent of isolates were resistant to at least one first-line drug.[50]

Although drug resistance presents a significant problem, most studies of treatment failure agree that the problem is predominantly one of designing and implementing programs that meet the needs of those afflicted. Until that happens, a diagnosis of tuberculosis will lead too rarely to curative treatment.[51] In one large town in southern Haiti, fully 75 percent of all patients had abandoned treatment by six months after diagnosis, and over 93 percent had abandoned treatment within one year.[52] Since short-course therapy did not exist at the time of this study, we must assume that the majority of patients in this series were left with partially treated disease.

What follows describes in some detail PIH/ZL's efforts to implement a tuberculosis-control program that takes into account the crippling poverty that so often plays a central role in determining who does or does not benefit from interventions. It was also important that the program avoid the "either-or" approach that has led some health advocates to adopt a Luddite stance. This position holds that it is acceptable to defer tuberculosis treatment while the "root causes" of the disease are addressed through development projects. But health policy is not a zero-sum game. One of the lessons learned in rural Haiti is that effective tuberculosis-specific interventions are both urgent and inexpensive and should not be regarded as somehow detracting from the broader development efforts that might well serve to reduce tuberculosis incidence.

Building a Tuberculosis-Control Program

Twenty years ago, Zanmi Lasante's catchment area included settlements scattered around the reservoir created by the Péligre Dam. In those years, as we were seeking to build community-based care and clinics and a hospital, the chief distinction we made was whether or not we could rely on a community health worker, or *accompagnateur*, to complement the efforts of facility-based clinicians. But we were also committed to keeping these facilities open to all those who might show up. Thus, Sector 1 of the catchment area ringed the lake and was home to approximately twenty-five thousand individuals, almost all of them peasants living in small villages; in each of these settlements, we had trained *accompagnateurs*. Sector 2, more loosely demarcated, consisted of a large number of outlying villages and towns contiguous to Sector 1.

Although patients in both sectors were offered the same clinical services (consultations with a physician, lab work, and all medication for about 80 cents), those in Sector 2 were not served by community health workers, nor did they benefit from activities sponsored by ZL such as women's health initiatives, vaccination campaigns, water protection efforts, and adult literacy groups. These interventions, implemented by *accompagnateurs*, had proven to be a powerful means of addressing malnutrition, diarrheal disease, measles, neonatal tetanus, and malaria. Through the community activities, the health workers were able to identify the sick and refer them to the clinic, where they received all antituberculous medications free of charge, thanks to the struggling national TB program, which was seeking NGO partners to help with implementation. (Isoniazid, ethambutol, pyrazinamide, and streptomycin were then on formulary at the clinic.)[53]

Although ZL clinicians were effective in identifying patients with pulmonary tuberculosis, it became clear during the late 1980s that detection of new cases did not necessarily lead to cure, in spite of the clinic's policy of waiving even the 80-cent fee for any patient diagnosed with tuberculosis. In December 1988, following the deaths from tuberculosis of three HIV-negative patients, all in their forties, staff met to reconsider how the care of these individuals had been managed. How had we failed to prevent these deaths?

Responses to this question—all of them claims of causality—varied. Some community health workers felt that tuberculosis patients who had poor outcomes were the most economically impoverished and thus the sickest. Others, including physicians and most nurses, attributed poor compliance to widespread beliefs that tuberculosis was inflicted through sorcery, which led patients to abandon biomedical therapy. Still others hypothesized that patients lost interest in chemotherapy after ridding themselves of the symptoms that had initially caused them to seek medical advice.

Over the next two months, PIH/ZL devised a plan to improve services to patients with tuberculosis and to test these discrepant hypotheses. Briefly, the new program embraced the goals of finding cases, offering adequate chemotherapy, and providing close follow-up. Although contact screening and BCG vaccination for infants were included in the program, the greatest concern was the care of smear-positive and coughing patients, whom many considered the most important source of community exposure.

The new program was designed to be aggressive and community-based, relying heavily on *accompagnateurs*—paid community health workers trained to provide medical and psychosocial support for their neighbors—for close follow-up. It was also designed to respond to patients' appeals for nutritional assistance and other forms of social support. All residents of Sector 1 diagnosed with pulmonary or extra-pulmonary tuberculosis would be eligible to participate in a treatment program featuring—during the first month following diagnosis—daily visits from their village health worker. These patients would receive financial aid of $30 per month for the first three months and would also be eligible for nutritional supplements.

Further, these patients were to receive a monthly reminder from their village health worker to attend clinic. Travel expenses (for example, renting a donkey) would be defrayed with a $5 honorarium when they arrived for a clinic visit. If a Sector 1 patient did not attend, someone from the clinic—often a physician or an auxiliary nurse—would visit the no-show's house. A series of forms, including a detailed initial interview schedule and home-visit reports, regularized these arrangements and replaced the relatively limited forms used for other clinic patients.

During the initial enrollment period, between February 1989 and September 1990, fifty Sector 1 patients were diagnosed with smear-positive tuberculosis and enrolled in the program.[54] Forty-eight had pulmonary tuberculosis. Seven individuals also had extrapulmonary tuberculosis (for example, tuberculosis of the spine), and two had cervical lymphadenitis ("scrofula") as their sole manifestation of tuberculosis. During the same period, the clinical staff diagnosed pulmonary tuberculosis in 213 patients from outside Sector 1. Many of these patients were from Sector 2, although a few had traveled even greater distances to seek care at the clinic; at least 168 of these individuals returned to the clinic for further care. The first fifty of these patients to be diagnosed formed the comparison group by which the efficacy of the new interventions would be judged. They were a "control group" only in the sense that they did not benefit from the community-based services and the financial aid and social support; all Sector 2 patients continued to receive "free" care—that is, without any users' fees at the point of diagnosis and care. It turned out that there were many hidden costs to the sick and their families.

To test hypotheses regarding associations between patients' beliefs and clinical outcomes, all patients were interviewed regarding their own explanatory models and their experience of tuberculosis.[55] The mean age of the patients (forty-two years) and the sex ratio (both groups had significantly more women than men) did not vary significantly between the two groups.[56] But indirect economic indicators (for example, years of school attended, ownership of a radio, access to a latrine, a tin roof rather than a thatched roof) suggested that patients from Sector 2 may have been slightly less poor than those from Sector 1. This is not surprising, as several of the villages in Sector 1 are squatter settlements dating from the year the valley was flooded.

Table 6.1 summarizes the findings of this study of "health care delivery," as we were terming the modest effects. The following discussion offers a detailed explanation.

Mortality. One patient from the Sector 1 group died in the year following diagnosis, although she did not die from tuberculosis. Six patients from Sector 2 died, all from tuberculosis; one of these was a young woman also seropositive for HIV.

Sputum Positivity. The clinical staff attempted to examine sputum for acid-fast bacilli (AFB)[57] approximately six months after the start of therapy as well as whenever patients developed recrudescent symptoms. No patients from Sector 1 were sputum-positive at six months. One young woman did become sputum-positive during a pregnancy in the subsequent year; she was infected with HIV and relapsed or was reinfected with a second strain of tuberculosis. Of the Sector 2 cohort, nine patients had demonstrable acid-fast bacilli in their sputum about six months after the initiation of therapy.

TABLE 6.1 CHARACTERISTICS OF TUBERCULOSIS
IN SECTOR 1 VERSUS SECTOR 2 PATIENTS

	Sector 1	Sector 2
All-cause mortality (eighteen months follow-up)	1 (2%)	6 (12%)
Sputum-positive for AFB after six months of treatment	0	9 (18%)
Persistent pulmonary symptoms after one year of treatment	3 (6%)	21 (42%)
Average weight gained/patient/year (lbs.)	9.8	1.9
Return to work after one year of treatment	46 (92%)	24 (48%)
Average number of clinic visits/patient/year	11.6	5.4
Average number of home visits/patient/year	32	2
HIV co-infection	2 (4%)	3 (6%)
Number denying the role of sorcery in their illness	6 (12%)	9 (18%)
One-year disease-free survival	50 (100%)	24 (48%)

Persistent Pulmonary Symptoms. After a year of treatment, a thorough history and physical exam screened for persistent pulmonary symptoms such as cough, shortness of breath (dyspnea), and hemoptysis. Only three patients of the Sector 1 group reported such symptoms, and two of them had developed asthma during their convalescence. Twenty patients in Sector 2, however, continued to complain of cough or other symptoms consistent with persistent or partially treated tuberculosis. One additional patient in this group was an asthmatic without radiographic or other evidence of persistent tuberculosis.

Weight Gained. Monitoring body weight revealed marked differences between the two sector groups. Correcting for fluctuations associated with pregnancy, Sector 1 patients gained an average of nearly ten pounds during the first year of their treatment. Patients from Sector 2 had an average weight gain of about two pounds.

Return to Work. The vast majority of patients from both groups were peasant farmers or market women whose families relied on their ability to perform physical labor. It is especially notable, then, that one year after diagnosis, forty-six of the Sector 1 patients stated that they were able to return to work. In Sector 2, fewer than half (twenty-four patients) were able to do so.

Clinic Visits. As patients were given one month's supply of medication with each visit, ZL staff strongly encouraged monthly clinic visits, which served as an indirect measure of a patient's adherence to therapy. In the Sector 1 group, the one-visit-per-month ideal was nearly achieved: these patients, who received a small sum for travel expenses, averaged 11.6 visits per year. Patients in the control group averaged 5.4 visits per year.

Home Visits. The treatment protocol then called for at least 30 grams of intramuscular streptomycin over the first two months of therapy, and community health workers were asked to administer these injections to the patients living in Sector 1. Most patients from Sector 2 had their streptomycin administered by local *pikiris,* or injectionists. (Some lived near licensed practical nurses and received this drug in other clinics.) This is perhaps the chief reason that the number of home visits by members of the ZL staff was far higher in the Sector 1 group than in the Sector 2 group: thirty-two visits in the former versus two visits in the latter.

HIV Seroprevalence. The rate of HIV seroprevalence was not substantially different between the two groups. Only two patients from Sector 1 showed serologic evidence of HIV infection; both had lived in urban Haiti for extended periods. One of these patients became smear-positive for acid-fast bacilli during a pregnancy that occurred more than a year after she completed her initial course of therapy. She was treated with a new multidrug regimen and remained asymptomatic some sixty months after her initial tuberculosis diagnosis. In the Sector 2 group, similarly, three patients were seropositive for HIV, and all had lived in greater Port-au-Prince.

Etiologic Conceptions about Illness. Previous ethnographic research had revealed extremely complex and changing ways of understanding and speaking about illness among rural Haitians.[58] Open-ended interviews with patients in both groups permitted staff to delineate the dominant explanatory models used by members of both groups. Because some had hypothesized that a belief in sorcery would lead to higher rates of noncompliance, the staff took some pains to address this issue with each patient. The results showed that, although few from either group would deny the possibility of sorcery as an etiologic factor in their own illnesses, there was no discernible relationship between avowed adherence to such beliefs and a patient's degree of compliance with a biomedical regimen. The PIH/ZL effort demonstrated the relative insignificance of patients' understandings of etiology, when compared to access to financial aid and social support, such as food packages.

Cure Rate. In June 1991, forty-eight of the Sector 1 patients remained free of pulmonary symptoms. Two patients with a persistent cough or dyspnea did not meet radiologic or clinical diagnostic criteria for tuberculosis (both had developed bronchospastic disease). Therefore, the clinical staff judged that none had active pulmonary tuberculosis, giving the participants a cure rate of 100 percent. One of these patients, as noted earlier, was co-infected with HIV but remained asymptomatic sixty months after her initial diagnosis of tuberculosis. We could not locate all the patients from Sector 2, but of the forty patients examined at more than one year after diagnosis, only twenty-four could be declared free of active disease based on clinical, laboratory, and radiographic evaluation. (Six patients from this group had died during the course of this study.) Even if the four patients lost to follow-up had in fact been cured, that would have left twenty-six others dead or with signs and symptoms of persistent tuberculosis—a cure rate of, at best, 48 percent.

In short, the small group of patients fared better when they were beneficiaries of the program that reduced *structural* barriers to care. Deep local knowledge, coupled with careful social analysis, led the ZL staff to recognize the salience of structural explanations in discerning causes of treatment failure. It also helped doctors, nurses, and administrators to better understand their patients' everyday struggles. They redoubled their efforts in the tuberculosis-control program, working to remove barriers to care. ZL offered funds for transportation to the clinic, gave food supplements to patients and their families, and asked community health workers not only to monitor daily consumption of medication but also to assess the obstacles that patients encountered in accessing care. In some cases, ZL provided housing and paid school fees for patients' children in order to ensure that each household had sufficient resources for nutrition and that patients could come to the health center for appointments. The results of such intervention spoke for themselves—deaths from tuberculosis dropped to nearly zero for those participating in this program. We published our findings in 1991, taking pride in having introduced the term "donkey rental fees" to the medical literature.[59] More importantly, this modest project helped move discussions away from immodest claims of causality about treatment failure. It was not the patients' "beliefs" that led to poor outcomes but rather an ineffective and costly—to the patient—delivery system that led to failure. Community-based care with "wraparound" social support relying on *accompagnateurs* became the standard of care for PIH/ZL tuberculosis programs, which also sought to strengthen the national programs so that they could achieve similar results.

From Tuberculosis to AIDS

This early work was not the only time that PIH/ZL would be confronted with culturalist explanations of ill health in Haiti—for example, that sorcery or ignorance, not poverty, had led to the deaths of tuberculosis patients—and other immodest claims of causality (whether Haitian or imported). The emergence of AIDS in Cange, first identified there by ZL staff in 1986, posed a new set of challenges for the beleaguered population. When the first AIDS drugs became available in the mid-1990s, skeptics claimed that they were too expensive for poor people. Others argued that stigma would prevent people living with AIDS from seeking care at all and that providers should therefore focus solely on education and prevention. And there was stigma and fear: We initially found that even with the introduction of HIV testing in the clinic, only around 20 percent of pregnant women agreed to be tested.

Stigma was a barrier, but not an insurmountable one. In 1994, Zanmi Lasante acquired ATZ and later nevirapine for the prevention of mother-to-child transmission of HIV. Once an effective preventative was offered, testing among pregnant women jumped to nearly 90 percent. Testing is integral to HIV prevention—knowledge of test results can guide decision-making—and clinic staff noted that prevention outcomes improved substantially once they had the key deliverables (tests, counseling, key drugs, condoms, and so on) on hand. Stigma lessened when antiretroviral drugs became available for the prevention of mother-to-child transmission.[60]

But one key intervention remained absent: triple-combination antiretroviral therapy (ART), which was, in the United States and Europe, transforming AIDS from a fatal illness into a chronic disease. Although the 1996 Vancouver International AIDS Conference made a nod to equity—with its theme "One World, One Hope"—AIDS drugs remained out of reach in poor countries around the globe, including in Haiti and across Africa. By the mid-1990s, Zanmi Lasante had built, ward by ward, a full-fledged hospital in Cange, with primary care services, a women's clinic, dozens of inpatient beds, surgical services, and interventions for a wide array of illnesses. The hospital was by then filled with patients admitted with a diagnosis of AIDS or found, in the course of hospitalization for various causes, to be infected with HIV.

Having cut its teeth in a squatter settlement in which nothing would have been termed "sustainable" or "affordable" or "feasible," the team launched the HIV Equity Initiative in 1998, procuring the costly anti-retroviral medications required by the sickest patients in Cange and surrounding villages. The care delivery model was built on ZL's earlier experiences with tuberculosis treatment: to reduce structural barriers to care, ZL continued comprehensive social support, such as covering transportation and food costs and having community health workers provide directly observed therapy.[61]

PIH/ZL ran up against significant opposition. Some policymakers argued that cultural factors would disrupt AIDS treatment in poor countries, leading to inconsistent therapy and thereby increasing the risk of developing drug resistance. As chapter 5 noted, the head of the U.S. Agency for International Development dismissed the idea that ART could be provided in Africa, asserting in testimony before the U.S. Congress in 2001 that Africans "do not know what watches and clocks are. They do not use Western means for telling time."[62] But these too were immodest claims of causality: ZL soon recorded some of the highest rates of ART adherence in the world.[63]

The program also had unintended positive effects elsewhere in the clinic and hospital. For one, it boosted morale: the process of watching someone who had been near death get better rapidly—the "Lazarus effect"—was uplifting for family members, friends, other patients, and clinical staff. Hospital beds once occupied by AIDS patients suffering slow deaths from opportunistic infections opened up, as AIDS became a disease treated at home with the help of *accompagnateurs* or in ambulatory clinics. Patients on ART returned to work and to caring for their children, few of whom were infected. Indeed, the much-feared epidemic of pediatric AIDS dwindled as prevention of mother-to-child transmission was scaled up in Cange and elsewhere.

Within a few years of its launch, the HIV Equity Initiative showed that AIDS prevention and care could be mutually reinforcing. Furthermore, providing AIDS treatment improved the overall systems of care delivery—processes such as more efficient drug procurement and avoidance of stockouts, for example—in the Cange hospital and clinics. As the staff grew and began providing more complex services to an increasing patient load, ZL staff redesigned and rebuilt the hospital to increase the efficiency of patient flow and care. By the late 1990s, fifteen years after conducting their first needs assessment, Partners In Health and Zanmi Lasante had built a community-based, clinic-supported, hospital-linked health care model capable of, if not always successful at, delivering high-quality services in rural Haiti, which was without electricity or paved roads or modern sanitation (although these were to come). The early success of the HIV Equity Initiative countered immodest claims that complex health interventions, such as supervised administration of ART, could not be delivered in resource-poor settings.[64] Similar, if more vertical, efforts were launched in urban South Africa.[65]

In 2001, this modest initiative helped lead to the Harvard "Consensus Statement on Antiretroviral Treatment for AIDS in Poor Countries,"[66] which called for widespread roll-out of integrated AIDS prevention and care and served as one key example in arguments that sparked the world's largest global health initiatives: the Global Fund to Fight AIDS, Tuberculosis and Malaria[67] and the U.S. President's Emergency Plan for AIDS Relief.[68] These small victories also reinforced advocacy efforts for universal access to AIDS treatment, culminating with the World Health Organization's "3 by 5" initiative, which set the goal of treating three million people with ART by 2005.[69] Meanwhile, the PIH/ZL team faced its own scale-up challenges as did the health authorities in Haiti's underfunded and understaffed public sector.

Scaling Up in Rural Haiti

Despite the slogan of the 1978 Declaration of Alma-Ata (described in chapter 4), the year 2000 was not marked by celebrations of health care for all. It was, rather, the year that AIDS surpassed tuberculosis as the leading infectious killer of young adults worldwide.[70] Haiti was no exception. The PIH/ZL team could not effectively wage a community-based war against these scourges from a single squatter settlement. Scaling up would require efforts to build new facilities or rebuild the existing ill-supplied and poorly staffed—and mostly empty—public clinics and hospitals in rural Haiti. (Similar challenges were faced in urban areas where the GHESKIO team, led by Dr. Jean Pape, had for years sought to link improved service delivery to research and training.)[71] Nor could the team based in Cange respond adequately to the overwhelming number of patients arriving each day in the over-crowded courtyards of the place patients had taken to calling "the village of medicine."

By the early 2000s, however, available resources for HIV/AIDS programs had increased substantially (as chapter 5 details). Could funding designated for specific disease-control efforts be leveraged to boost primary care and strengthen public-sector health systems, as had proven possible in Cange? Could access to integrated care be significantly expanded? Could the model developed in Cange be replicated within central Haiti's public-sector institutions?

Haiti was the first country to receive funding from the Global Fund to Fight AIDS, Tuberculosis and Malaria. Haiti's coordinating body—an in-country committee that manages Global Fund grants throughout the nation—was convened by First Lady Mildred Aristide, who asked that the first meeting be held in Cange. As part of the initial grant, the government asked that Zanmi Lasante expand to three new sites, including Lascahobas, a small city in central Haiti, a couple of hours from Cange. But ZL faced a dilemma: they sought to strengthen comprehensive health care services, while the Global Fund sponsored AIDS programs exclusively. Could ZL take a disease-focused (or "vertical" program, to use public health jargon) and make it simultaneously "horizontal" (one that strengthens primary health care broadly)?

Under the direction of Dr. Fernet Léandre and PIH physicians Serena Koenig and David Walton, both with Boston's Brigham and Women's Hospital, a Zanmi Lasante team began working in Lascahobas in August 2002. What they found initially was all too common for a rural public health system left in neglect by the state for decades:

> Our preliminary assessment found the Lascahobas public clinic to be nearly empty in the morning and closed by noon. We found a demoralized staff (there were no doctors) with very little in the way of tools. As for HIV prevention and care, no services were being offered at all: the absence of serologic tests meant that even voluntary counseling and testing and prevention of mother-to-child transmission were unavailable. On paper, at least, diagnosis and care of tuberculosis were provided free of charge to patients. But in the year preceding scale-up, only nine cases of tuberculosis had been diagnosed in Lascahobas, and roughly half of these were lost to follow-up. Incidence data from the Cange region would have predicted closer to 180 patients each year presenting with active tuberculosis.[72]

The ZL team went to work, staffing the Lascahobas clinic and offering comprehensive treatment for HIV using the same protocol followed at Cange. This strategy was based on a number of core principles, summarized in the accompanying box. The results were rapid and remarkable: testing uptake boomed, improving case detection; hundreds of patients who needed ART were soon in treatment. This transformation is best captured graphically, in figures 6.4 and 6.5.

Moreover, transformations were evident in other areas of health care as well, as demonstrated in figures 6.6, 6.7, 6.8, and 6.9. (In figure 6.7, the dramatic spike in tuberculosis case detection is an example of the "first pass effect": disease-endemic regions without access to treatment

Health Care Delivery Model

Strengthening Access to Primary Health Care. A strong foundation of primary care enables treatment of specific diseases, including complications of childbirth and also chronic diseases, from AIDS to diabetes. Most people seek care because they feel sick, not because they have a particular disease. When quality primary care becomes available, communities can develop new faith in their local health systems, increasing use of general medical services as well as services for more complex diseases. PIH thus seeks to integrate infectious-disease interventions into a broad range of basic health and social services.

Providing Health Care and Education for the Poor. User fees decrease attendance at clinics and schools, especially in settings where the burdens of poverty and disease are greatest. PIH works to ensure that cost does not prevent access to primary health care and education for the poor.

Relying on Community Partnerships. PIH's programs involve community members at all levels of assessment, design, implementation, and evaluation. Community health workers *(accompagnateurs)* may be family members, friends, or even patients who provide health education, refer people who are ill to a clinic, deliver medicines—often directly observed therapy—and offer social support to patients in their homes. Community health workers do not supplant the work of doctors or nurses; they interface between the clinic and the community. In recognition of the critical role they play, they are compensated for their work.

Addressing Basic Social and Economic Needs. Achieving good health outcomes requires attending to people's social and economic

see an initial increase in the number of cases detected when treatment becomes available.)

The encouraging improvements achieved at Lascahobas were not unique; similar improvements were documented at each of the public facilities ZL helped to rehabilitate across the Central Plateau. (The new Lascahobas clinic is pictured in figure 6.10.) By the end of 2009, Zanmi Lasante was serving more than 1.1 million people through ten public-sector health facilities; each delivered comprehensive services in line with the model of care pioneered in Cange. When the January 2010 earthquake struck, ZL's Haitian staff, numbering more than ten

---

needs and overcoming structural barriers to care. Through community partners, PIH works to improve access to food, shelter, clean water, sanitation, education, and economic opportunities.

Working in the Public Sector. A vital public sector is often the best way to bring health care to the poor. While nongovernmental organizations play a valuable role in addressing short-term needs, only public-sector health systems can ensure universal and sustained access. Governments are the only institutions capable of conferring a right to health care on their citizens. Rather than establishing parallel systems, PIH works to strengthen and complement existing public-sector health infrastructure.

Focusing on Women and Children. The health of women and the health of future generations are intertwined. Women and children are sometimes less likely than men to receive household resources for adequate nutrition and health,[1] and thus we must pay particular attention to their needs, from the design of health infrastructure to social support programs, to ensure equitable access to care.

Harnessing Technology and Communications. New innovations in medical informatics can improve health care delivery systems in rich and poor settings. PIH has implemented electronic medical records, which assist in data collection and patient monitoring, and other technologies—including communications technologies—to rationalize supply-chain management, laboratory informatics, and patient transfers.

Disseminating Lessons Learned. The science of global health delivery is nascent but growing. Information dissemination allows health providers to learn from the successes and failures of colleagues around the globe.

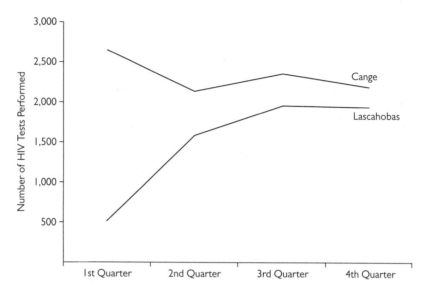

FIGURE 6.4. Voluntary HIV testing in Cange and Lascahobas, July 2002 through September 2003. Source: David A. Walton, Paul E. Farmer, Wesler Lambert, Fernet Léandre, Serena P. Koenig, and Joia S. Mukherjee, "Integrated HIV Prevention and Care Strengthens Primary Health Care: Lessons from Rural Haiti," *Journal of Public Health Policy* 25, no. 2 (2004): 137–158.

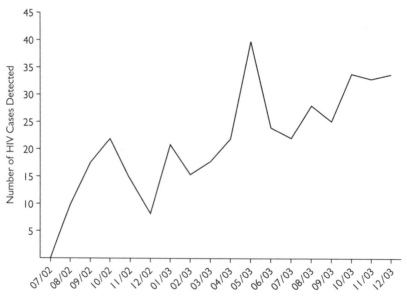

FIGURE 6.5. HIV case detection (number of HIV-positive serologies) in Lascahobas, July 2002 through December 2003. Source: David A. Walton, Paul E. Farmer, Wesler Lambert, Fernet Léandre, Serena P. Koenig, and Joia S. Mukherjee, "Integrated HIV Prevention and Care Strengthens Primary Health Care: Lessons from Rural Haiti," *Journal of Public Health Policy* 25, no. 2 (2004): 137–158.

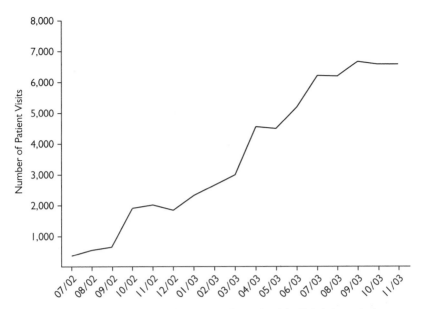

FIGURE 6.6. Ambulatory patient visits to the primary health clinic in Lascahobas, July 2002 through November 2003. Source: David A. Walton, Paul E. Farmer, Wesler Lambert, Fernet Léandre, Serena P. Koenig, and Joia S. Mukherjee, "Integrated HIV Prevention and Care Strengthens Primary Health Care: Lessons from Rural Haiti," *Journal of Public Health Policy* 25, no. 2 (2004): 137–158.

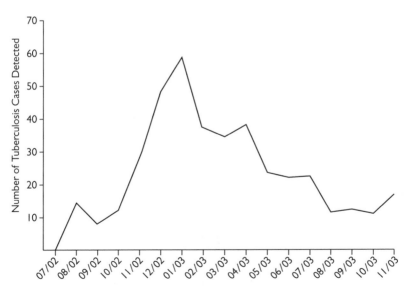

FIGURE 6.7. Tuberculosis case detection in Lascahobas, July 2002 through November 2003. Source: David A. Walton, Paul E. Farmer, Wesler Lambert, Fernet Léandre, Serena P. Koenig, and Joia S. Mukherjee, "Integrated HIV Prevention and Care Strengthens Primary Health Care: Lessons from Rural Haiti," *Journal of Public Health Policy* 25, no. 2 (2004): 137–158.

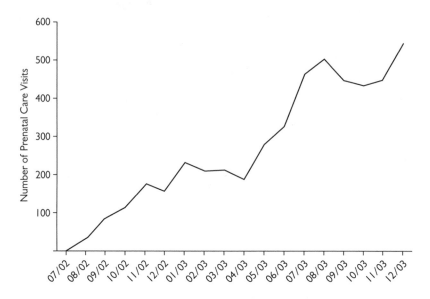

FIGURE 6.8. Prenatal care visits to the clinic in Lascahobas, July 2002 through December 2003. Source: David A. Walton, Paul E. Farmer, Wesler Lambert, Fernet Léandre, Serena P. Koenig, and Joia S. Mukherjee, "Integrated HIV Prevention and Care Strengthens Primary Health Care: Lessons from Rural Haiti," *Journal of Public Health Policy* 25, no. 2 (2004): 137–158.

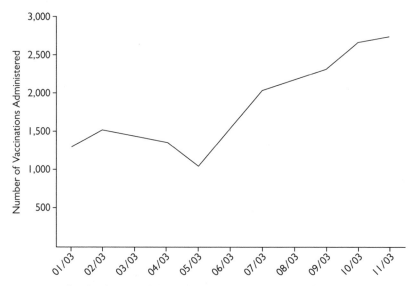

FIGURE 6.9. Vaccinations administered in Lascahobas, January 2003 through November 2003. Source: David A. Walton, Paul E. Farmer, Wesler Lambert, Fernet Léandre, Serena P. Koenig, and Joia S. Mukherjee, "Integrated HIV Prevention and Care Strengthens Primary Health Care: Lessons from Rural Haiti," *Journal of Public Health Policy* 25, no. 2 (2004): 137–158.

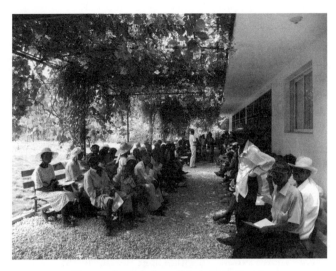

FIGURE 6.10. The new Lascahobas clinic in 2010. Courtesy David Walton.

thousand, mobilized rapidly, coordinating Port-au-Prince's damaged General Hospital and running a series of health clinics in the tent cities that soon filled every open space in Haiti's capital. (See the final section of this chapter for a more detailed account of ZL/PIH's efforts in the aftermath of the earthquake.) Shortly after the quake, at the request of the Haitian government, PIH began construction of the largest hospital in its history (and one of the largest in Haiti): the Mirebalais Hospital, a three-hundred-bed, solar-powered, world-class facility in the middle of central Haiti, which will serve as a national training and referral center.

As ZL was expanding across central Haiti, PIH was also expanding beyond Haitian shores. The following section takes a closer look at one such project, known as Inshuti Mu Buzima—Partners In Health in Rwanda. The idea was not to shift our focus from *accompagnateurs* and clinics to academic medical centers but, rather, to embed a teaching hospital in a delivery system that stretched from homes and villages, where chronic disease is managed, to modern safe facilities.

FROM HAITI TO RWANDA

Although Rwanda and Haiti are separated by geography, history, culture, and political economy, they have sufficient similarities to war-

TABLE 6.2 HEALTH AND DEVELOPMENT INDICATORS IN RWANDA AND HAITI, 2008

2008 Indicator	Rwanda	Haiti
Mortality rate for children under the age of five	112 per 1,000 live births	72 per 1,000 live births
Life expectancy at birth	50 years	61 years
Adult literacy rate	65%	62%
Gross national income per capita	US$410	US$610
Adult HIV prevalence rate	2.8%	2.2%

SOURCE: UNICEF, "At a Glance: Haiti," www.unicef.org/infobycountry/haiti_statistics.html; and UNICEF, "Rwanda: Statistics," www.unicef.org/infobycountry/rwanda_statistics.html.

rant comparison. Both are mountainous countries of approximately 10 million people living in an area roughly equal in size to the state of Maryland. Both are predominantly rural and agrarian; both have been exporters of tropical produce such as coffee. Both struggle with ecological degradation, although deforestation is far more widespread in Haiti. They also share a history of structural violence: poverty, unemployment, foreign meddling, postcolonial instability and violence, and a significant burden of disease.

In 2008, health and development indicators in Rwanda were generally slightly worse than in Haiti, as summarized in table 6.2. And the situation was certainly far worse in 1994, when Rwanda was engulfed by genocide and war. At the close of 1994, Rwanda lay in ruins. Many of its hospitals and clinics had been damaged or destroyed; others were simply abandoned. A large portion of the health workforce had been killed or was in refugee camps. These settlements were thinned by cholera and other "camp" epidemics and by a rising tide of AIDS, tuberculosis, and malaria. Child mortality was the highest in the world; malnutrition was rampant. Many development experts were ready to write the small nation off as a lost cause, a failed state, a hopeless enterprise. Today, Rwanda is the only country in sub-Saharan Africa on track to meet each of the health-related Millennium Development Goals by 2015. More than 93 percent of Rwandan infants are inoculated against eleven vaccine-preventable illnesses, up from 25 percent against five diseases in the year after the genocide. Over the past decade, death during childbirth has declined by more than 60 percent. Deaths attributed to AIDS, tuberculosis, and malaria have dropped even more steeply, as have deaths registered among children under the age of five. There's still a long way to go, but these are some of the steepest declines in mortality ever documented, anywhere and at any time, as we have concluded in reviewing these data. [73]

Rwanda's climb back toward peace and prosperity, including building one of the best health systems on the continent, is increasingly touted as a development success story.[74] As was true in Haiti, the relationship between Rwanda's troubled history and the health of its population demands an analysis that is geographically broad and historically deep in order to understand this progress.

History in Brief

The history of Rwanda remains contested. The popular press tends to overemphasize Rwanda's "tribes": the Hutu and the Tutsi. But claiming a clear ethnic or tribal divide obscures great social complexity whose roots are found in Rwanda's history and political economy. Unlike many other countries in the region (for example, Kenya, Uganda, or Tanzania) precolonial Rwanda was a single kingdom with a single language, Kinyarwanda.[75] Although precolonial histories of Rwanda rely heavily on oral traditions, it is widely accepted that the identities "Tutsi" and "Hutu" existed in the insular Nyiginya kingdom, which encompassed much of modern-day Rwanda before the first European colonial administrative office was established by Germany in 1897.[76] Scholars still debate the arrival of Tutsi pastoralists—possibly during the fifteenth century—to a region already inhabited by a distinct Hutu population.

Whether or not there were two truly distinct populations, these identities were fluid in the centuries preceding colonization, based more on socioeconomic status and vocation than physical characteristics.[77] "Tutsi" was initially an ethnonym used by part of Rwanda's herder community; "Hutu," as described by historian Jan Vansina, "was a demeaning term that alluded to rural boorishness or loutish behavior[,] used by the elite."[78] The term "Hutu" later evolved into a denotation for agriculturalists.[79] Social mobility was common between Hutus and Tutsis, as was intermarriage; of note, the Kinyarwanda word *kwihutura* ("Tutsization") denotes accrual of wealth and a new social identity as a Tutsi.[80] The term "tribe," as used by anthropologists, does not apply to the people of Rwanda. Contrary to popular accounts of "age-old animosity" between Hutu and Tutsi, there is little evidence of systematic violence between the two groups during the precolonial era.[81]

European colonists reified these identities into eugenic constructs.[82] Few Europeans had set foot in Rwanda when Germany "won" the country as a colonial holding at the Berlin Conference in 1885. When they arrived in the densely populated kingdom, German colonists made a strategic calculation to institutionalize inequality as a form of control: by forging an alliance with the Tutsi rulers of the kingdom's existing court and administrative system, the Germans could maintain control remotely without fear of unified nationalist insurrection. The divide was reinforced during an 1897 insurrection, when an anti-Tutsi movement gained momentum in the northwest part of the country.[83]

The Belgians, who later "won" the territory from the Germans after World War I, buttressed this *realpolitik* "divide and conquer" strategy with racial ideology and pseudoscience. Belgian scientists, armed with scales and measuring tapes and calipers, measured Rwandans' physical features and propagated theories of racial distinction: Tutsis, they claimed, were tall, with "noble," aquiline, Caucasoid facial features; Hutus were short with "coarse," "bestial" features such as wider noses. The Belgians used these ethnic distinctions to further the "Hamitic hypothesis" of European race theorists Giuseppe Sergi and Charles Gabriel Seligman, who claimed that the Tutsis were among the descendants of pastoralist Caucasians from the Middle Eastern "Hamites."[84] Emerging European political ideologies and conflicts were also brought to bear on the myths and mystifications about social identity in colonial Rwanda. Monsignor Léon Classe, the first bishop of Rwanda, allied the Roman Catholic Church with the Belgian strategy, warning that any effort to replace Tutsi rulers with "uncouth" Hutus "would lead the entire state directly into anarchy and to bitter anti-European communism."[85]

In 1933, the Belgian administrators conducted a census and issued ethnic identity cards; every Rwandan was labeled Hutu (83 percent), Tutsi (16 percent), or Twa (1 percent).[86] The identity cards served to decrease the possibility of Hutus becoming Tutsis; Tutsis gained more exclusive access to education in Catholic schools and to administrative and political jobs. Journalist Philip Gourevitch argues that in this apartheid colonial state, "'ethnicity' became the defining feature of Rwandan existence," and "the idea of a collective national identity was steadily laid to waste."[87]

Decades of systematic exclusion from political and economic power instilled resentment in the Hutu majority, who began calling for social revolution. After World War II, Belgium's colonial administration was placed under the trusteeship of the United Nations, and international pressure to move the country toward independence increased. A group of Hutu intellectuals published the *Hutu Manifesto* in 1957, a tract that embraced the Hamitic myth by arguing that because the Tutsis were foreign invaders, Rwanda should be ruled by the Hutu majority.[88]

In the years preceding their departure (and after the Tutsi elite began to espouse nationalist ideals of independence), the Belgian administrators reversed allegiance from the Tutsis to the Hutus, claiming newfound respect for the historically oppressed. Belgian colonel Guy Logiest fancied himself a champion of democratization, citing "a desire to put down the arrogance and expose the duplicity of a basically oppressive and unjust aristocracy."[89] In 1959, when an uprising led by Hutu revolutionaries left ten thousand Tutsis dead, Belgian troops stood by while Colonel Logiest denied a request from Rwanda's king to deploy an army against the revolutionaries. The following year, Logiest replaced Tutsi chiefs with Hutus and presided over communal elections in which Hutus won an overwhelming majority of the top posts. Organized violence, arbitrary arrests, and expropriation of Tutsi property led an estimated tens of thousands of Tutsis to flee into exile.[90]

The Republic of Rwanda was officially established in 1962. The ruling Hutu elite used violence and divisive rhetoric to portray the Tutsis as the cause of the persistent, grinding poverty in which most of the population continued to live.[91] Yet even with the country's discriminatory policies, violent massacres, and limited access to social services, some in the international development community came to hail Rwanda as a stable democracy and model of development. International aid, which accounted for more than 70 percent of public expenditures between 1982 and 1987, strengthened the regimes of presidents Kayibanda (1962–1973) and Habyarimana (1973–1994), even as they concentrated much of Rwanda's wealth into the hands of a small group of Hutu elites. Infrastructure programs supported by World Bank loans disproportionately benefited northern Rwanda, including President Habyarimana's home province of Gisenyi.[92] International technical advisors devised development projects run through the government's top-down administrative framework.[93] But by focusing on indicators of mortality and GDP, the aid community could claim some progress in Rwanda, even as the tiny country became the continent's third-largest weapons importer.[94]

In the early 1990s, the Habyarimana regime began arming and training Hutu militias while stoking the rhetoric of ethnic hatred via radio broadcast. Nevertheless, donor governments, most notably that of France, continued to provide aid to the regime. The population, including most of the Hutu majority, grew increasingly impoverished as coffee prices plummeted in international markets. The government continued to use the Tutsi minority as a scapegoat for the pauperization of the majority.

After President Habyarimana's plane was shot from the sky on April 6, 1994, Hutu militias carried out a systematic genocide. Over the course of one hundred days, nearly 1 million Tutsis and moderate Hutus were killed.[95] Although the genocide was carefully planned— lists of targets were read over the radio—the killing itself was decentralized. One study estimates that between 14 and 17 percent of the adult male Hutu population participated in the slaughter.[96] The country was devastated; most of its infrastructure was destroyed. At the behest of the United States and other world powers, a small UN protection force led by General Romeo Dallaire was first forbidden from protecting the Rwandan population and then hastily withdrawn.[97]

In the wake of the killings came massive internal and external displacement. As the Rwandan Patriotic Front (RPF), a military force led by Tutsi refugees invading from Uganda, ousted the Hutu militias, nearly 2 million refugees (mostly Hutus) fled the country. In bordering eastern Zaïre (now the Democratic Republic of the Congo), the humanitarian community, seeking to reduce the suffering of the refugees, established huge refugee camps. But these places of refuge soon became sites for perpetuating the violence, as the leaders of the genocide used the camps as a base to gather their forces and continue the killing, within the camps and across the border in Rwanda. The humanitarian aid groups at first failed to discern the situation and then were unable to respond in an effective way.[98] Fiona Terry, a former humanitarian relief worker, notes that expatriate aid groups found airbills for arms imports *into* the camps from the United Kingdom, South Africa, Israel, Albania, China, and elsewhere.[99] The humanitarians also presided over a cholera outbreak in the camps that claimed some twelve thousand lives.[100] The few foreign military interventions dispatched to the area proved equally inept or worse. In June 1994, for example, the French deployed peacekeeping troops to Rwanda. Yet Gourevitch and other observers report that while the killing stopped in regions overtaken by the RPF, it continued almost unabated in the southwestern region held by French forces.[101] It would be difficult to come up with a more vivid example of the unintended consequences of purposive social action. And this mayhem was precisely the consequence intended by some within the camp and in other settings in which the architects of the genocide sought refuge.

In the aftermath of the genocide, Rwanda began the process of rebuilding. Paul Kagame, the leader of the RPF who became president in 2000, quelled the remaining political violence within Rwanda's borders. The transitional government abolished the labels "Hutu" and "Tutsi" and the ethnic ID cards of the colonial and postcolonial eras.[102] The challenge of adjudicating guilt or innocence, and of meting out justice, was enormous; Rwanda's poorly equipped prisons were full to bursting for years, and the criminal justice system had itself participated in, or been undone by, the genocide. Many of the alleged perpetrators of murder were repatriated to their communities after being tried before community courts known as *gacaca*, which sentenced community service more frequently than imprisonment.[103]

Although still a recipient of foreign aid, Rwanda has announced the goal of becoming an aid-independent, middle-income country by 2020.[104] A densely populated, landlocked nation subject to the vicissitudes of international prices for its few exports, Rwanda is now seeking to develop a knowledge-based economy focused on services and to establish itself as the information-technology hub of East Africa. (Singapore and South Korea have been cited as its development models.) To that end, Rwanda has joined the East African Community (a regional free-trade organization), changed its official second language from French to English, and invested heavily in science and technology education and broadband lines. The number of university students increased from five thousand in 1991 to forty-four thousand in 1999.[105] Between 1995 and 2010, per capita GDP nearly quadrupled.[106] The disbursal of public funds is increasingly transparent, and public officials are held to rigorous standards of accountability.

Rwanda is not without its critics, including those who denounce the state's restrictions on free speech. But although postcolonial and postgenocide tensions remain high in Rwanda, the current government has managed to usher in stability and growth. All things considered, few would disagree that Rwanda has made remarkable progress since 1994. It is perhaps in the arena of health care delivery and building health that Rwanda's greatest improvements have been registered. A model of health care focusing on reaching the poor majority in rural regions similar to that described in central Haiti—linking community-based intervention to a system of public clinics and district hospitals—is one reason why.

PIH in Rwanda: Inshuti Mu Buzima

In 2002, the Clinton HIV/AIDS Initiative (now the Clinton Health Access Initiative of the William J. Clinton Foundation) and Partners In Health, already collaborating in Haiti, began to discuss expanding to sub-Saharan Africa. Yet with ongoing work in Russia, Peru, the United States, and other countries, in addition to growing responsibilities in Haiti, Partners In Health staff worried about becoming stretched too thin.

Nevertheless, at the invitation of the Rwandan government, Partners In Health began working in the Eastern Province of Rwanda in 2005. PIH would work closely with the public sector: PIH-supported facilities would be staffed by clinicians and managers from Boston, Haiti, and elsewhere but also by Ministry of Health employees. New and renovated hospitals and clinics would also belong to the ministry. PIH's pilot programs would inform national scale-up if proven effective. Over the long term, the Ministry of Health would gradually assume full control of the PIH-supported sites; PIH sought to "work itself out of a job" by founding a Rwandan sister organization committed to addressing, over the long term, the health problems of rural Rwandans, most of whom still lived in poverty.

Inshuti Mu Buzima ("partners in health" in Kinyarwanda) would come to resemble Zanmi Lasante more closely than many of PIH's other sister organizations. Whereas PIH in Russia focused almost exclusively on tuberculosis among prisoners, and PIH in urban Peru focused almost exclusively on tuberculosis, PIH in Rwanda sought to prove that comprehensive primary health care (including care for AIDS, tuberculosis, and malaria) could be delivered effectively and equitably in two rural resource-poor districts. These districts were home to a half-million residents but no doctors before PIH's arrival. NGOs were based mostly in cities and towns and had little implementation capacity in the small villages where so many lived. The head of the National AIDS Control Commission at the time pointed out that with more than 150 AIDS-related nongovernmental organizations in Rwanda, fewer than 150 people were on AIDS therapy outside the capital city of Kigali. An estimated 100,000 Rwandans needed such care. Along with the Ministry of Health and other partners, including UNICEF and the

Global Fund to Fight AIDS, Tuberculosis and Malaria, PIH planned to scale up AIDS treatment and testing while also helping the Ministry of Health build a comprehensive public-sector health system in the region.

These plans were met with skepticism and objections among some authorities—the same objections made when Zanmi Lasante began enrolling patients on ART in 1998. Some claimed that AIDS stigma would prevent people from getting tested; others argued that ART was too expensive or too complicated to roll out on the scale PIH and the Rwandan Ministry of Health planned. But we doubted the plausibility of these claims, given Zanmi Lasante's experience in launching the HIV Equity Initiative in Haiti. Physicians and program managers from Zanmi Lasante, including Dr. Fernet Léandre, went to Rwanda to help recruit and train community health workers, nurses, doctors, pharmacists, and program managers.

In April 2005, Inshuti Mu Buzima (IMB) began working in an abandoned hospital in Rwinkwavu, a village accessed by an unpaved road near the Tanzanian border. The hospital, once supported by a Belgian mining company, was mostly deserted and inhabited by squatters; a few nurses treated a handful of ambulatory patients each day. The hospital walls were covered with graffiti, proclaiming messages such as "AIDS will finish off those of you who we do not kill."[107]

While rebuilding infrastructure—a new laboratory, a larger and well-stocked pharmacy, an operating room, which are pictured in figure 6.11—the IMB staff expanded community- and facility-based care. Before IMB's arrival, fewer than one hundred patients were on antiretroviral treatment at the six facilities in its catchment area. In its first year, IMB enrolled more than one thousand people into a program of ART, using the community-based model pioneered in central Haiti: every patient was paired with a paid community health worker, or *accompagnateur*, usually a neighbor, who made daily or twice-daily home visits to observe the ingestion of medications and ensure that patients had access to food (each patient receiving ART was entitled to food packets for the first six months of therapy), housing, transportation, schooling for children, and other forms of psychosocial assistance. All services were provided at no cost to patients. As in Haiti, availability of treatment sparked an increase in HIV testing: by 2008, facilities supported by IMB had tested more than eighty thousand people for HIV infection. That same year, a survey of 223 people on community-based ART for two years at IMB-supported sites found that 98 percent had suppressed viral loads (>500 copies/mL).[108] In comparison, a meta-

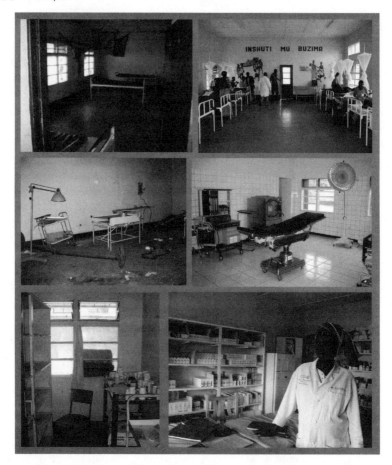

FIGURE 6.11. Rwinkwavu District Hospital in Rwanda, before and after the IMB scale-up: the inpatient ward (top), the operating theater (center), and the pharmacy (bottom).

analysis of ART in Europe and North America found that only 75 to 85 percent of patients had a similar viral load suppression in response to treatment.[109] Moreover, staff and community members were surprised and heartened when patients with advanced AIDS and tuberculosis, malnourished children, and cancer patients were restored to health—the "Lazarus effect" again. Patients came from across Rwanda, and from neighboring countries, to receive care at IMB-supported facilities.

Paying community health workers has been a subject of much debate among global public health experts and among public-sector leaders with small health budgets. PIH has shown, in Haiti and Rwanda as in

Peru and Russia, that paid community health workers can significantly improve adherence to therapy. To answer questions about cost, the Clinton Foundation examined IMB's expenditures in 2006, finding that paid *accompagnateurs* accounted for 9.3 percent of IMB's labor costs and 4.2 percent of overall operating costs. The study estimated that paying a health worker to accompany every AIDS patient in Rwanda would cost $3 to $5 per capita per year.[110] This figure does not account for the savings generated by adherence to first-line medications—second-line antiretrovirals are much more expensive—much less the gains in survival. Moreover, by compensating community health workers, health projects can create meaningful jobs for the poor. This benefits not only the individuals but also their families, communities, and local economies. The debate about paying community health workers continues, stemming, in large part, from the lack of available funds to compensate paraprofessionals in the health sector in Rwanda and elsewhere.

Claims of cultural barriers to community-based care were common at first among foreign observers, who doubted the utility of *accompagnateurs* in a society riven by genocide only a decade earlier. But such claims were also exaggerated. The Ministry of Health has commenced a large-scale national recruitment and training program for community health workers; forty-five thousand have already been deployed across the country.[111] It is the building of an equitable system of care, one that stretches not only across the nation but also from hospital to health center and into patients'—and potential beneficiaries'—homes that accounts for much of Rwanda's success in breaking the cycle of poverty and disease. Success in health care delivery (like that in the economic sector, which helps fuel it) required the hard work and passion of many NGOs and generous funding from many partners. But it required most of all the coordination of such efforts by a public sector bent on having them add up to more than the sum of their parts and to serve to strengthen the national health system.

It should be noted that the Rwandan Ministry of Health and Inshuti Mu Buzima have learned from each other over the years, since the missions are different but complementary—a "preferential option for the poor" is not always the same as building a social safety net for all, rich or poor or in between. The struggle to train and stipend community health workers is one example. Modes of building out insurance schemes, and the role of user fees, are another. In 2006, the Ministry of Health announced the national implementation of a community-based *mutuelle* health insurance scheme. The Rwandan government mandates that every citizen purchase health insurance. Annual premiums vary by region, but in the rural districts in which PIH works, membership costs 1,000 Rwandan francs (slightly less than US$2) per year. For members, the copayment for most primary care visits is 150 RWF (about US$0.27); for hospitalizations, patients pay 10 percent of the cost of drugs, consultations, and procedures.[112] Those who have not subscribed to *mutuelles* bear the full costs at the point of care. By the end of 2008, the Ministry of Health reported that 95 percent of Rwandans were enrolled in a *mutuelle*.[113]

In contrast, IMB has since 2005 offered free care at the six sites it supports. Realizing that much of the population in its catchment area was too poor to afford premiums and that point-of-care fees constitute significant barriers to care among the destitute sick, IMB did not seek to recover costs from patients themselves. Yet the Rwandan government sought a unified health financing system, and the *mutuelles* scheme had expanded access to care compared to the erstwhile user fee cost-recovery system. Following the Ministry of Health's lead, in 2006 IMB facilities adopted the *mutuelle* system. In keeping with the ministry's standards, patients presenting for HIV counseling and testing, antiretroviral therapy, tuberculosis care, or prenatal visits are not charged copayments. IMB also pays premiums and copayments for people whom local leaders deem too poor to pay.[114] IMB contributes additional funds to the coffers of *mutuelle* accounts in its catchment area to support free care for children under five years old and patients presenting for malaria diagnosis or care. IMB also set up facilities to eliminate the ancillary costs of *mutuelle* enrollment, such as obtaining a picture on an insurance card. Hence many, but not all, copayments were waived at IMB sites.

Despite IMB's efforts to reduce the cost burden on patients, copayments remain a barrier to care even among those enrolled in *mutuelles*. A recent evaluation found, for example, that although the *mutuelle* system increased coverage, those in the poorest quintile continued to face catastrophic health expenditures and suffer from decreased access to care because of copayments.[115]

IMB has, from the beginning, sought to avoid the pitfalls of foreign aid, which were showcased during the Rwandan genocide and its aftermath. In contrast to the technocratic and anti-participatory culture of aid projects in pre-1994 Rwanda,[116] IMB's efforts are embedded in local communities; priorities are identified and reassessed by *accompagnateurs* and other community members. The program main-

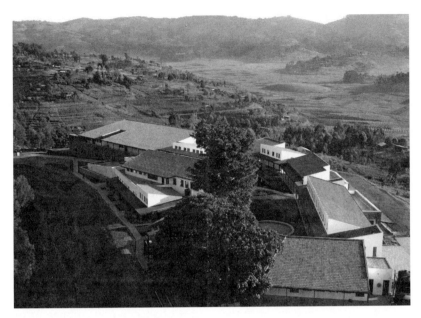

FIGURE 6.12. Butaro Hospital, Rwanda.

tains only a light expatriate presence: 99 percent of IMB staff members
are Rwandan, though expatriates live and work on the campuses of
the rural health facilities in Kirehe, Rwinkwavu, and Butaro. Finally,
IMB strives to avoid the technocratic reductionism that characterized
the early 1990s international development community in Rwanda by
approaching health from a biosocial perspective. It seeks to address the
social and economic barriers to good health in addition to the biologic
ones; it helps patients attain better housing and sufficient food, just
as it prescribes correct therapeutic regimens for them. This approach
seeks not only to improve health and education and aggregate economic growth indices but also to recognize the dignity of some of
Rwanda's poorest people.

In 2007, the Rwandan Ministry of Health asked IMB to expand to
Burera, a district in the north of Rwanda slightly less poor than the
districts in which IMB already worked. In 2008, IMB began supporting fifteen health centers throughout the district and broke ground on a
new district hospital. Built by local workers, the hospital was designed
to minimize airborne infection and optimize patient flow between
wards. Butaro Hospital was officially opened in January 2011; it serves
as a model for other districts (see figure 6.12).

By March 2011, IMB had expanded to support or operate three hospitals and thirty-six health centers in three of Rwanda's thirty districts. Approximately six thousand patients were on ART in those three districts. An open-source system of electronic medical records, first piloted for AIDS patients at IMB sites, was adopted by the Ministry of Health for use at all public-sector health facilities. Most important, perhaps, IMB had built a long-term partnership to accompany the Rwandan government in designing, implementing, and refining its innovative District Health System Strengthening Framework, which draws on IMB's model of care delivery. As in central Haiti, this model linked hospitals and clinics to rural communities with the help of community health workers. It is a platform able to deliver care for acute and chronic disease, regardless of whether their etiologies are held to be communicable or noncommunicable. What works for AIDS should work just as well for epilepsy, congestive heart failure, schizophrenia or other major mental illness, or diabetes.[117] Community health workers can also improve the quality of follow-up care for cancer and trauma patients, just as they enhance the success of vaccination campaigns or family planning for those seeking it.

Significant challenges remain in scaling up community-based care nationwide. Even if the Rwandan government endorsed compensating community health workers, it might not be able to afford supporting a new cadre of public servants. Such a decision might even disqualify Rwanda from international sources of credit by running afoul of policies restricting the size of the national civil service. Providing food to patients who receive ART also remains, in global public health circles, contentious and attracts little funding. Some international funders continue to counsel governments to recover costs from patients through point-of-care fees, warning of the dangers of frivolous use of medical services as a moral hazard, even in regions where multiple barriers have long kept patients from accessing care.

IMB's work in Rwanda has demonstrated that the patient outcomes achieved in rural Haiti are replicable in African nations with stable governments committed to expanding access to health care for the rural poor. Since it began working in Rwanda in 2005, Partners In Health has also established similar, if smaller, programs in rural Lesotho and Malawi. It has deployed the same model to improve outcomes among patients with cancers, mental illnesses, and other chronic diseases, including epilepsy, heart disease, and diabetes. (See chapter 11 for a discussion of recent efforts to combat noncommunicable diseases and surgical diseases.) Sister organizations have adopted the PIH model

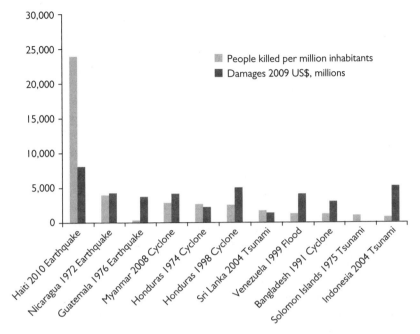

FIGURE 6.13. Loss of life and economic damages in major disasters: The 2010 earthquake in Haiti in comparison. Source: Eduardo A. Cavallo, Andrew Powell, and Oscar Becerra, *Estimating the Direct Economic Damage of the Earthquake in Haiti,* Inter-American Development Bank Working Paper, Series IDB-WP-163, February 2010.

to deliver comprehensive health care in Burundi and in Liberia.[118] In each case, but especially in Rwanda, close collaboration with the public sector has helped to ensure that the efforts of PIH and its partners can be scaled up and sustained over the long term—as long, that is, as there are health problems afflicting the poor and marginalized.

FROM RWANDA BACK TO HAITI: AFTER THE 2010 EARTHQUAKE

On January 12, 2010, a magnitude 7.0 earthquake devastated Haiti, particularly the capital, Port-au-Prince. Estimates of the death toll ranged from 220,000 to 316,000; more than 300,000 were injured.[119] Some believe that 60 percent of all federal, administrative and economic infrastructure was destroyed. An estimated 2.3 million people—including 302,000 children—were displaced from their homes.[120] The destruction in Haiti, in terms of both loss of life and economic loss, surpassed that of any other natural disaster in recent decades (as figure 6.13 demonstrates).[121]

The quake took a heavy toll on public health and education infrastructure. Eighty-four of 393 health facilities in the region were damaged or destroyed, including 20 hospitals. The General Hospital, the national teaching and referral hospital, was badly damaged. The collapse of the adjacent nursing school killed two entire classes of nursing students and their teachers, who were in the midst of an exam.[122] It was a profound blow to the already understaffed Haitian health workforce. Additionally, 23 percent of all schools in Haiti were affected, including 80 percent of the schools in Port-au-Prince. The destruction of so many government buildings and the deaths of many public-sector workers further crippled the Haitian government's ability to respond to the disaster.[123]

One of the largest humanitarian relief efforts in history was registered in Haiti after the earthquake. Bilateral and multilateral donors pledged $5.4 billion, and more than half of U.S. households contributed to the humanitarian response.[124] Zanmi Lasante staff responded within hours, helping to keep the General Hospital up and running, launching clinics in four of Port-au-Prince's internally displaced persons (IDP) camps, and providing care for thousands of victims who made it out of the city to the Central Plateau. Though Zanmi Lasante is not a relief organization, its Haitian staff and decades of experience providing health care in Haiti put the organization in a good position to help. Thousands of other medical, surgical, and public health professionals traveled to Haiti to join the humanitarian effort.

While countless lives were saved in the weeks following the earthquake, local and international relief teams faced tremendous challenges attempting to care for the wounded in health facilities that were decrepit and under-resourced even before the quake. The earthquake can be understood as an "acute-on-chronic" event:

> Haiti has long faced social and economic problems, and its medical and public-health challenges are rooted in these problems. To these chronic problems the earthquake added an acute crisis: "acute-on-chronic" in medical jargon. Whether looking at health, education, potable water, or safe and affordable housing, similar conclusions could be drawn: first, great weakness in the public sector makes it exceedingly difficult to deliver basic services at significant scale; second, not enough of the pledged earthquake relief reached those in need through mechanisms that might address this central weakness. In other words, Haiti's acute-on-chronic problems were not effectively dealt with by the development and reconstruction machinery in spite of many good intentions and extraordinary generosity.[125]

The reconstruction process has proven even more challenging. By the close of 2012, approximately $3.01 billion, or 56 percent of the recovery funds pledged for 2010–2012 by bilateral and multilateral donors, had been disbursed. But only 10 percent of this aid has been channeled to the Haitian government or Haitian institutions.[126] (Although low, 10 percent is an improvement from the 0.3 percent of humanitarian aid that went to the Haitian government immediately following the quake.) Thousands of foreign contractors and NGOs have worked in parallel without much coordination. Many resettlement and reconstruction initiatives were stalled. The establishment of the Interim Haiti Reconstruction Commission—a multilateral body co-chaired by Haiti's prime minister to monitor and coordinate foreign assistance after the earthquake—sought to improve transparency and direct funds toward key recovery projects, but the challenges before it were immense.[127] Its mandate expired in 2011. Two and a half years after the quake, published estimates concluded that more than 350,000 remained internally displaced in makeshift camps.[128] To make matters worse, an outbreak of cholera—a disease undetected in Haiti for over a century—erupted in October 2010. The epidemic soon became the world's largest in recent history; years of underinvestment in clean water and sanitation fueled its rapid spread.[129]

Despite their divergent sociopolitical contexts, can parallels be drawn between Rwanda in the aftermath of the 1994 genocide and post-earthquake Haiti? Both countries suffered massive loss of life and significant internal—and, in the case of Rwanda, external—displacement. Both events were acute-on-chronic: crises natural and unnatural amid histories of widespread poverty, weak or predatory governments, and underdeveloped health and education infrastructure. Both countries also confronted the double-edged sword of international aid: sorely needed relief and recovery efforts and investment tempered by the unintended consequences of aid that is often inefficient and poorly coordinated and that sometimes weakens local capacity by bypassing the governments and institutions of its intended beneficiaries.

Several lessons drawn from Rwanda's progress in rebuilding infrastructure, achieving stability, and cultivating economic development are worth noting as Haiti continues down the long road to recovery. First, Rwanda has been steadfast about transparency and accountability in the government, which has aided the efficacy of its own programs and helped attract sustained foreign investment. Second, Rwanda established clear national development plans, which have

182 of the name

promoted coordination among donors and implementing partners. Regular progress reviews assess aid effectiveness and hold implementing partners accountable.[130] NGOs that are unwilling to work in accordance with the government's plans are sometimes asked to leave the country. Third, development strategies that help the poor have aimed to reduce inequality through infrastructure investments and efforts to achieve universal access to health care and education in previously neglected rural communities, such as those served by Partners In Health. The Rwanda government has also institutionalized gender equity in its civil service. It recently passed Sweden as the country with the highest percentage of female civil servants in the world.[131]

Though Rwanda remains poor by international standards, its government offered financial assistance to support the humanitarian response in Haiti. The Rwandan Ministry of Foreign Affairs has also established an Office of South-South Collaboration to facilitate intergovernmental cooperation. A number of Haitian government officials have visited their counterparts in Rwanda to learn about its rebuilding strategy and share expertise. In late 2010, Partners In Health established an independent Haiti-Rwanda Commission to help share lessons about recovery from disasters, natural and unnatural, and to better address extreme poverty.

The partnership between Haiti and Rwanda is just one example, among many, of South-South collaboration. Similarly, the work of Partners In Health in these countries is just one example, among many, of effective health care delivery in resource-poor settings. Our hope is that these cases highlight key characteristics of global health delivery that may be reproducible elsewhere. The next chapter builds on many of the themes discussed here by introducing the notion of a science of global health delivery.

SUGGESTED READING

Farmer, Paul. *Haiti after the Earthquake.* New York: PublicAffairs, 2011.
———. *Infections and Inequalities: The Modern Plagues.* Berkeley: University of California Press, 1999.
———. *The Uses of Haiti.* Monroe, Maine: Common Courage Press, 1994.
Farmer, Paul, Cameron T. Nutt, Claire M. Wagner, Claude Sekabaraga, Tej Nuthulaganti, Jonathan L. Weigel, Didi Bertrand Farmer, Antoinette Habinshuti, Soline Dusabeyesu Mugeni, Jean-Claude Karasi, and Peter C. Drobac. "Reduced Premature Mortality in Rwanda: Lessons from Success." *British Medical Journal* 346 (February 9, 2013): 20–22.

Gourevitch, Philip. *We Wish to Inform You That Tomorrow We Will Be Killed with Our Families: Stories from Rwanda*. New York: Farrar, Straus and Giroux, 1998.

Government of Rwanda, Ministry of Health; Partners In Health; and Clinton Foundation. *Rwanda Rural Health Care Plan: A Comprehensive Approach to Rural Health, November 2007*, 30–36.

Hallward, Peter. *Damming the Flood: Haiti and the Politics of Containment*. London: Verso, 2010.

Lu, Chunling, Brian Chin, Jiwon Lee Lewandowski, Paulin Basinga, Lisa R. Hirschhorn, Kenneth Hill, Megan Murray, and Agnes Binagwaho. "Towards Universal Health Coverage: An Evaluation of Rwanda *Mutuelles* in Its First Eight Years." *PLoS ONE* 7, no. 6 (2012): e39282.

Mamdani, Mahmood. *When Victims Become Killers: Colonialism, Nativism, and the Genocide in Rwanda*. Princeton, N.J.: Princeton University Press, 2001.

Rich, Michael L., Ann C. Miller, Peter Niyigena, Molly F. Franke, Jean Bosco Niyonzima, Adrienne Socci, Peter C. Drobac, Massudi Hakizamungu, Alishya Mayfield, Robert Ruhayisha, Henry Epino, Sara Stulac, Corrado Cancedda, Adolph Karamaga, Saleh Niyonzima, Chase Yarbrough, Julia Fleming, Cheryl Amoroso, Joia Mukherjee, Megan Murray, Paul Farmer, and Agnes Binagwaho. "Excellent Clinical Outcomes and High Retention in Care among Adults in a Community-Based HIV Treatment Program in Rural Rwanda." *Journal of Acquired Immune Deficiency Syndromes* 59, no. 3 (2012): e35–42.

Trouillot, Michel-Rolph. *Haiti, State against Nation: The Origins and Legacy of Duvalierism*. New York: Monthly Review Press, 1990.

Uvin, Peter. *Aiding Violence: The Development Enterprise in Rwanda*. West Hartford, Conn.: Kumarian Press, 1998.

Vansina, Jan. *Antecedents to Modern Rwanda: The Nyiginya Kingdom*. Madison: University of Wisconsin Press, 2004.

Walton, David A., Paul E. Farmer, Wesler Lambert, Fernet Léandre, Serena P. Koenig, and Joia S. Mukherjee. "Integrated HIV Prevention and Care Strengthens Primary Health Care: Lessons from Rural Haiti." *Journal of Public Health Policy* 25, no. 2 (2004): 137–158.

Wilentz, Amy. *The Rainy Season: Haiti—Then and Now*. New York: Simon and Schuster, 2010.

7

Scaling Up Effective Delivery Models Worldwide

JIM YONG KIM, MICHAEL PORTER, JOSEPH RHATIGAN,
REBECCA WEINTRAUB, MATTHEW BASILICO, CASSIA VAN
DER HOOF HOLSTEIN, PAUL FARMER

The previous chapter explored the health care delivery model of Partners In Health, Zanmi Lasante, and Inshuti Mu Buzima in the rural reaches of Haiti and Rwanda. Working in the public sector, PIH and its sister organizations have helped transform patient care and improve the overall health of people living in impoverished areas. PIH is one among many organizations that have discovered ways to deliver high-quality health services in resource-poor settings. But is its model generalizable? In this chapter, we step back to consider general principles of global health delivery.

We begin with the Global Health Delivery Project at Harvard, an academic collaboration seeking to discern and promulgate principles of effective health care delivery. The chapter examines a strategic framework developed by this group and offers a series of examples from the project's case studies. The remainder of the chapter then broadens the focus, exploring the promise of health systems strengthening, a strategy that extends the GHD framework to the regional or national (or global) level. After a brief review of the health systems of several countries, the chapter concludes by turning to one of the essential components of health care delivery: the necessary human resources. Throughout, we aim to synthesize key lessons that practitioners and policymakers have learned, with the goal of introducing the emerging science of global health delivery.

PRINCIPLES OF EFFECTIVE GLOBAL HEALTH DELIVERY

The Global Health Delivery Project is a partnership between the schools of business, medicine, and public health at Harvard and the Brigham and Women's Hospital. The project took shape to help fill the knowledge gap about the delivery of health care services in resource-poor areas. Many global health programs targeting these areas have proved successful, yet there has been little systematic analysis of how such programs deliver quality care. What is missing, in other words, is a science of global health delivery. In response, GHD is developing a series of case studies drawn from countries ranging from Iran to Kenya to Brazil to Indonesia on topics such as measles vaccination, antimalarial drug production, and HIV counseling and testing. Although the field is young, its analysis is instructive. Here we consider four salient principles that, taken together, offer a strategic framework for effective global health delivery:

Adapting to local context

Constructing a care delivery value chain

Leveraging shared delivery infrastructure

Improving both health delivery and economic development

Adapting to Local Context

Local factors, such as climate, labor market characteristics, and demographic trends, pattern the burden of disease and access to health care in a given setting. As chapter 6 explains, the strategy of Partners In Health has, from the beginning, been guided by local knowledge. Awareness of specific structural barriers to accessing care in Cange— unemployment, insufficient access to food and clean water, shoddy health infrastructure, high transport costs, and poor housing, to name just a few—informed its *accompagnateur*-based care delivery model and its strategy of providing wraparound social services. Such programmatic innovations were in many ways the foundation of Partners In Health and Zanmi Lasante's clinical performance.

How do programs adapt to the local context? Assessing the local contours of disease burden is an essential first step: disease prevalence and modes of transmission often vary greatly within countries and regions. For example, in 2003, Kenya's HIV prevalence rate was an estimated 6.7 percent nationally, but the prevalence rates in its provinces ranged from nearly o percent (North Eastern Province) to 15.1 percent (Nyanza Province).[1] Within Nyanza Province, there were (and are) also large differences in prevalence among major cities and between cities and rural areas. Recognizing geographic differences in prevalence rates is essential to any health delivery strategy.

Politics, without fail, also influences the provision of care and accessibility of services. Instability, insecurity, or predation can have far-reaching effects on health care delivery and can jeopardize the work of providers. Haiti is a case in point: as chapter 6 details, a history of elite control and political turmoil disrupted and undermined efforts to strengthen the national health system. Furthermore, public health is predicated on the provision of public services. The public sector is often the only health provider for the poor. Public goods like potable water and clean air are necessary inputs for the good health of a population; in their absence, waterborne diseases like typhoid and pollutant-associated diseases like asthma may become more common. Clean water is also required for formula feeding children of HIV-positive mothers, who are counseled to avoid breastfeeding; in poor settings that lack water security, additional interventions such as water purification technologies are needed for successful formula feeding.

Economic conditions also play a significant role in determining access to care and the burden of disease. Although the links between poverty and health are well known,[2] understanding the precise, local mechanisms by which poverty and inequality in part shape the patterns of disease and the availability of care are key starting points for the science of global health delivery. Patients who cannot afford transportation to a local clinic, for example, may need additional resources to borrow a car or, in remote rural areas, rent a donkey;[3] the destitute sick may also need help with child care or food for their families.

Social and cultural factors, such as gender disparities and disease-related stigma, influence the local landscape of health care. The health needs of marginalized populations—such as the squatters Zanmi Lasante began serving in Cange in the 1980s, or commercial sex workers in Mumbai, India[4]—often go unaddressed by health providers. The stigma associated with particular diseases, such as mental illnesses or neglected tropical diseases, may prevent patients from seeking care.[5] In such situations, health providers may need to intensify and expand their case-finding efforts and provide care with even greater confidentiality to gain the trust of patients. Local religious practices can also affect care-seeking and service delivery: in Haiti, for example, diseases such as tuberculosis and AIDS have long been attributed, at times, to sorcery.[6] Such alternate etiologies can lead individuals to eschew biomedical solutions.

These are just a few examples of local context that must be considered. Because every local situation is different, it is impossible to enumerate a checklist of considerations that are relevant everywhere. But it is important to underscore the centrality of *ethnography* and *discernment* as starting points for global health delivery. The challenge for

---

Case Brief 1. Polio in Uttar Pradesh: Local Context Matters

Poliomyelitis, an enterovirus spread by fecal-oral transmission, can cause paralysis. Fortunately, inexpensive vaccines have been available since the 1950s. By 1985, however, vaccine coverage in India was still below 50 percent of the population.

In the 1990s, the Indian government significantly expanded its polio eradication efforts by instituting National Immunization Days. On a national level, the program achieved impressive results: more than 100 million children were vaccinated, and coverage exceeded 94 percent.[1]

Despite the campaign's success in reducing polio cases nationally (as shown in map 7.1), vaccination rates remained poor in parts of the country. By the end of the decade, officials noted that vaccine coverage in a number of districts in the province of Uttar Pradesh was under 20 percent. Ethnographic investigation indicated that residents did not consider polio a leading health concern; many asked why polio was being targeted instead of other pressing health needs.[2] A predominantly Muslim province in a Hindu-majority nation, Uttar Pradesh had a legacy of skepticism toward outside intervention. Family planning and immunization campaigns in the province a decade earlier had been construed by some as an attempt to sterilize Muslim communities, fueling distrust of health care personnel.[3] The province is also one of India's poorest, and it faces a high burden of diarrheal disease, which significantly reduces the oral polio vaccine's efficacy.[4]

In 2002, Uttar Pradesh experienced a resurgence of polio.[5] Variable achievements of the national campaign in this province illustrate the role of local factors in mediating the delivery of health services, and community-based adjustments to the campaign have succeeded in eliminating polio from India since 2011.

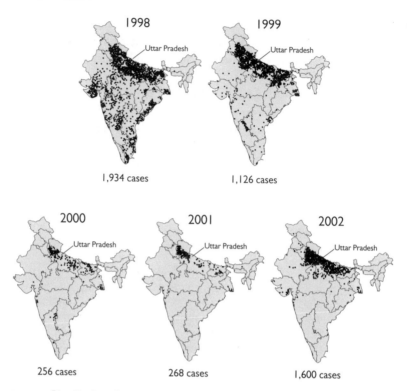

MAP 7.1. Distribution of polio cases in India, 1998–2002. Source: Andrew Ellner, Sachin H. Jain, Joseph Rhatigan, and Daniel Blumenthal, "Polio Elimination in Uttar Pradesh," HBS no. GHD-005 (Boston: Harvard Business School Publishing, 2011), Global Health Delivery Online, www.ghdonline.org/cases/; data from National Polio Surveillance Project, www.npspindia.org/.

practitioners is to conduct ethnographic research and discern which aspects of the local context matter and to adapt programs accordingly.

This approach may diverge from global public health policy. For example, although the World Health Organization (WHO) and other international health authorities did not (and often do not) recommend compensating community health workers, Zanmi Lasante has found that paid *accompagnateurs* provide first-rate home-based care for complex afflictions such as tuberculosis, AIDS, and certain malignancies.[7] Habits and protocols generated in one context may become institutionalized—to use Peter Berger and Thomas Luckmann's term (explained in chapter 2)—among global public health authorities and thus diverge from the complexity of local contexts. Global policies can be helpful in offering strategies and standards for care delivery, but they must be adapted to local contexts to minimize unintended negative consequences.

Constructing a Care Delivery Value Chain

The second principle of effective health delivery involves choosing and adapting health interventions based on *value for patients,* defined as overall health outcomes per cost.[8] This definition differs from the standard practice of considering the cost-effectiveness of isolated interventions. For example, care delivery for HIV/AIDS involves the primary activities of prevention, testing and screening, staging, delaying progression, initiating antiretroviral therapy, continuous disease management, and management of clinical deterioration. By adapting a value-based approach, program design reflects this overall set of activities and the links—information and resource flow, to name a few—between them. A value-based approach emphasizes the integration of interventions, creating a shared delivery infrastructure.

The care delivery value chain (CDVC) is a conceptual tool that optimizes value for patients across the myriad steps in the delivery of care. The CDVC considers care as a *system,* not as discrete interventions. For a given medical condition, the CDVC maps out the relevant health delivery activities, highlighting the flow of care and the links between different providers and services. The CDVC thus cultivates a systemic analysis of value creation that defines a medical condition as an interrelated set of circumstances. Based on the principle that patients receive greater value when different interventions work in concert, a CDVC allows program managers to optimize this value as the delivery of health care and the health interventions become more integrated.

As illustrated in figure 7.1, every CDVC begins with monitoring and prevention; progresses through diagnosing, preparing, intervening, and rehabilitating; and ends with monitoring and managing. Monitoring and prevention include tracking a patient's condition, assessing risk, and taking steps to prevent or reduce the seriousness of illness or injury. The activities following monitoring and prevention support management of the medical condition over time to sustain desired results and minimize reoccurrence. Three additional categories of supporting activities cut across each stage of the care cycle: informing and engaging, measuring patient progress, and accessing the site of care. These activities help bind the care cycle together; this

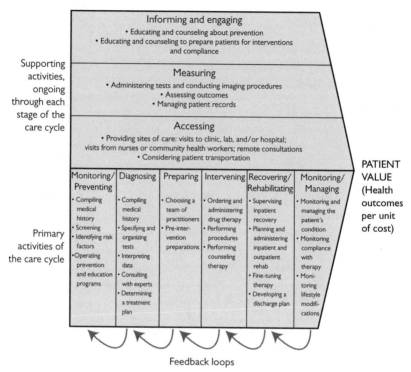

Supporting activities, ongoing through each stage of the care cycle

Primary activities of the care cycle

PATIENT VALUE (Health outcomes per unit of cost)

Feedback loops

FIGURE 7.1. The care delivery value chain. Adapted from Michael E. Porter and Elizabeth Olmsted Teisberg, *Redefining Health Care: Creating Value-Based Competition on Results* (Boston: Harvard Business Review Press, 2006).

integrated perspective is essential to managing prevention and treatment efforts.

By highlighting that the value of a specific intervention is linked to the entire health system, the CDVC reflects a broad, biosocial conception of health care delivery. By identifying factors such as patient access to information and treatment, and other external indicators that are especially crucial in resource-limited settings and are often beyond the considerations of today's provider organizations, the CDVC provides a framework within which providers can analyze the totality of the care delivery process and also examine service facilities, design geographic expansion, improve existing metrics, and analyze costs. While most medical providers have delineated, however implicitly, the distinct activities in managing a patient's condition, the CDVC provides a common language for understanding and potentially improving the overall system of care delivery.[9]

Case Brief 2. AMPATH HIV Care: A Care Delivery Value Chain

In 1989, the Indiana University School of Medicine in the United States and the Moi University School of Medicine in Kenya launched a joint project in Kenya's Western Province that aimed to expand health services and to train American and Kenyan clinicians. For several years, the program offered mainly primary care services. By the late 1990s, however, it became clear that the partnership could not meet the province's health needs without providing HIV care. The main teaching hospital recorded eighty-five AIDS deaths in 1992; by 2000, there had been more than one thousand.

In response, they created the Academic Model for Prevention and Treatment of HIV/AIDS (AMPATH), which rolled out an AIDS prevention and treatment program targeting various points in the disease cycle. AMPATH providers offered HIV counseling and testing, antiretroviral therapy, and treatment of opportunistic infections, including tuberculosis. The program referred patients to oncology care (Kaposi's sarcoma is among the most common opportunistic infections across sub-Saharan Africa), provided reproductive health services, and delivered antenatal care to reduce HIV transmission between mother and child. It also offered food and social support for patients in great need. To tackle the many afflictions associated with AIDS—opportunistic infections, sexually transmitted infections, poverty, stigma—AMPATH developed a package of integrated interventions, including prevention, diagnosis, treatment, and clinical management of complications. What began with a single patient scaled up to more than one thousand in the first three years (see figure 7.2); by 2008, the program had a cumulative enrollment of more than sixty-eight thousand patients and operated seventeen centers. AMPATH had become the largest provider of antiretroviral treatment in Kenya.

Nonetheless, a 2007 survey indicated that 85 percent of residents in AMPATH's catchment area were unaware of their HIV status. The AIDS patients AMPATH identified received excellent care, but others remained beyond its reach; the program's services were insufficiently addressing HIV transmission. A pilot project called Home-Based Counseling and Testing was begun, which provided door-to-door information, testing, and counseling. The project reached 95 percent of the 19,054 eligible residents, 96 percent of whom received HIV tests. By 2010, AMPATH had expanded this service throughout the catchment area; knowledge of HIV status increased markedly, as did patient volume. Expanding services at the front end of the care delivery value chain—knowledge of HIV status and counseling about preventing transmission—helped AMPATH enroll more than 120,000 people in treatment by 2011.[1]

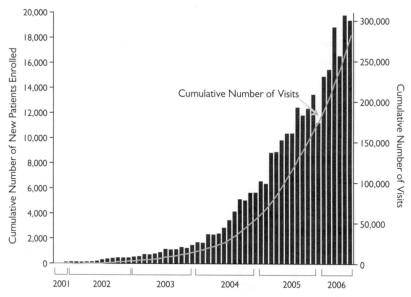

FIGURE 7.2. AMPATH HIV program scale-up: Cumulative visits and number of new patients, 2001–2006. Adapted from Peter Park, Arti Bhatt, and Joseph Rhatigan, "The Academic Model for the Prevention and Treatment of HIV/AIDS," HBS no. GHD-013 (Boston: Harvard Business School Publishing, 2011), Global Health Delivery Online, www.ghdonline.org/cases/.

Leveraging Shared Delivery Infrastructure

Many different interventions require the same health infrastructure for effective delivery. For example, although treatments for malaria and trypanosomiasis have disparate syntheses, biochemical properties, and dosages, they both rely on procurement systems, a robust supply chain, financing, management, clinical staff, and treatment facilities.

Most successful global health programs make it a point to leverage shared delivery infrastructure wherever possible, which brings clear advantages for both providers and patients. Providers save time and resources by using the same hospitals and clinics, modes of transport, laboratories, and supply chains to deliver multiple interventions at once. For example, harmonizing the storage and distribution of numerous different medications in a single pharmacy requires fewer staff and resources than having separate pharmacy systems for each intervention. Indeed, leveraging shared delivery infrastructure across a range of interventions can generate economies of scale and greater efficiency for the health system as a whole.[10]

Patients also benefit from shared delivery infrastructure. Many people present at health facilities without knowing what illness—or, as is often the case in settings of poverty, illnesses—they have. Clinics that can deliver a range of services, from primary health care to specialty care for leading causes of morbidity and mortality, will be better pre-

---

Case Brief 3. BRAC's Rural Tuberculosis Program: Shared Delivery Infrastructure

BRAC (formerly known as the Bangladesh Rural Advancement Committee) has promoted rural economic development since shortly after Bangladesh gained its independence in 1971. Before long, BRAC leadership realized the links between health care and development; they began investing in local health delivery systems by training a cadre of female community health workers, called *shasthya shebikas*. The *shebikas* implemented grassroots health education programs and taught community members how to dispense medications for minor medical needs. BRAC provided ongoing training as well as logistical and clinical support for the *shebikas*, each of whom served 250 to 300 households.

In the early 1980s, BRAC staff identified tuberculosis (TB) as among the most pressing health needs in rural Bangladesh. Beginning in a district of 250,000 people, BRAC set up a pilot program of TB control based on the existing network of *shebikas*. During regular home visits, *shebikas* screened for TB and conducted active case-finding, referring suspected cases to treatment facilities and counseling patients with confirmed TB to help them adhere to therapy. After patients completed treatment, *shebikas* were paid. BRAC also integrated this program into the government health system: public-sector facilities provided medicines and laboratory capacity whenever possible. Where there was not sufficient public-sector capacity, BRAC set up its own laboratories according to government guidelines. The *shebikas* followed the protocol of the government's National Tuberculosis Programme, including treatment and reporting procedures.

BRAC's TB program was hailed as a success and expanded to ten *upazilas* (subdistricts) in 1991; by 2006, it served a catchment area with more than 83 million residents. That year, BRAC treated 87,000 TB patients and recorded a cure rate of 92 percent. Today, BRAC's work is widely regarded as a paradigm of TB control. Its model—based on BRAC's large network of trained and paid *shebikas* and integrated with the public-sector health system—exhibits the substantial benefits of leveraging shared delivery infrastructure in global health delivery.[1]

pared to respond to diverse patient needs. A patient co-infected with tuberculosis and HIV—in 2000, some 30 percent of tuberculosis cases in sub-Saharan Africa were attributed to HIV infection[11]—will be best served by a clinic that tests for HIV and refers to tuberculosis services next door. Even with proper referrals, patients have an easier time accessing needed services when care is integrated and centralized. Especially outside tertiary care centers, shared delivery infrastructure is simpler and less expensive for patients to navigate.

Improving Both Health Delivery and Economic Development

In rich and poor countries alike, poverty and inequality are often chief risk factors of ill health. The concept of structural violence, described in chapter 2 and elsewhere, highlights some of the mechanisms by which large-scale social forces become embodied as disease and disability among the poor and otherwise vulnerable.[12] A crucial objective in itself, poverty reduction is also fundamental to building a strong health system: no health system can provide high-quality care to all those who need it—over the long term—without modern infrastructure, a robust workforce, a decent school system, water and sanitation systems, and a working economy.[13] Conversely, the health of a nation's population is an important precondition to sustainable development.[14] Preventable and treatable diseases like AIDS and tuberculosis thin workforces and civil services;[15] children who do not receive treatment for parasitic worms—not to mention malnutrition, diarrheal diseases, and respiratory diseases—suffer long-term developmental deficits that are later manifested as skill deficits and lower wages among adults.[16]

There is thus synergy between health delivery and economic development. Prudent global health delivery maximizes the spill-over effects that can foster economic growth. Procuring locally produced goods strengthens demand, for example; hiring local staff whenever possible and promoting job creation can help reduce unemployment. Strengthening physical infrastructure (roads, bridges) and public works (water, sanitation, electricity) can improve health care delivery while also facilitating economic transactions. In addition to easing ambulance passage and enabling supply chain logistics, road improvements in rural areas can boost trade and make labor markets more dynamic. In other words, well-designed global health programs can harness a positive feedback loop between poverty reduction and health system strengthening.

These four principles of global health care delivery—adapting to local context, constructing a care delivery value chain, leveraging shared delivery infrastructure, and improving both health delivery and economic development—offer a strategic framework to guide program design and resource allocation. They are, however, only a first step

Case Brief 4. A to Z Textile Mills Ltd.: Improving Health and the Economy

Insecticide-treated bed nets (ITNs) have been shown to reduce malaria transmission when used regularly and mended or replaced periodically. An initial effectiveness study performed in the Gambia in 1991 suggests that use of these bed nets reduced mortality among children under the age of five by up to 60 percent.[1]

In 2000, international malaria-control organizations committed to scaling up the use of bed nets, but utilization rates have remained somewhat low. One problem was that when ITNs were first developed, the nets needed to be retreated with insecticide every six months. More recently, manufacturers such as Sumitomo Chemical Company in Tokyo have developed insecticidal bed nets that remain effective for at least three years. Sumitomo's product is called Olyset. In 2006, the Roll Back Malaria Partnership—a multilateral coalition formed in 1998 to intensify and coordinate global efforts against malaria—called for 80 percent coverage with long-lasting insecticidal bed nets among vulnerable populations by 2010.

In order to increase access to bed nets and to boost local production capacity, Sumitomo chose to partner with public- and private-sector ventures in sub-Saharan Africa. Instead of restricting manufacturing to its own factories, for example, Sumitomo partnered with A to Z Textile Mills Ltd., in Arusha, Tanzania. One of Africa's largest ITN producers, A to Z had been producing bed nets for over a decade (6 million in 2002 alone). After partnering with Sumitomo, A to Z expanded annual production to more than 19 million royalty-free Olyset nets in 2008. When demand continued to outstrip production, Sumitomo and A to Z entered into a 50/50 joint venture to build an additional factory north of Arusha (see figure 7.3). Together, these efforts created more than 5,300 salaried jobs—90 percent of which went to women—and supported an estimated 24,000 people in the surrounding community. Partnering with A to Z also reduced Sumitomo's shipping and distribution costs. This success story highlights the potential synergy that exists between the health and business sectors.[2]

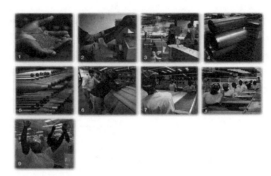

FIGURE 7.3. The Olyset manufacturing process at A to Z Textile Mills Ltd., Arusha, Tanzania. (1) Master batch, (2) melting granules, (3, 4) yarn extrusion, (5) spooling, (6) knitting, (7) cutting, (8) sewing, and (9) quality control. Adapted from William Rodriguez and Kileken ole-MoiYoi, "Building Local Capacity for Health Commodity Manufacturing: A to Z Textile Mills Ltd.," HBS no. GHD-009 (Boston: Harvard Business School Publishing, 2011), Global Health Delivery Online. http://www.ghdonline.org/cases/. Courtesy A to Z Textile Mills Ltd, Arusha, Tanzania.

toward building a robust science of global health delivery, which will require further research on innovative approaches.

The next section examines the challenge of scaling up model systems. Are the lessons gleaned from these case studies generalizable? What does health systems strengthening look like on a national or global scale?

HEALTH SYSTEMS STRENGTHENING

Defining Health Systems

Building resilient health systems that provide high-quality, comprehensive care for every person who needs it is a difficult, complex, and resource-intensive task; it takes years, if not decades, to do it well. But this remains, to many practitioners, the holy grail of global health work.[17] Although most of the examples considered here are confined to the health sector, the efficacy of health systems at large hinges on social policies, public works, environmental conditions, economic development, and many other factors. While improving health care delivery

The WHO Health System Framework

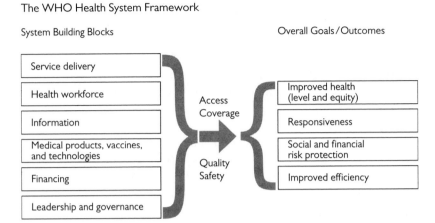

FIGURE 7.4. The health system framework outlined by the World Health Organization. Source: World Health Organization, *Everybody's Business: Strengthening Health Systems to Improve Health Outcomes* (Geneva: World Health Organization, 2007), 3.

and implementing health-sector reforms can address many specific causes of morbidity and mortality, improving the health of a population in the long run also demands large-scale social change.

Health systems are made up of the institutions and personnel charged with providing health care and improving health within a given area. A 2007 report by the WHO, *Everybody's Business: Strengthening Health Systems to Improve Health Outcomes,* highlights six essential building blocks of functioning health systems: service delivery; the health workforce; information; medical products, vaccines, and technologies; financing; and leadership and governance (see figure 7.4).[18]

Former Secretary of Health of Mexico Julio Frenk extends this definition by noting the dynamic relationship between a health system and the population it serves:

In a dynamic view, the population is not an external beneficiary of the system; it is an essential part of it. This is because, when it comes to health, persons play five different roles: (i) as patients, with specific needs requiring care; (ii) as consumers, with expectations about the way in which they will be treated; (iii) as taxpayers and therefore as the ultimate source of financing; (iv) as citizens who may demand access to care as a right; and most importantly, (v) as co-producers of health through care seeking, compliance with prescriptions, and behaviors that may promote or harm one's own health or the health of others. The importance of this perspective is that it opens the door to population-side interventions to improve the health system.[19]

By considering the many roles patients play in health systems, Frenk eschews a unidirectional depiction of health care moving from providers to patients. Good health systems, he argues, draw on the populations they serve to deliver better care. Families, for example, are often the principal caregivers in the management of chronic disease, especially for the elderly.[20] The *accompagnateur* and *shebika* models of Zanmi Lasante and BRAC, respectively, offer two other examples of integrating local communities into health care delivery. The next section examines approaches that integrate contributions from both providers and patients to strengthen health systems.

The Diagonal Approach

Though most global health practitioners and policymakers share the long-term goal of strengthening health systems, many prioritize more targeted interventions in the short term. This debate echoes the debate over primary health care versus selective primary health care discussed in chapter 4: advocates of a *vertical* approach favor disease-specific interventions, while advocates of a *horizontal* approach favor primary care improvements and investments in health systems.

The polio eradication effort illuminates this distinction. Since 1988, the WHO, UNICEF (the United Nations Children's Fund), the Rotary Foundation, and, more recently, the Bill and Melinda Gates Foundation have driven an ongoing campaign to eradicate polio with oral vaccine. Globally, reported cases dropped from more than thirty-five thousand in 1988 to fewer than seven hundred in 2003.[21] (As one example, India's polio vaccination campaign was described in the previous section and illustrated in map 7.1.) In the decade since, despite renewed attention and many millions of dollars, between one and two thousand cases have been recorded annually in several countries in West and Central Africa; in 2009, twenty-three previously polio-free countries were reinfected due to imports of the virus. Today, persistent pockets of transmission in northern Nigeria and on the border between Afghanistan and Pakistan are the focus of polio eradication interventions.[22] Polio vaccination is a paradigmatic vertical intervention: eradicating polio would prevent people from suffering from this disabling and deadly illness ever again; it would be a credit to modern medicine. But why pour millions of dollars into combating a disease that causes only a few thousand cases and several hundred deaths each year, critics ask, when other infectious killers like AIDS, TB, malaria, and the neglected tropical diseases—not to mention noncommunicable diseases, mental disorders, maternal mortality, and other global health priorities—claim millions of lives per year?[23] Alternatively, why focus on individual diseases at all, when health systems could be strengthened to combat polio, AIDS, and whatever comes along next?

A different way of conceptualizing this trade-off between vertical and horizontal interventions is the *diagonal approach*. Julio Frenk and others argue that disease-specific interventions, when delivered well, can also strengthen health systems.[24] In other words, vertical programs can also be horizontal ones. Chapter 6 explores how TB and AIDS treatment, coupled with comprehensive care and wraparound services, improved primary health care in Haiti's Central Plateau.[25] Partners In Health and Zanmi Lasante used TB and AIDS efforts as a wedge to strengthen the local health system. Frenk noted a similar phenomenon in Mexico when the government initiated a conditional cash transfer program called *Opportunidades* (Opportunities). To be eligible for a cash transfer, families needed to demonstrate that their children were regularly attending school and had received a package of basic health care, including growth monitoring, nutritional supplementation, and treatment for common infectious diseases—all of which could be deemed vertical interventions. But implementing *Opportunidades* among the poor improved health indicators—maternal mortality dropped, for example—and fostered a better functioning health system across the board.[26] These and other examples of the diagonal approach demonstrate that, when guided by sound principles of global health delivery (such as those outlined earlier), health initiatives can respond to particular causes of mortality and morbidity while also strengthening health systems more generally.

The Role of the Public Sector

In rich and poor countries alike, governments play an important role in providing health care services—especially for poor and vulnerable populations who often fall through the cracks of private-sector health care markets. As chapter 4 describes, the privatization of health sectors during the structural adjustment era in the 1980s and 1990s undermined access to care among the poorest people in a number of developing countries.[27] Even moderate user fees can prevent the poor from accessing health services;[28] and when private health care providers lack consumers (patients), they tend to relocate to markets in which they can recoup costs. Hence the concentration of private providers in urban centers in developing countries: for example, in recent years there have been three CAT scanners in Haiti, all in private-sector health facilities in the capital, Port-au-Prince.[29]

Such market failures in health care are well known.[30] Many policymakers and practitioners agree that if health systems are to provide comprehensive services that reach the poor, on a large scale and over time, governments must play a leading role. The 2005 Paris Declaration on Aid Effectiveness and the 2008 Accra Agenda for Action both recommended that global health initiatives work in conjunction with, if not directly through, the public sector. More than 150 national governments, major bilateral and multilateral donor agencies, and nongovernmental organizations ratified these documents.[31]

What are the advantages of strengthening public-sector health systems in developing countries with democratic governments? First, governments are the only institutions capable of enshrining—and providing—health as a *right*. International covenants such as the Universal Declaration of Human Rights might declare a right to health in principle, but they can do little in the way of implementation.[32] Only governments can guarantee that all their citizens have access to the health services necessary to live full lives in good health. Second, democratic governments are generally more *accountable* to their citizens than non-state health care providers are to those they serve. Nongovernmental organizations (NGOs), for example, are dependent on and accountable to their funders. If a major donor withdraws support for AIDS programs that supply contraceptives to commercial sex workers, NGOs who depend on that donor may be forced to cut such services, even if the population they serve will be worse off as a result.[33]

Governments, in contrast, are less vulnerable to the whims of donors; they can design programs according to evidence and local needs instead of the fads du jour of global health. They are therefore charged with providing a broad *scope* of health services instead of specific interventions supported by donors. Governments are also expected to provide services for their citizens in the long term—beyond the ebb and flow of foreign aid. Public-sector health systems are thus often more *sustainable* than private efforts. When funding dries up and NGOs pack their bags, the government remains.

Governments are also typically best positioned to provide services

TABLE 7.1 ADVANTAGES OF PUBLIC-SECTOR HEALTH SYSTEMS IN DEMOCRACIES

Rights	Only states can guarantee rights, including the right to health
Accountability	Governments are accountable to their citizens, and democracies have avenues for citizen participation; most NGOs are ultimately accountable to donors
Scope	Public-sector systems are responsible for meeting all the health needs of their citizens, as opposed to delivering a single intervention
Sustainability	Public-sector services tend to persist; even robust NGOs can eventually lose their funding
Scale	Public-sector systems have the broadest reach and are often the only source of potential care for the most vulnerable
Efficiency	The economies of scale harnessed through shared delivery infrastructure are greatest for the largest system, the public sector
Coordination	With a national outlook, the public sector is positioned to balance needs and minimize duplication of efforts
Global commitment	The Paris Declaration on Aid Effectiveness (2005) and the Accra Agenda for Action (2008) commit to public-sector ownership and maximum utilization of country delivery systems in efforts to expand health systems

on a large, or indeed national, *scale,* which can ensure that vulnerable populations like the rural poor are not left out. Given that there are latent economies of scale in health care delivery, governments, by nature of their mandate and their reach, are poised to harness these *efficiencies* by building robust national health systems. Additionally, governments can *coordinate* and integrate the efforts of diverse health providers to ensure that care is delivered efficiently and equitably throughout a given country. Without nationwide delivery strategies, private-sector health care providers may cluster in wealthy urban areas and forfeit the economies of scale that come with collaboration and health systems strengthening. An estimated ten thousand NGOs work in Haiti, for example; with better coordination, as former prime minister Garry Conille called for, such efforts might amount to more than the sum of their parts.[34] By integrating public and private health care efforts through shared delivery infrastructure, governments can foster more efficient and equitable health systems. Table 7.1 summarizes eight reasons why working through the public sector in democratic nations is the prudent approach.

Examples of Effective Public-Sector Health Systems

The Indian state of Kerala has achieved impressive health outcomes by building a strong public-sector health system. Although private-sector health initiatives have expanded since the mid-1980s, public programs coordinate the state's health system and account for the majority of health care provision and training. The Keralan public-sector approach prioritizes prevention, immunizations, and infant and maternal care alongside curative care.[35] (In contrast, many market-based health systems, such as that of the United States, underperform in preventative care.) Kerala also invests heavily in education—including health education—and female literacy rates are higher in Kerala (87 percent) than in other parts of India and most of the developing world.[36]

This model has realized good health outcomes and low costs: Kerala spent $28 per capita on health in 2000 and recorded an infant mortality rate of 14 per 1,000 births and life expectancies of seventy-six years for women and seventy for men.[37] In contrast, the United States spent $4,703 per capita on health in 2000 and recorded an infant mortality rate of 7 in 1,000 births and life expectancies of eighty for women and seventy-four for men.[38] Moreover, thanks to Kerala's universal health care scheme, its citizens have, by many estimates, some of the best access to services in the developing world, even in rural areas.[39] For example, 97 percent of Keralan mothers deliver their babies in hospitals or other institutions.[40]

Critical to the Keralan model is high social-sector spending: 15 percent of the state budget was allocated to health and 25 percent to education throughout the 1990s.[41] These high percentages are a function of the government's small overall budget; per capita spending figures highlight how little investment is needed to realize good health outcomes when an efficient national health system is in place. There are, of course, trade-offs and complexities associated with Kerala's model. The state has India's highest suicide rate; additionally, as access to care increased, so did reported morbidity.[42] As Amartya Sen suggests, the latter finding likely reflects the lack of reporting capacity before health services were scaled up.[43] Such biosocial complexities, which have been explicated at length elsewhere,[44] are endemic to global health work. Nonetheless, Kerala exemplifies some of the benefits of a strong public-sector health system.

Although Cuba can be a polarizing case, its health system has long won acclaim, even from unlikely admirers such as the former president of the World Bank, James Wolfensohn. By many standards, Cuba has some of the best health indicators in the developing and developed world.[45] The national health system provides free care—especially primary health care and preventative services, just as the Keralan system does—for all Cuban citizens.[46] The cornerstone of the national health service is the *médico de familia,* the family doctor, who, like a general practitioner, provides primary care services and acts as a gatekeeper to specialized services.[47] Thanks to national training programs across the country, Cuba boasts more than 65,000 doctors for a population of 11 million, a rate of about one doctor per 175 people. (The United States has one doctor per 375 people.)[48] Even the rural reaches of Cuba are serviced by physicians and nurses and dedicated health facilities. In fact, Cuba has long been a net exporter of skilled health professionals. After the 2010 Haiti earthquake, the Cuban medical brigade was among the largest and most dedicated foreign aid efforts. It has also proved to be among the longest-lasting: although the great majority of NGOs and foreign relief teams long ago departed the country, a large portion of the Cuban brigade remains in Haiti, actively engaged in controlling cholera and strengthening that country's beleaguered health system.[49] Like the system in Kerala, the Cuban model has its drawbacks, most notably its association with the country's oppressive communist government. But the components of its model are not unique to a communist system: any government could adopt a family doctor approach or increase emphasis on preventative and primary care.

As chapter 6 describes, Rwanda has also emerged as a model of national health system strengthening. The Rwandan Ministry of Health adopted a community-based approach to tackling AIDS and many other leading causes of mortality and morbidity, and the ministry encouraged coordination and integration by mandating that non-state providers work within the country's national strategies.[50] In fact, Minister of Health Dr. Agnes Binagwaho often bars foreign initiatives from Rwanda if they do not work in conjunction with the public-sector health system. This policy has helped Rwanda's health system become more efficient and equitable; the efforts of multiple providers, through partnerships, have exceeded expectations. Rwanda's health indicators have improved dramatically: mortality among children under five dropped from 196 per 1,000 in 2000 to 103 per 1,000 in 2007.[51] Rwanda is one of the only developing countries within reach of providing universal antiretroviral treatment coverage for people with AIDS.[52]

The U.S. Health System

With its state-of-the-art facilities and cutting-edge procedures, the U.S. health system has been described as "the most advanced system of care in the world."[1] But it is also burdened with unsustainably rising costs and great disparities in access to quality care. The United States, despite its great wealth and capability, is the only high-income Western nation that does not guarantee universal health insurance.[2] Some 50 million people went without health insurance in 2010,[3] although the 2010 Affordable Care Act is projected to reduce this number. Stratified by age and income, the uninsured have a 25 percent higher mortality risk in future years compared to individuals who do have insurance. The Institute of Medicine estimates that eighteen thousand Americans die prematurely each year for want of timely care.[4] Such gaps occur predominantly among the poor. Health care is regarded as a commodity rather than a right, and it is therefore rationed based on ability to pay for the majority of Americans.[5] Unlike countries that ration health care explicitly—a practice many Americans vocally oppose—price rationing simply excludes those who can't afford it.

In addition to concerns about access and equity, the U.S. health system is also beset by inefficiencies.[6] Despite spending $8,300 per person on health care in 2010—more than double the median per capita expenditures of other high-income countries—aggregate health outcomes in the United States are frequently lackluster.[7] Several indicators are worse than those in other high-income countries: the WHO's *World Health Report 2000* ranked the U.S. health care system thirty-seventh in the world, for example.[8] Though cross-country comparisons must be used with caution,[9] the United States's middling rankings are disquieting: in 2006 it was ranked thirty-ninth for infant mortality, forty-third for adult female mortality, forty-second for adult male mortality, and thirty-sixth for life expectancy.[10]

Although at times it may seem like the language of global health delivery and that of U.S. health care reform have little in common, in the past few decades health care delivery strategies have been imported from developing countries to the United States—examples of "reverse innovation"—often improving health outcomes among vulnerable populations while cutting costs. Chapter 11 describes several such examples and provides a more in-depth analysis of the U.S. health system.

These and many of its other gains in part stem from a strategy of building a strong national health system.[53]

An approach that focuses on public-sector health system strengthening will not suit all settings. In fragile or predatory states, governments may have neither the will nor the capacity to provide health services for their citizens; in such places, nonstate providers sometimes serve as the caregivers of last resort. Nonetheless, NGOs and other private providers have found it possible and fruitful to work with governments in many challenging settings, including Haiti, where political instability and anemic public-service provision have been the norm. In particular, local governments may have greater continuity of leadership and overall stability than national governments, which face more frequent—and typically more fevered—election cycles. Corruption, one of the most commonly touted arguments against working with governments in developing countries, can also be less endemic at the district level. Moreover, charges of corruption are usually meant to end, not start, a conversation about how to strengthen local institutions and health care delivery capacity. Working with public-sector ministries, although difficult, offers an opportunity to strengthen the infrastructure of transparency and accountability in the governments of developing countries. Corruption is often enabled by a lack of computer-based bookkeeping, accountants, and trained civil servants—or even a lack of reliable electricity, in some cases.[54] Chapter 10 argues that *accompanying* local institutions, public and private, offers a compelling approach for global health work and foreign assistance in general.

But accompaniment is a long way from the status quo. Public-private partnerships in global health efforts remain uncommon in the early twenty-first century. Although some countries, such as Rwanda, have worked to harmonize nonstate health care initiatives with state programs, most developing nations have parallel public and private health systems. For example, NGOs, which provide a substantial portion of the health services available in such settings, rarely work in conjunction with the public-sector health system. Without coordination, parallel systems of care can lead to inefficiencies, uneven access to services, and gaps in the standard of care.[55] In some cases, private providers, including NGOs, can unwittingly undermine public-sector health initiatives by offering high salaries that distort the labor markets for health care workers.[56] Further, NGOs and other foreign initiatives, accountable to their donors, bring their own priorities, which often diverge from government priorities and national strategies.

But NGOs can also partner with local and national governments and work through public-sector health systems to strengthen health care delivery capacity. One successful practitioner of this approach has been the Clinton Health Access Initiative (CHAI, formerly the Clinton HIV/AIDS Initiative), which, among other things, seeks to strengthen public-sector health systems by improving supply chain management, rural health infrastructure, laboratory systems, and training platforms for health care workers. CHAI's stated goal is "to work ourselves out of a job," by building local government capacity in the health sector.[57] This approach accords with the Accra Agenda for Action and the Paris Declaration on Aid Effectiveness. Although not suited for all contexts, global health practitioners would do well to seek public-private partnerships capable of strengthening national health systems in the long term.

HUMAN RESOURCES FOR HEALTH

Human resources are a key component of health systems. No health system can function without well-trained and fairly compensated doctors, nurses, laboratory technicians, pharmacists, social workers, community health workers, and the many other types of personnel necessary to deliver care effectively and equitably to all who need it. Yet there are far too few health care workers around the world. According to the WHO, there is a global shortfall of more than 4 million health care workers; the organization estimates that an additional 2.4 million workers will be needed to meet the Millennium Development Goals (explored in chapter 11).[58] Both developed and developing countries face such deficits, though they are more acute in the latter.[59] The ratio of health care workers to population size illustrates the disequilibrium: the United States has an average of 24.8 health care workers per 1,000 people; in Africa, the ratio is 2.3 per 1,000.[60] There are also significant regional inequalities. Malawi has 260 medical doctors and a population of 13 million; rural areas often lack a single doctor per several hundred thousand people.[61] The scarcity of health personnel means that many clinics and hospitals are unable to deliver timely, quality care. In Ghana, one report found that 77 percent of health facilities were unable to provide 24-hour emergency services, including maternal care for women in childbirth.[62]

Building a robust health care workforce around the world will require new institutions for medical education and improvements to those that already exist. There are only sixty-six medical schools on the entire African continent, which has a population of more than 1 billion people.[63] In 2008, African medical schools produced some eight thousand doctors, many of whom emigrated to wealthier countries for better pay and job stability.[64] Historically, government-run medical and nursing schools have trained the majority of health professionals in developing countries; but recently private schools have begun to play a larger role. In the eastern Mediterranean region, for example, the private sector accounted for 10 percent of all medical training institutions in 1980 and for nearly 60 percent in 2005.[65] Much of this private-sector growth is attributable to social-sector spending reductions encouraged during the structural adjustment era. Ultimately, greater investment by both governments and private institutions is necessary to reach the WHO target of building a "pipeline [spanning] primary, secondary, and tertiary education institutions and health services facilities that produce a range of workers from auxiliaries to technicians and professionals."[66] The cost of bridging this training gap over a twenty-year period is, on average, an estimated $88 million per country per year, which would demand increasing health expenditures by $1.60 per person per year.[67]

In addition to training more doctors and nurses and pharmacists, "task shifting" initiatives can help address the human resources shortfall. A 2008 study found that the quality of integrated management of childhood illness varied little among providers of different training levels in four countries.[68] Trained community health workers in particular can provide a range of essential services, such as home-based care and directly observed therapy for complex diseases like AIDS and multidrug-resistant tuberculosis and certain malignancies.[69] As chapter 4 describes, community-based primary care, such as that provided by barefoot doctors in China and rural doctors in India, has proven to be effective and low-cost for decades. Partners In Health's efforts, from Haiti to Peru to Rwanda to Russia to the United States, also follow a community health worker model.[70]

Training large numbers of community health workers can be accomplished rapidly at a low cost. Based on the Millennium Villages Project, which works in ten sub-Saharan African countries, Columbia University's Earth Institute developed a plan to train an additional 1 million community health workers in Africa—a ratio of 1 community health worker per 650 people in rural Africa—for $6.56 per person served, or $2.3 billion per year (including existing government and donor expenditures). Replicating such efforts in other parts of the developing world would help to improve health system capacity. The Earth Institute report asserts: "The importance of CHWs [community health workers] is not a new realization. Now is the time to align CHWs with broader health system strengthening efforts at the primary care level, improve CHW financing, and broadly disseminate recent advances in technology, diagnostics and treatment to support community-based health workers."[71] Complementary to professional training programs, community-based training initiatives are essential for bridging the health care worker gap—and for strengthening health systems in general.

But improving and expanding training capacity in poor countries will not solve the crisis in human resources for health. The shortage of health care workers is exacerbated by the phenomenon of "brain drain": doctors and nurses and other health professionals frequently migrate within and between countries to seek out higher salaries or more favorable work conditions. The data can be discouraging: Zambia retained only 50 out of 600 doctors trained there since 1970; Zimbabwe retained 360 out of 1,200 doctors trained there in the 1990s; Ghana retained 267 out of 871 medical personnel trained there from 1993 to 2002.[72] Health professionals often migrate for work because under-resourced health systems offer meager salaries and lack the tools and technologies they were trained to use. Such environments are deeply demoralizing for health care workers of all stripes. "Before training we thought of doctors as supermen. . . . [Here] we are only mortuary attendants," said one physician working in a beleaguered hospital in Kenya.[73]

NGOs and private practitioners in urban centers typically offer higher salaries than national health systems. Lack of opportunities or facilities can draw health care workers from rural areas and toward urban settings.[74] Shortages of health care workers in rich countries—magnified by the increasing health needs of aging populations—also attract doctors and nurses from poor nations. About one in five physicians in the United States is foreign-trained. The United States authorizes 50,000 special visas for foreign nurses annually, while some 150,000 applicants are rejected from U.S. nursing schools every year.[75] Recruiters for hospitals in wealthier countries are often allowed to advertise directly to medical professionals in developing countries.[76] It is difficult not to hold certain rich countries partly accountable for the flight of health professionals from the developing world. Complicit countries, including the United States, could help reduce the pull factors motivating the brain drain by expanding domestic nursing and medical schools to meet rising demand without importing doctors and nurses from abroad.

Reversing the brain drain will require substantive reforms and investments by countries poor and rich. Health professionals are of course entitled to seek better opportunities and options. To retain medical practitioners, developing countries must be able to offer competitive salaries, fringe benefits (such as discounted housing), and a professional medical environment that includes modern health facilities (intensive care units, operating rooms), adequate supplies of medications and diagnostic tools, a sizable support staff, and continuing medical education and training programs. One study found that nonfinancial incentives such as training, study leave, and professional support were among the most important factors affecting retention across four sub-Saharan African countries. In other words, the best way to keep doctors and nurses from moving to wealthy areas is health systems strengthening: when health professionals are compensated fairly, surrounded by well-trained colleagues, and have access to modern medical tools and facilities, many choose to stay in the countries in which they were trained.[77]

Without investing in training and health infrastructure across the developing world, and reforming the institutional architecture that pulls health professionals from poor settings to rich ones, the brain drain will likely continue to debilitate health systems in poorer countries. It reduces the supply of doctors and nurses, and it forfeits the investment—most of it made by cash-poor governments—that went into training such personnel in the first place. The effects of the brain drain therefore fall on ministries of health, which are often accused of not spending enough on health,[78] even though some have budgets no bigger than the budget of a single hospital in the United States.[79] Such effects fall hardest, of course, on the poor, who live in precisely the places where health professionals are unable to find satisfying work conditions. The brain drain thus illustrates how economic disparities and other large-scale social forces pattern the health of populations around the globe; in short, it exemplifies structural violence.

CONCLUSION

This chapter has explored the nascent science of global health delivery, which seeks to identify and scale up effective models of health care delivery around the world. The Global Health Delivery Project has provided several basic principles of health care delivery: adapting to the local context, designing systems of care that maximize value to patients, leveraging shared delivery infrastructure, and improving both health delivery and economic development. It has also provided case studies of these principles in action, highlighting programmatic features that improve or undermine the quality of health care delivery. The chapter also examined health system strengthening on a national and transnational scale and pointed to the *diagonal approach* as a compelling strategy for responding to specific causes of mortality and morbidity while also strengthening provision of primary health care services. The final section then looked at human resources for health, one key component of health systems strengthening and a telling example of the ways in which global political economy structures the fault lines of global health.

One theme that has recurred throughout the chapter is the biosocial complexity endemic to global health work. The next chapter builds on this theme by analyzing some of the difficulties associated with developing metrics of disease burden and other quantitative tools in the context of two complex—and critical—global health challenges: mental illness and multidrug-resistant tuberculosis.

SUGGESTED READING

Berwick, Donald M. "Disseminating Innovations in Health Care." *Journal of the American Medical Association* 289, no. 15 (2003): 1969–1975.

Ellner, Andrew, Sachin H. Jain, Joseph Rhatigan, and Daniel Blumenthal. "Polio Elimination in Uttar Pradesh." HBS no. GHD-005. Boston: Harvard Business School Publishing, 2011. Global Health Delivery Online, www.ghdonline.org/cases/.

Frenk, Julio. "The Global Health System: Strengthening National Health Systems as the Next Step for Global Progress." *PLoS Medicine* 7, no. 1 (2010): e1000089.

Garrett, Laurie. "The Challenge of Global Health." *Foreign Affairs* 86, no. 1 (2007): 14–38.

Grimshaw, Jeremy, and Martin P. Eccles. "Is Evidence-Based Implementation of Evidence-Based Care Possible?" *Medical Journal of Australia* 180, no. 6, suppl. (2004): S50–S51.

Kim, Jim Yong, Paul Farmer, and Michael E. Porter, "Redefining Global Health Care Delivery," *Lancet* (20 May 2013).

Kim, Jim Yong, Joseph Rhatigan, Sachin H. Jain, Rebecca Weintraub, and Michael E. Porter. "From a Declaration of Values to the Creation of Value in Global Health: A Report from Harvard University's Global Health Delivery Project." *Global Public Health* 5, no. 2 (2010): 181–188.

May, Maria, Joseph Rhatigan, and Richard Cash. "BRAC's Tuberculosis Program: Pioneering DOTS Treatment for TB in Rural Bangladesh." HBS no. GHD-010. Boston: Harvard Business School Publishing, 2011. Global Health Delivery Online, www.ghdonline.org/cases/.

Murray, Christopher. "A New Institute for Global Health Evaluations." *Lancet* 369, no. 9577 (2007): 1902.

Park, Peter, Arti Bhatt, and Joseph Rhatigan. "The Academic Model for the Prevention and Treatment of HIV/AIDS." HBS no. GHD-013. Boston: Harvard Business School Publishing, 2011. Global Health Delivery Online, www.ghdonline.org/cases/.

Porter, Michael E., and Elizabeth Olmsted Teisberg. *Redefining Health Care: Creating Value-Based Competition on Results*. Boston: Harvard Business Review Press, 2006.

Quigley, Fran. *Walking Together, Walking Far: How a U.S. and African Medical School Partnership Is Winning the Fight against HIV/AIDS*. Bloomington: Indiana University Press, 2009.

Raviola, Giuseppe, M'Imunya Machoki, Esther Mwaikambo, and Mary Jo DelVecchio Good. "HIV, Disease Plague, Demoralization, and 'Burnout': Resident Experience of the Medical Profession in Nairobi, Kenya." *Culture, Medicine, and Psychiatry* 26, no. 1 (2002): 55–86.

Roberts, Marc J., William Hsiao, Peter Berman, and Michael R. Reich. *Getting Health Reform Right: A Guide to Improving Performance and Equity*. New York: Oxford University Press, 2008.

Rodriguez, William, and Kileken ole-MoiYoi. "Building Local Capacity for Health Commodity Manufacturing: A to Z Textile Mills Ltd." HBS no. GHD-009. Boston: Harvard Business School Publishing, 2011. Global Health Delivery Online, www.ghdonline.org/cases/.

Sanders, David, and Andy Haines. "Implementation Research Is Needed to Achieve International Health Goals." *PLoS Medicine* 3, no. 6 (2006): e186.

Stilwell, Barbara, Khassoum Diallo, Pascal Zurn, Marko Vujicic, Orvill Adams, and Mario Dal Poz. "Migration of Health-Care Workers from Developing Countries: Strategic Approaches to Its Management." *Bulletin of the World Health Organization* 82, no. 8 (2004): 595–600.

World Health Organization. *Everybody's Business: Strengthening Health Systems to Improve Health Outcomes*. Geneva: World Health Organization, 2007.

———. *World Health Report 2006: Working Together for Health*. Geneva: World Health Organization, 2006.

8

The Unique Challenges of Mental Health and MDRTB

Critical Perspectives on Metrics of Disease

ANNE BECKER, ANJALI MOTGI, JONATHAN WEIGEL, GIUSEPPE RAVIOLA, SALMAAN KESHAVJEE, ARTHUR KLEINMAN

This chapter examines two topics that warrant closer examination: mental health and multidrug-resistant tuberculosis (MDRTB). Pairing these topics is unusual, but both offer fertile ground for exploring some of the tensions and challenges endemic to global health scholarship and practice. Both mental health and MDRTB are urgent priorities worldwide and yet often attract little attention among practitioners, researchers, policymakers, and funders of global health efforts. Both are associated with a significant share of the annual global toll of disability-adjusted life years (DALYs)—a metric of disease burden that this chapter considers in depth. Yet why are mental health and MDRTB often confined to the sidelines? How do they contribute to a political economy of disease neglect?

On another level, mental health and MDRTB resist straightforward categorization in conventional global health metrics. Is it possible to quantify the manifold expressions of neuropsychiatric distress? If not, how should programs be designed and resources allocated to reduce the burden of mental illness around the globe? MDRTB is a highly contagious, airborne, and often deadly infection—a public health practitioner's worst nightmare—but is also complicated and expensive to treat. How might cost-effectiveness analysis fully account for the challenges posed by MDRTB? How does the risk of resurgent MDRTB epidemics rank among global scourges? We hope this chapter will help readers develop a better understanding of these two complex and often neglected priorities, while employing theoretical perspectives considered throughout this book and thus further highlighting the need for a critical sociology of global health.

THE "ODD CASE" OF MENTAL HEALTH

Mental health has an uneasy relationship with traditional international health and global health discourses.[1] Although tens of millions of people suffer from mental disorders worldwide, the health care resources allocated to respond to the associated morbidity, distress, and impairment are disproportionately low, as table 8.1 demonstrates. Perhaps as a reflection of Cartesian dualism—"mind over matter"— mental disorders are often placed in a separate category from medical disorders affecting other organ systems.[2] Whereas physical ailments are routinely and widely accepted as objective realities, many laypersons regard the symptoms of neuropsychiatric disorders as subjective experiences and therefore less firmly grounded in the medical domain.[3] Mental distress can manifest itself along a gradient of suffering that is not easily recognized as a discrete illness or included within conventional biomedical classifications of disease. The "odd case" of mental health therefore vividly illustrates the complexities (and shortcomings) of extant metrics for disease burden.

Readers may be more familiar with mental health issues in urban and suburban areas of rich countries such as the United States, where reports of increasing incidence of depression and prescription of psychotropic medications are common in the popular press.[4] Aggregate statistics demonstrate a 76 percent increase in the reported prevalence of depression in the United States from 1980 to 2000.[5] Use of antidepressants such as fluoxetine (Prozac) and paroxetine (Paxil) tripled from 1988 to 2000, and it is estimated that in any given month 10.6 percent of women and 5.2 percent of men in the United States use an antidepressant.[6]

The rapid rise of documented mental health conditions, especially depression, has led some to suggest that, in many cases, the U.S. health establishment medicalizes normal sadness. Allan Horwitz and Jerome Wakefield, for example, argue that "the recent explosion of putative depressive disorder, in fact, does not stem primarily from an actual increased incidence of this condition. Instead it is largely a product of conflating the two conceptually distinct categories of normal sadness and depressive disorder."[7] In scrutinizing the increase in psychotropic drug use, commentators in the popular press have also suggested that

TABLE 8.1   DISEASE BURDEN OF MENTAL DISORDERS
COMPARED TO RESOURCE ALLOCATION

	Burden of Mental Disorders (Percentage of DALYs)[a]	Percentage of Budget Allocated to Mental Health[b]
Low-income countries	7.88	2.26
Lower-middle-income countries	14.50	2.26
Higher-middle-income countries	19.56	4.27
High-income countries	21.37	6.88
All countries	11.48	3.76

SOURCE: Shekhar Saxena, Graham Thornicroft, Martin Knapp, and Harvey Whiteford, "Resources for Mental Health: Scarcity, Inequity, and Inefficiency," *Lancet* 370, no. 9590 (2007): 883.
[a]PERCENTAGE of disability-adjusted life years (DALYs) attributable to mental disorders. DALYs are defined as the sum of the years of life lost as a result of premature mortality in the population and the years lost as a result of disability for incident cases of mental disorders.
[b]MEDIAN values for the percentage of countries' total health budgets allocated to mental health.

pharmaceutical companies profit by supporting research that expands the territory of indications for their products and by promoting "me-too" drugs.[8] The relocation of grief and sadness, arguably emotional states that can fall well within social norms, to the medical domain demonstrates the need for careful critique—among health practitioners, policymakers, and regulators, not to mention patients—of how modern health systems can be co-opted by economic and political interests.[9]

But it is misleading that stories about therapeutic excess tend to dominate the public conversation; mental illness in fact represents one of the largest causes of unchecked suffering in the United States and throughout the world. For example, a 2005 study found that 27 percent of the adult population in Europe had experienced at least one mental disorder in the previous twelve months.[10] Sizable ethnic and socioeconomic disparities shape patterns of help-seeking, access to care, and therapeutic outcomes for mental disorders in the United States, Europe, and most high-income countries.[11] If anything, neuropsychiatric morbidity is underdiagnosed and antidepressants are underutilized in rich and poor countries alike.[12]

Moreover, many low-income countries experience high psychiatric morbidity. In 2004, the World Health Organization (WHO) found that East and Southeast Asia had the world's highest rate of neuropsychiatric disability per capita.[13] Studies attribute 12 to 15 percent of the global burden of disease to neuropsychiatric disorders (especially chronically disabling depression), a greater share than that attributed to global infectious diseases, such as tuberculosis, or to chronic diseases, such as cancer and heart disease.[14] Put another way, mental and neurological illnesses account for 26.8 percent of all years lived with disability in low- and middle-income countries alone.[15]

These figures may underestimate the true burden of psychiatric illness, however, because of the complexity of quantifying and reporting mental illness globally. For example, symptoms of neuropsychiatric distress and help-seeking behaviors are often less visible and less reported among vulnerable groups such as women and adolescents.[16] The scarcity of specialty mental health services—and the concentration of available services in urban centers—also makes it extremely difficult to generate prevalence estimates in low- and middle-income countries. Additionally, estimates based on universalizing criteria for mental disorders, such as those listed in the *Diagnostic and Statistical Manual of Mental Disorders V (DSM-V)*—the American Psychiatric Association's widely used classification manual—have uncertain validity within populations other than those for which they were developed (mainly European and American populations). These diagnostic criteria have potentially limited clinical utility across diverse cultural and social contexts, given the phenomenologic variation in psychiatric presentation and the culture-specific rhetoric used to signal distress.

Conventional public health metrics also fail to account for the risk of co-morbidities associated with mental illness. A series of 2007 studies published in *The Lancet* mapped out how mental illness—depression, substance abuse, suicide, post-traumatic stress disorder—clusters with physical illness.[17] The researchers found, for example, that mental disorders increase the risk of both communicable diseases such as TB and sexually transmitted infections and noncommunicable diseases such as coronary heart disease, stroke, and diabetes.[18] Conversely, many physical diseases, such as AIDS and malaria, were found to increase the risk of developing mental disorders.[19] These vicious clusters of disease illustrate the importance of integrating mental health services into health systems. The authors of the *Lancet* series end by reasserting a proposition first argued in the World Health Organization's 2001 *World Health Report:* "there can be no health without mental health."[20]

Of the estimated 400 million mentally ill individuals worldwide, the majority of those with serious mental disorders do not receive the care they need.[21] For many, this lack of access stems from poverty. Indeed, inadequate access to care compounds the elevated risk of mental illness faced by the poor. In a 2003 study, Vikram Patel and Arthur Kleinman conclude that "the experience of insecurity and hopelessness, rapid social change, and the risks of violence and physical ill-health may explain the greater vulnerability of the poor to common mental disorders."[22] Hunger and malnutrition, inadequate living and working conditions, urban crowding, and rural isolation also contribute to the greater risk of mental illness faced by poor populations around the world. In other words, structural violence predisposes the poor to mental distress.[23] In *World Mental Health: Problems and Priorities in Low-Income Countries,* anthropologist Robert Desjarlais and colleagues trace the social mechanisms underpinning this relationship:

> These problems [such as chronic hunger, sexual exploitation, and pervasive underemployment], rooted in everyday structure of societies, can take as great a toll on mental health as does the acute stress of a major life crisis such as bereavement, with which mental health professionals are more familiar. To think about mental health, then, one must consider a range of interrelated forces that, at first glance, might not appear to be "psychiatric" problems.[24]

In other words, many of the same social and economic circumstances that predispose the global poor to infectious and chronic physical diseases also predispose them to mental illness.

Socially marginalized groups bear the brunt of the disease burden. Women, for example, experience a disproportionate share of chronic psychiatric morbidity. Because they traditionally work long hours without adequate compensation and often receive less social support than men, women face multiple social vulnerabilities associated with neuro-psychological distress.[25] Such gender-based risk is manifest in mental health disparities in China, for example, where women's suicide rate is 25 percent higher than that of men (see the box on page 220). Children living in poverty are also at heightened risk. Developmental attrition (stemming chiefly from malnutrition), lack of education, child labor, and child prostitution—these are just a handful of the harmful early-life experiences that elevate the risk of chronic mental disorders among young people. The WHO estimates that between 10 and 20 percent of children and adolescents are affected by psychiatric problems, which account for five of the top ten causes of morbidity among those age five and older.[26] Suicide rates are often highest among young people. In fact, suicide is the first or second leading cause of death among fifteen- to thirty-four-year-olds in China and a number of European countries; it is

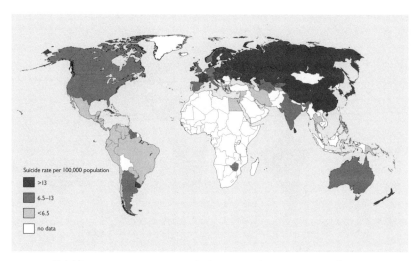

Suicide rate per 100,000 population

■ >13

■ 6.5–13

□ <6.5

□ no data

MAP 8.1. Suicide rates per 100,000 population, 2007. Courtesy Bamse/Wikimedia Commons; data courtesy World Health Organization.

the third leading cause of death for this age group in the United States.[27] High rates of suicide also afflict elderly populations in China, Japan, and many other countries. Furthermore, shortcomings in knowledge of mental health continue to be an ongoing challenge; for example, the suicide rate data for many countries, particularly in Africa and Southeast Asia, are often lacking or of questionable quality (see map 8.1).

In some cases, the stigma and vulnerability attached to neuropsychological disease can lead to violations of basic human rights. "The stigma of mental illness is so great that the mentally ill are unable to gain employment, finish schooling, marry, live independently, or have their care paid for by insurance companies," write Vikram Patel and colleagues.[28] They describe one particularly horrifying incident known as the "Erwadi Tragedy," in which more than twenty mentally ill patients perished in a fire at an Indian healing temple because they had been chained to their beds.[29] Disturbing examples of stigma attached to psychiatric disorders are, of course, in no short supply in developed countries, too. Patel and colleagues argue that, as with other health-related stigmas, the fear and discrimination directed toward the mentally ill derive from ignorance and neglect. When a disease is poorly understood and left untreated, they contend, there is a greater chance that society will blame the victim; as mental health information and

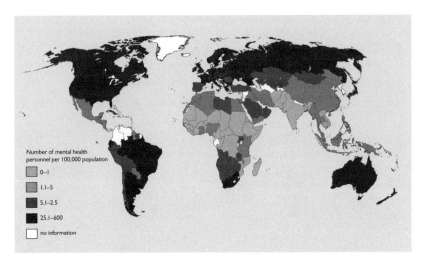

Number of mental health
personnel per 100,000 population

☐ 0–1
☐ 1.1–5
■ 5.1–2.5
■ 25.1–600
☐ no information

MAP 8.2. Human resources for mental health: Psychiatrists, psychologists, nurses, and social workers per 100,000 population, 2005. Source: Shekhar Saxena, Graham Thornicroft, Martin Knapp, and Harvey Whiteford, "Resources for Mental Health: Scarcity, Inequity, and Inefficiency," *Lancet* 370, no. 9590 (2007): 880.

treatment programs have been deployed, reported stigmas have correspondingly decreased.[30]

Reversing the status quo of neglect for the mentally ill would demand substantial resources and political commitment. Most poor countries spend only a few cents per person per year on mental health services. Mental health professionals are also in short supply in many of these countries, as map 8.2 illustrates: there are only twenty trained psychiatrists working in all of Tanzania, a country with a population of 44 million, where total expenditures on mental health average US$0.05 per person per year.[31] Comparing this figure to the $104 billion spent on mental health and substance abuse in the United States in 2001—a mere 7.6 percent of total health expenditures—paints a sobering picture of the uneven landscape of global mental health.[32]

Nonetheless, a rising tide of compelling evidence suggests that mental health care can be effectively and inexpensively integrated into health systems despite sizable implementation barriers. Desjarlais and colleagues, for example, document successful community-based treatment programs in South America:

> One means of filling the gap between resources and needs is to train primary health care workers in identifying and treating the mental health problems [of patients]. A preliminary training course developed for primary

care workers and nurses in Colombia and Ecuador confirmed that local health workers can provide needed mental health care to their patients. With initial training using basic screening techniques, the primary care workers were better able to determine the emotional state of victims and to recommend appropriate care.[33]

The Nepal Community Mental Health Project also shows the promise of integrating mental health services into health systems.[34] When the program began in 1984, Nepal had twenty-two psychiatrists in the entire country; only three worked outside the capital, Kathmandu. The project began by training local health workers to assess and treat basic mental disorders in four remote Himalayan districts that had almost no available mental health care. According to Sarah Acland, who wrote a case study on the project, "The aim of the mental health program was to bring mental health care to the rural poor by integrating services into the already extant community health system. This was to be achieved by training health workers in the recognition and management of mental and neurological disorders."[35] By 1993, the health posts counted 421 active patients and reported thousands of patient visits, involving 4,878 cases of epilepsy, 557 cases of psychosis, and 1,124 cases of depression.[36] By delivering mental health services through existing health infrastructure—however fragile—the program made strides toward reducing neuropsychiatric disability at low cost.

A number of mental health programs have adopted a similar community-based approach. In the 1960s and 1970s, Thomas Lambo and colleagues launched a village-based care program for the mentally ill in Nigeria, which yielded promising results.[37] A national treatment program in Chile also reduced the prevalence of depression, according to some indicators, by integrating services into existing primary health care delivery efforts.[38] Because of the co-morbidities between mental and physical diseases, such efforts can be mutually reinforcing. Community-based mental health programs have provided treatment in rural Haiti for years.[39] After the January 2010 earthquake caused widespread neuropsychiatric distress, some providers responded to the need. For example, Zanmi Lasante's mental health and psychosocial program rapidly expanded from just three psychologists to seventeen, and from twenty social workers (and assistants) to fifty.[40] The needs remain great, but partnerships with the Haitian Ministry of Health have been forged to strengthen Haiti's national mental health treatment and training capacity.

Amid increasing reports of mental health treatment programs like those mentioned here, the WHO released its *Mental Health GAP Action Programme* in 2010 to encourage delivery of services for mental, neurological, and substance-use disorders in developing countries.[41] Basic treatment packages for such disorders can be implemented at low cost in resource-poor settings in conjunction with task-shifting programs that engage community health workers in care delivery.[42] If scaled up, such approaches could do much to reduce the burden of mental illness around the globe.[43]

Despite these promising advances, uncertainty and debate remain

Suicide in China

One tragic consequence of neglecting mental health services is suicide.[1] However, Kleinman, Patel, and others explain how context-specific social and economic forces—and not just mental illness—shape the local profile of suicide in different settings.[2] China offers a particularly sobering picture of how such forces can lead to hopelessness and death.

The WHO estimates that there are 14 cases of suicide per 100,000 people in China annually.[3] Others question the validity of government-reported statistics and calculate the rate as 28.72 per 100,000 (or more than 320,000 per year).[4] In either case, this is one of the world's highest rates and the fifth greatest cause of death in the country.[5] The problem is especially grave among young people ages fifteen to thirty-four, for whom suicide is the leading cause of death (19 percent of all deaths), and among women, whose suicide rate is 25 percent higher than that of men. This latter figure represents a departure from the global norm, in which the suicide rate averages 3.5 times higher for men than for women (see, for example, figure 8.1).[6] In China, 90 percent of suicides occur in rural areas. Taken together, these statistics suggest that young women living in rural areas are at greatest risk of suicide. Even with the challenges of translating and quantifying mental distress across cultures, all available indicators paint a stark portrait of a rural population in China facing a heavy burden of mental illness without much access to care.

Why is suicide risk structured along these demographic and geographic lines? The rapid social and economic transformations of modern China constitute the backdrop against which individuals—most often young women in rural areas—commit this desperate act.[7] More than 150 million internal migrants, mostly men, moved from rural to urban areas, weakening the support system for married women who have children and elderly parents to care for. Also, the health

about how to reduce chronic psychiatric morbidity. Arthur Kleinman's longstanding critique of medicalization raises important questions for any proposal seeking to scale up mental health services—or health care of any kind—among underserved populations:

> This process of *medicalization* is responsible for certain of biomedicine's most controversial attributes. Biomedicine's sector of influence continues to grow as more and more life problems are brought under its aegis.

of China's population has been transformed on many fronts over the past three decades of market-oriented reforms: mental disorders such as depression and substance abuse increased, as did AIDS, sexually transmitted diseases, and violence. Such social upheaval is a known risk factor for mental illness.[8]

In China, privatization changed health care delivery from a "solidarity-based" insurance scheme to "individual-based" insurance. This sudden policy shift shocked the system: rural hospitals and clinics were emptied of patients who could not pay the required fees. The community-based care model, long a trademark and strength of the Chinese health system, struggled in the new consumer system.[9] Even when desperate individuals overcame the stigma associated with mental illness, they often could not find prompt, affordable, and quality care. Poor emergency care services in rural areas, combined with access to lethal means—pesticides used in agriculture, for example—also contribute to the high suicide rate.[10] Some estimate that fewer than 40 percent of suicides in China are associated with diagnosable mental illnesses.[11]

The low social status of women in Chinese society may help to explain the gendered burden of suicide in that country. Stories of female infanticide and a general prejudice against women and girls are not unfamiliar.[12] Amartya Sen's 1992 article "Missing Women" highlights the insidious effects of gender bias in many developing countries. Despite a natural tendency for men to have higher mortality rates than women, women have the higher rates in some low- and middle-income countries. Sen attributes this inverted ratio to the lack of care, support, and attention females receive in countries such as China, India, and Pakistan. By calculating the difference between the real and estimated population ratios, Sen postulates that, in 1992, 48 million women were "missing" in China.[13] It would be difficult to come up with a better example of how structural violence becomes embodied in marginalized individuals.

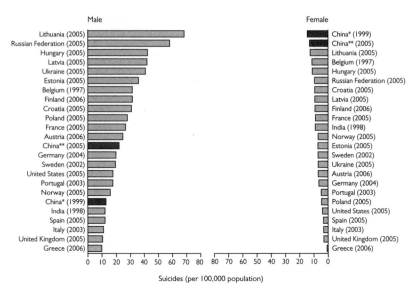

FIGURE 8.1. Suicide rates in selected countries, by gender. The dates in parentheses indicate the year of the most recent statistics available as of 2008. Source: China-Profile, "Suicide Rates in China, Selected European Countries, and the USA, 2008," www.china-profile.com/data/fig_suicide-rates_1.htm; data courtesy World Health Organization.

Alcoholism, other forms of drug abuse, obesity, aging, child abuse, violence—all are presently articulated as health (or mental health) conditions. Medicalization leads us to search for their genetic roots, to assess other individual risk factors, and of course to quest for treatments; yet, while giving the sufferer the sick role, medicalization can stigmatize as well as protect; it can institute a misguided search for magic bullets for complex social problems; and it can obfuscate the political and economic problems that influence these behaviors.[44]

Kleinman, a psychiatrist, examines post-traumatic stress disorder (PTSD) as an example of the medicalization of suffering. Without doubting the importance of the services provided to people who have endured political or wartime trauma, Kleinman notes how such trauma is neatly packaged (and commodified) as a disease—as PTSD—within the *DSM*. "You cannot bill third-party payers for coming to the aid of those who have experienced political trauma," he writes. "You can bill them for a major depressive disorder, any one of the anxiety disorders, or PTSD. Every conceivable psychological problem is listed in the *DSM* as a disease, precisely because treating disease is authorized for remuneration, whereas responding to distress is not. Thus, there is a political economy to the use of the disease concept."[45]

It is essential to consider such critiques in efforts to improve the quality of psychiatric diagnosis and care. They are not intended to discourage the use of psychiatric services or modern medicine as a whole; these concerns are often coupled with advocacy of global health equity and expanding access to mental health services around the world.[46] Kleinman's point, echoed in chapter 2 and throughout this volume, is that global health practitioners and scholars must cultivate habits of critical self-reflection to best prepare themselves for the biosocial complexities endemic to this line of work.

Another challenge in global mental health is that research on mental illness in non-Western countries is seriously under-represented in high-impact psychiatry journals. A 2001 survey found that more than 90 percent of all literature published in the six leading international psychiatric journals derived from Euro-American societies.[47] In his 2010 book *Crazy Like Us: The Globalization of the American Psyche,* Ethan Watters elaborates on Kleinman's critiques to examine the ways Western mental health practices can complicate the recognition of culture-specific expressions of mental distress and disability. Watters artfully brings to the mainstream a body of literature built by cultural psychiatrists and medical anthropologists.[48] Global dissemination of classification paradigms drawn from the *DSM* can have the unintended effect of restricting the forms of psychiatric distress clinicians diagnose around the world to illness presentations common among Euro-American populations. Watters explains this phenomenon, in part, as a product of globalization: anorexia nervosa patients with symptoms similar to those of patients in the United States appeared in Hong Kong in the mid-1990s, for example.[49] He joins others in suggesting that the reductive biologic view of mental illness embraced by Western medicine narrows the range of phenomenologic representations of neuropsychiatric distress diagnosed in the clinic. Even in Europe and the United States, phenomenologic outliers are often excluded from clinical trials, unrecognized in clinical settings, and not effectively treated with available therapeutic strategies.[50]

These examples draw attention to the challenges of classifying illness across borders, not to mention developing interventions with broad clinical utility across diverse contexts. To achieve effective and culturally appropriate therapeutic adaptation and innovation, Kleinman argues, clinical medicine must be integrated with local knowledge and practice concerning illness and health. Nonetheless, beneath the diverse manifestations of mental illness are certain biological processes that are mediated by context-specific social forces.[51] Serious psychiatric disorders such as depression and schizophrenia are recognizable (and sometimes treatable) around the world, even if they differ in their course and convey different meanings depending on the local context.[52]

From a sociology-of-knowledge perspective, the hegemony of Euro-American definitions of mental illness reveals how history and political economy pattern both institutionally authorized "objective" understandings of disease and the "subjective" illness experience of individuals.[53] The diffusion of medical knowledge validated by the WHO or the American Psychiatric Association into individual subjectivities spreads around the globe, illustrating Michel Foucault's concept of biopower (see chapter 2). These are *disciplining* processes, as Foucault notes: human bodies and subjectivities are defined, and redefined, in ways mediated by the flow of power and knowledge within and between societies.

The *DSM,* for example, has been revised multiple times since its initial publication in 1952; the fifth edition is due to be published in mid-2013. Each iteration rewrites, to a certain extent, our understanding of how certain signs, symptoms, and experiences of emotional distress fit within or track as disorders: some behavioral patterns are deemed newly pathological, others reclassified as normative. The first *DSM,* for example, included homosexuality as a category of mental disorder. Although it was removed in 1974, this notorious section demonstrates the extent to which "scientific" efforts to categorize mental illness are vulnerable to politics and prejudice. Such controversies over the *DSM*'s content continue to this day.

The collective authors of the *DSM* endeavor to ground their decisions in rigorous empirics. But the profound biosocial complexity of mental illness makes such a task—one that is undoubtedly necessary to increasing the effectiveness and equity of global mental health care—fraught with problems. Any effort to formulate distinct categories and types of mental illness at some point reduces and reifies the manifold subjective experiences of neuropsychiatric distress according to one set of norms. Nonetheless, tools to classify and measure psychiatric morbidity—even imperfect ones—are essential to understanding the burden of mental disorders and mobilizing the political will and resources to help reduce the attendant suffering.

THE DALY: STRENGTHS AND LIMITATIONS

Introducing the DALY

One such tool is the *disability-adjusted life year,* or DALY: a metric of disease burden that captures more nuance and complexity than extant summary measures such as mortality and morbidity statistics. The DALY quantifies an individual's loss of health resulting from a specific disease or injury: "the present value of the future years of disability-free life that are lost as the result of the premature deaths or cases of disability occurring in a particular year."[54] After designing this metric, health economist Christopher Murray and colleagues were themselves surprised to learn that using DALYs to analyze the global burden of disease revealed mental illness to be among the greatest causes of disability throughout the world.[55]

Murray's team developed the concept of disability-adjusted life years in the early 1990s. The DALY was designed as a composite indicator of disease burden resulting from disability (morbidity) and early death (mortality). This analytic tool enabled scholars and policymakers to identify the relative contributions of discrete diseases to the overall global disease burden, which helps guide prioritization and resource allocation in global health.[56] Designing this metric led Murray and his colleagues to complex ethical and practical questions. How does one quantify the amount of suffering from an illness for a year relative to not being alive for that year? How does one compare morbidity and mortality for a young boy in a rich country to that for an elderly woman in a poor country?

To enable comparisons among diverse illness experiences, the researchers asked an independent panel of experts to weight different classes of disability on a scale of 0 to 1, where 0 is equivalent to full health and 1 is equivalent to death.[57] Table 8.2 presents some of the conclusions drawn by this panel. These classifications are still used to compare years of life lost from injury to mortality.

Murray's team also developed an age-weighting mechanism, in which the relative value of healthy life increases from birth to age twenty-five

TABLE 8.2   DALY DISABILITY CLASSES AND SEVERITY WEIGHTING

Disability Class	Severity Weighting	Indicator Conditions
1	0.00–0.02	Vitiligo on face, weight-for-height <2 standard deviation
2	0.02–0.12	Watery diarrhea, severe sore throat, severe anemia
3	0.12–0.24	Radius fracture in stiff case, infertility, erectile dysfunction, rheumatoid arthritis, angina
4	0.24–0.36	Below-the-knee amputation, deafness
5	0.36–0.50	Rectovaginal fistula, mild mental retardation, Down syndrome
6	0.50–0.70	Unipolar major depression, blindness, paraplegia
7	0.70–1.00	Active psychosis, dementia, severe migraine, quadriplegia

SOURCE: Christopher J.L. Murray and Alan D. Lopez, eds., *The Global Burden of Disease: A Comprehensive Assessment of Mortality and Disability from Diseases, Injuries and Risk Factors in 1990 and Projected to 2020* (Cambridge, Mass.: Harvard University Press, 1996), 40.

and then declines slowly throughout old age (see figure 8.2).[58] When calculating the global burden of disease, this age-weighting system can be used; researchers cite a "broad social preference" to value the life of a young adult more than that of a child or an older adult.[59] Commentators point out that this algorithm closely follows the relationship between age and economic productivity: ages associated with greater potential for economic productivity are assigned a higher value than those associated with less potential.[60] Given evidence of different life expectancies for men and women, Murray and his colleagues chose to assume a life expectancy for women that is 2.5 years longer than that for men. They decided not to use measures of other relevant social dimensions beyond age and gender to determine the amount of life lost to disability or mortality.[61] Hence, for example, the impact of illness on families is not included in the metric, although it is a well-established social sequela of many diseases.

The intended uses of the DALY, Murray emphasizes, guided its design. He identifies four uses for the DALY: setting health care priorities, setting research priorities, identifying disadvantaged groups in need of targeted health interventions, and enabling better evaluation of interventions.[62] Indeed, two important applications of the DALY are analyzing the transnational burden of disease and allocating resources based on cost-effectiveness analysis. The Global Burden of Disease

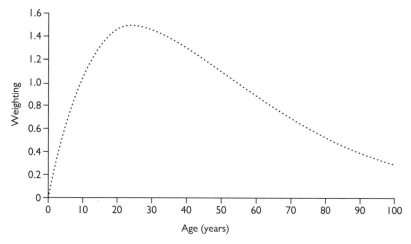

FIGURE 8.2. An age-weighting mechanism that can be used in calculating the global burden of disease. Source: Christopher J. L. Murray, "Quantifying the Burden of Disease: The Technical Basis for Disability-Adjusted Life Years," *Bulletin of the World Health Organization* 72, no. 3 (1994): 436.

Study, commissioned by the World Bank in 1992 and updated first in 1996 and again in 2000, was an impetus for the creation of the DALY and its first major use. A well-known report by Murray and Alan Lopez, *The Global Burden of Disease,* which assessed mortality and disability for the year 1990 using DALYs, has since become widely used by policymakers, practitioners, and researchers. In particular, the report drew attention to the fact that the vast majority of premature death and disability occurs in poor countries. Much to the surprise of its architects, it also revealed that tuberculosis, mental disorders, and road-traffic accidents were three of the leading causes of DALYs in 1990.

Perhaps the most significant use of the new data generated by Murray and his team describing the global burden of disease was the World Bank's 1993 *World Development Report,* for which Murray's work had been commissioned in the first place. Discussed at length in chapter 4, the report enshrined cost-effectiveness analysis as a principal tool for policymaking and determining the allocation of resources in global health. (Some of the implications of the use of cost-effectiveness analysis are considered later in this chapter.)

Given the multiple parameters informing the calculation of DALYs— including the prevalence of numerous diseases—researchers often lack adequate data, especially from rural, resource-poor settings; in these cases, DALYs are modeled using data from other places deemed comparable. Sometimes such extrapolation requires a leap of faith: DALY estimates for most of sub-Saharan Africa, for example, have been calculated using data from South Africa alone.[63] Those familiar with the diversity of disease patterns and illness experiences across the African continent regard such simplifications with ample suspicion. In addition, even when data are available, validity may be uncertain, as the reporting capacity in many resource-poor settings is extremely limited.

But simplification was inevitable in developing a universal metric like the DALY. Despite its shortcomings, the DALY has opened new and critical terrain in global health scholarship and practice, drawing attention to neglected diseases, including mental disorders, and rationalizing the allocation of health resources. Indeed, the DALY enhanced the accuracy of burden of disease estimates, which guide health policymakers and practitioners. In one case, health officials in Morogoro, Tanzania, used the DALY in conjunction with other instruments to improve the allocation of health resources in the country when additional funding became available. Figure 8.3 illustrates the result: expenditures were more closely matched with the principal sources of disease burden.

In 2000, Murray's team used the DALY to rank health systems around the world according to the cost-effectiveness of their health expenditures.[64] The rankings, which listed France first and the United States thirty-seventh, surprised many health experts and, in some cases, provided impetus for reform. Health ministries, for example, could use Murray's rankings to demand more resources.[65] Julio Frenk, then the minister of health of Mexico, invoked the rankings to build support for a universal health insurance program that would provide medical care for the poor.[66] Six years later, researchers found, again using Murray's metrics, that the new program had increased access to care among the poor and reduced expenditures for catastrophic conditions in the country's health system.[67] The DALY facilitated cost-effectiveness calculations that served as catalysts for, and indicators of, health care reform to benefit those in greatest need of services.

Unpacking the DALY

The contributions of the DALY to global health policy and practice are too numerous to count. Few would dispute that adopting the DALY

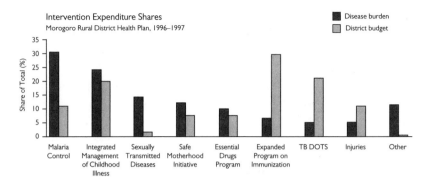

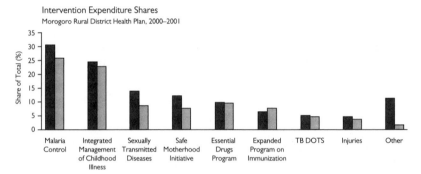

FIGURE 8.3. Estimated disease burden and corresponding health expenditures before and after analysis utilizing the DALY and other metrics, Morogoro, Tanzania. Adapted from Don de Savigny, Philip Setel, Harun Kasale, David Whiting, Graham Reid, Henry Kitange, Conrad Mbuya, Leslie Mgalula, Harun Machibya, and Peter Kilima, "Linking Demographic Surveillance and Health Service Needs—The AMMP/ TEHIP Experience in Tanzania," in *Proceedings of the MIM Africa Malaria Conference,* Durban, South Africa, March 1999.

has helped global health policy and practice become more evidence-based and more attentive to neglected diseases and populations. But it is important to be aware of the complexities associated with quantifying the burden of disease. Every context-independent disease metric is predicated on reducing the subjective and multifaceted experience of ill health into objective indicators. "When objective indexes are used," writes Arthur Kleinman, "they measure biological change as if it were fungible, separable from the experience of distress and the bearing of suffering."[68] Such separations can distort the lived experiences of patients. "In many contexts," Amartya Sen observes, "the perception itself is part of the ailment. Having a headache, or experiencing nausea or dizziness, can be seen as a disease in itself and not just a symptom of one."[69] The inherent subjectivity of the illness experience is, by definition, discounted by the DALY and other conventional metrics of disease burden.

Furthermore, in many cultures, suffering occurs interpersonally as much as, or perhaps more than, it is experienced by individuals—another register of the burden of disease to which the DALY is insensitive. Kleinman's concept of "social suffering" reflects the fact that the burden of disease—patterned by large-scale social forces—falls on families and communities just as it does on individuals:

> Social suffering results from what political, economic, and institutional power does to people and, reciprocally, from how these forms of power themselves influence response to social problems. . . . The trauma, pain, and disorders to which atrocity gives rise are health conditions; yet they are also political and cultural matters. Similarly, poverty is the major risk factor for ill health and death; yet this is only another way of saying that health is a social indicator and indeed a social process.[70]

The DALY considers only the years of disability-free life lost to individuals, thereby neglecting the impacts of disease encompassed by the concept of social suffering.

The specific mechanisms and assumptions of the DALY are worth examining in more detail. For example, what demographic characteristics should a metric of disease burden take into account when evaluating the benefits of a health intervention for a particular individual? Murray advocates restricting such calculations to age and gender. Indeed, his ability to gain acceptance for a metric that uses equal weighting—as opposed to the "willingness to pay" measure that favors the wealthy and is often used in welfare analysis by economists—is a laudable feat.[71] "Nearly everyone would agree," Murray asserts, "that attributes such as race, religion or political beliefs have no place in the construction of a health indicator." He offers this example: "the premature death of a forty-year-old woman should contribute equally to estimates of the global burden of disease irrespective of whether she lives in the slums of Bogotá or a wealthy suburb of Boston."[72] Certainly all individuals should be treated fairly by such a metric. But even if we agree that these individuals should not be compared on the basis of their productivity measured in dollars, we can still ask whether these two deaths are really alike. What if the forty-year-old woman served as the sole provider for her children and elderly parents (a not uncommon situation in parts of Colombia)? If suffering is understood as both an individual *and* a social phenomenon, as Kleinman suggests, the burden of this death on the community might be greater in certain ways than that of a suburban Bostonian woman who has a different set of responsibilities. The point is not that deaths in poor communities are more devastating than those in wealthy communities, but that the impact of ill health—such as the premature death of a forty-year-old woman— may vary substantially across time and place.

Perhaps as important as how the DALY treats diverse individuals as alike is how it treats them as unalike. Women and men, for instance, are assigned different survival potentials. "There appears to be a biological difference in survival potential between males and females," Murray writes. "Not all this difference is biological; a large share is due to injury deaths among young males and higher levels of risk factors such as smoking. If we examine high-income groups in low mortality populations, the gap in life expectancy between males and females narrows considerably."[73] Life choices related to income levels are certainly in part responsible for the different life expectancies. But the DALY's age-weighting scheme reifies the survival potential of men as lower than that of women, which could have a wide range of unintended consequences. If women have higher life expectancies, for example, their premature deaths are calculated as greater losses than the premature deaths of men; disease burden is thus found to be greater among female cohorts. Given this finding, policymakers might be inclined to direct more resources toward women's health issues, which could, in turn, further increase their survival potential. This mutually reinforcing cycle could hypothetically increase existing health disparities between men and women.

One of the most controversial elements of the DALY is its weighting of time lost due to premature death, especially when its authors calculate with reference to measures such as the cohort expected years of life lost (CEYLL).[74] Because CEYLL is determined by the projected life expectancy of an individual's presumed peers, or cohort—that is, persons living in the same country during the same era as the individual under consideration ("1900s–1950s USA females," for instance)—the time lost to a premature death in sub-Saharan Africa is measured as less than that lost to a premature death in the United States, where life expectancy is significantly higher than in much of Africa. Put another way, this application of the DALY weights the death of a thirty-year-old male in the United States as a greater loss in numerical terms—

and, implicitly, in normative terms—than the death of a thirty-year-old male in Africa. Though surely not the intention of the architects of these metrics, one potential implication of using geographically variable life expectancies is the allocation of resources to combat diseases that prematurely take the lives of those with the longest survival potential—such as the wealthy.

The algorithm of the DALY is thus freighted with complexity. Differential weighting by geography often distorts the nature of the disease burden in poor areas. In fact, as Sudhir Anand and Kara Hanson argue, choosing to exclude one's ability to cope with disease from the measurement of the DALY alters the very concept of disease burden: "The 'burden' of disease as defined by Murray . . . would seem to be closer to the aggregate quantity of ill-health than to the 'burden' as commonly understood. . . . If the goal were measurement of the actual 'burden' of illness, more information would be needed about the circumstances of individuals who experience ill-health (e.g., the support provided through public services, private incomes, family and friends) and not just their age and sex."[75] This "semantic quibble," they insist, actually has substantive moral implications: the DALY might disadvantage those least able to cope with disease, for example.

In order to avoid valuing a Nigerian life less than a Japanese life, policymakers use standardized maximum life expectancies when calculating DALYs, instead of cohort averages. These life expectancies are usually around eighty years (or more for women), much higher than the average life expectancy in many developing countries. Using these figures when calculating disease burden or the cost-effectiveness of an intervention, Anand and Hanson observe, "implicitly assumes that health interventions alone are capable of achieving an increase in life expectancy to these higher levels. It is clear that many non-health circumstances will also need to change for life expectancy to rise to the level used in the DALY calculations."[76] Here, again, metrics that measure only health-related variables can obscure the broader social determinants of health, not to mention the effects of large-scale social change on health outcomes.

The DALY does consider some social determinants of health, most notably by differential age weighting. "In all societies social roles vary with age," Murray writes. "The young, and often the elderly, depend on the rest of society for physical, emotional and financial support. Given different roles and changing levels of dependency with age, it may be appropriate to consider valuing the time lived at a particular age unequally."[77] In the DALY's formulation, a year of life at age two is worth only 20 percent of a year of life at age twenty-five (the age at which years are deemed most valuable); a year of life at age seventy is worth only 46 percent of this maximum value.[78] What Murray—and the DALY—neglects is the profound variation in the relation of age to social roles across diverse societies and populations. Among communities with many low-income families, young people often assume important work responsibilities from a very early age: without their labor, many family-owned farms, for instance, would be hard pressed to stay solvent. Moreover, in many communities, including high-income ones, the elderly often end up taking care of themselves, as opposed to being cared for by middle-aged people or government programs.

These examples beg the question: should a burden of disease metric weight individuals' lives in terms of their productivity? "The theory of human capital views individuals as a type of machine with costs of maintenance and expected output," Murray states. "The value of time at each age for this human production machine should be proportionate to productivity."[79] But should disability be measured as mainly a function of productivity or "limited human functionality"? Or should it also factor in pain and suffering and stigma and other consequences of disability and illness among individuals and communities? Why are certain characteristics with differential impact on health outcomes, such as age and gender, deemed relevant for inclusion in the DALY algorithm while others, such as individuals' community responsibilities, are excluded? Part of the answer concerns the values embedded in the DALY, such as maximizing productivity and thus economic development. Another question, then, is whether these are the right values with which to approach measuring the burden of disease. Any attempt to describe "health" or "disease burden" quantitatively by definition reduces the social complexity associated with such concepts. All we can do, Murray notes, is critically examine our metrics so that this reduction embeds the values deemed best for their intended use.

In light of these challenges, it is no surprise that the introduction and use of the DALY has had unforeseen consequences. One example concerns the global burden of mental illness: in the September 2007 issue of *The Lancet,* a number of scholars note that the estimates produced using the DALY "have drawn attention to the importance of mental disorders for public health." Indeed, mental disorders made up an estimated 14 percent of the global disease burden in 2007. In the same stroke, however, the authors critique the division of mental and physical illness: "because [Murray and colleagues] stress the separate contributions of mental and physical disorders to disability and mortality, they might have entrenched the alienation of mental health from mainstream efforts to improve health and reduce poverty. The burden of mental disorders is likely to have been underestimated because of inadequate appreciation of the connectedness between mental illness and other health conditions."[80] Surely the architects of the DALY did not intend to reify the distinction between mental and physical conditions. But such unintended consequences are inherent in global health and other complex social fields.

Because it can help researchers estimate the relative value of competing health interventions, the DALY has also, among other things, enabled the widespread use of cost-effectiveness as a basis for resource allocation. In the 1993 *World Development Report,* the World Bank endorsed cost-effectiveness as a key strategy to improve health in developing countries: "An important source of guidance for achieving value for money in health spending is a measure of the cost-effectiveness of different health interventions and medical procedures—that is, the ratio of costs to health benefits (DALYs gained)."[81] Because DALYs enabled a composite measure of the burden of disease, policymakers could compare the cost-effectiveness of different interventions with greater precision.

Despite its utility for understanding global disease burden and improving the allocation of resources in the health system, cost-effectiveness analysis can lead to unintended, and in some cases perverse, consequences. The next section considers one case in closer detail: the use (or misuse) of cost-effectiveness analysis to formulate policy for controlling multidrug-resistant tuberculosis in Peru.

MDRTB AND THE LIMITS OF COST-EFFECTIVENESS ANALYSIS

Tuberculosis is a treatable airborne infectious disease that claims more than 1.7 million lives each year. Multidrug-resistant tuberculosis (MDRTB)—caused by strains of *Mycobacterium tuberculosis* resistant to isoniazid and rifampin, two of the four first-line anti-tuberculosis drugs[82]—infects an estimated five hundred thousand people annually.[83] Although tuberculosis was virtually eliminated in Europe and the United States in the second half of the twentieth century, when short-course chemotherapy became available, epidemics in developing countries have continued largely unabated. Even today, during the golden age of global health, less than 1 percent of new MDRTB patients around the world receive treatment that would be considered standard-of-care in high-income countries.[84] The rest continue to spread drug-resistant disease until they die or, in rare cases, recover.

The causes and consequences of drug-resistant TB have been studied since the mid-twentieth century, and strategies for controlling MDRTB were introduced in the clinical literature in the early 1990s.[85] During a series of MDRTB outbreaks in the United States, a blueprint for its treatment was developed and rolled out: diagnosis with mycobacterial culture and drug-susceptibility testing, use of second-line anti-tuberculosis agents, infection control, and directly observed ingestion of medications. This strategy proved effective in controlling the outbreaks, and the Centers for Disease Control and Prevention (CDC) adopted this blueprint as the standard of care for MDRTB treatment in 1992.[86]

Meanwhile, the WHO had begun recommending DOTS (directly observed treatment, short-course) for tuberculosis treatment: patients were to be observed taking their medications—as recommended by the CDC guidelines, although in this case the medications were first-line drugs—to ensure adherence to the treatment regimen.[87] DOTS was deemed extremely cost-effective in the World Bank's 1993 *World Development Report,*[88] in accord with the emphasis on selective primary health care in international health circles during those years (discussed in chapter 4). However, for those who were not cured by their first course of medications, DOTS protocols called for retreatment with first-line therapy, even if the patients were found to have drug-resistant disease. This ran against the strategies that had been developed in the United States and elsewhere. To understand some of the effects of this policy in resource-poor settings, we can take a look at efforts to combat MDRTB in Peru.

In the late 1990s, global tuberculosis authorities praised the Peruvian National Tuberculosis Program—which was based on the DOTS approach—as a model for the region. WHO publications, such as the *TB Treatment Observer,* lauded the high cure rates achieved by the Peruvian program, while finding that pockets of drug-resistant disease were developing in other countries because of suboptimal implementation of the DOTS program.[89] At the time, drug-resistant disease was not held to be a ranking public health problem in Peru.

Staff at Socios En Salud, the Peruvian sister organization of Partners In Health, were therefore surprised to find patients presenting with MDRTB in the Carabayllo slum north of central Lima. An

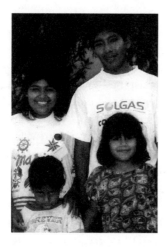

FIGURE 8.4. A "TB family" in Lima, Peru, whose plight starkly portrayed the limits of DOTS treatment. When this photograph was taken, the mother and father had active tuberculosis, and eight other family members either had TB or had died from it. When the standard DOTS regimen failed to improve the health of the father, who was infected with a multidrug-resistant strain of TB, he was labeled a defaulter and ordered to write an official note (shown here) stating that he had withdrawn himself from treatment. Photo courtesy of Partners In Health.

initial assessment of patients treated with DOTS who were still sick with active tuberculosis found that more than 90 percent tested positive for strains of MDRTB.[90] Some health authorities regarded these individuals as "problem patients" whose treatment had failed because they had not complied with the recommended DOTS treatment regimen. When one man named Chalo (pictured with his family in figure 8.4), who had likely acquired drug-resistant TB from a family member, failed to show signs of improvement, he was ordered to sign a document stating: "I am not going to take my therapy any more because it makes me feel sick, nauseated, and I am withdrawing from treatment."[91] (Chalo eventually received proper and curative treatment through Socios En Salud, though it is difficult to estimate how many thousands of others were not fortunate enough to receive the appropriate medical intervention.) Though such policies blamed patients for treatment failure, decades of clinical trials suggested that exclusive use of DOTS has little to no efficacy against drug-resistant strains.[92] This insight was reinforced by experience combating MDRTB outbreaks both in the United States and in countries of the former Soviet Union.

But instead of endorsing an MDRTB treatment strategy like the one the CDC developed in 1992, Peru's National Tuberculosis Program, at the recommendation of the WHO and the Pan American Health Organization, advised retreatment with DOTS for people who failed their first course.[93]

Why didn't global public health authorities recommend treating MDRTB with an effective regimen in resource-poor settings? Chapter 5 examined some of the immodest claims that in part prevented AIDS treatment from being scaled up in poor countries until the mid-2000s. In the 1990s, many public health experts made similar claims about multidrug-resistant tuberculosis, which requires expensive and complex therapeutic regimens that policymakers at the WHO and elsewhere judged unfit for resource-poor settings. In a 1996 report, the WHO concluded:

> *In developing countries, people with multidrug-resistant tuberculosis usually die because effective treatment is often impossible in poor countries.*[94]

The following year, the agency reiterated its conclusion, adding the cost of therapy to earlier concerns about weak health infrastructure:

> *MDRTB is too expensive to treat in poor countries; it detracts attention and resources from treating drug-susceptible disease.*[95]

These claims would be tested in the slums of Lima, Peru.

Using a model almost identical to that pioneered by Zanmi Lasante in Haiti (described in chapter 6), Socios En Salud built a "DOTS-Plus" treatment program, which added use of second-line medications, monitoring with sputum culture, drug-susceptibility testing, and directly observed individualized therapy to the existing DOTS regimen.[96] The initial cohort included seventy-five patients—many of whom had been recorded as DOTS defaulters or "problem patients"—with longstanding disease due to highly drug-resistant strains of tuberculosis.[97] (Infecting strains were resistant to a median of six drugs.) Patients initiated therapy between August 1996 and September 1999 and were treated for at least eighteen months with five or more drugs. The specific drug treatments were determined by the results of drug-susceptibility tests conducted at the Massachusetts State Laboratory Institute. Every patient was visited at least once per day by a community health worker, who observed the ingestion of medications, provided nutritional and financial support, and attended to other medical and psychosocial needs.[98]

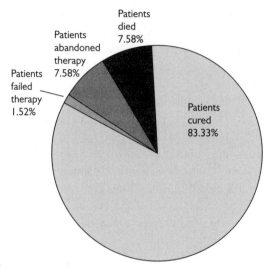

Total of seventy-five MDRTB patients

FIGURE 8.5. Outcomes for seventy-five "incurable" MDRTB patients in Peru, who were treated using the DOTS-Plus approach. Data from Carole Mitnick, Jaime Bayona, Eda Palacios, Sonya Shin, Jennifer Furin, Felix Alcántara, Epifanio Sánchez, Madeleny Sarria, Mercedes Becerra, Mary C. Smith Fawzi, Saidi Kapiga, Donna Neuberg, James H. Maguire, Jim Yong Kim, and Paul Farmer, "Community-Based Therapy for Multidrug-Resistant Tuberculosis in Lima, Peru," *New England Journal of Medicine* 348, no. 2 (2003): 119, 122.

As figure 8.5 dramatically illustrates, the program achieved a cure rate of 83 percent—as high as that reported in any hospital setting to date.[99] The seminal report on the U.S. MDRTB outbreaks in the late 1980s and early 1990s had documented favorable treatment outcomes in 65 percent of patients.[100] Furthermore, by moving treatment into the community, Socios En Salud was able to cut costs and reduce the risk of multidrug-resistant tuberculosis spreading nosocomially (in hospitals and clinics), without undermining the quality of therapy.[101] Although Socios En Salud encountered significant resistance at first, in subsequent years Peru's National Tuberculosis Program scaled up the DOTS-Plus model elsewhere in Lima and across Peru with favorable results.[102]

There was reluctance to heed the evidence of MDRTB outbreaks in

Peru not only among the staff of the National Tuberculosis Program but also—perhaps especially—among international public health authorities. Despite other examples of successful MDRTB treatment in Russia, Latvia, Estonia, and the Philippines, the WHO did not endorse the DOTS-Plus approach until the late 1990s—and only then after a substantial advocacy effort led by the CDC and Partners In Health, among others.[103] The Green Light Committee (GLC), a multi-institutional partnership launched as a working group in the WHO (and later supported by the WHO and the Stop TB Partnership), used a strategy of coordinated procurement and financing to achieve reductions in the cost of second-line tuberculosis drugs of up to 98 percent in the years 1997–1999.[104] The GLC reviews proposed MDRTB treatment projects and dispenses quality-assured medications and technical assistance to those it approves. By 2004, a total of 16,300 patients worldwide had been approved for full-course second-line therapy; by 2008, this figure had increased to 46,300.[105]

But approval isn't the same as implementation. In fact, between 2000 and 2009, only about 20,000 patients—of the more than 60,000 approved—were treated with quality-assured medicines through the GLC mechanism. In that same period, an estimated 5 million new MDRTB cases occurred worldwide; some 1.5 million people died.[106] Figure 8.6 illustrates the stark differential between those receiving treatment for MDRTB and those in need.

Progress has been slowed because of problems on several fronts. Although the GLC and others helped negotiate significant price reductions for certain second-line drugs, others remain expensive. Even for those drugs first on the negotiating table, costs have increased over the past decade—a typical five-drug MDRTB treatment regimen costs about $3,000 per patient per year—and their availability can be sporadic.[107] Moreover, too often technical assistance, such as advice about how to improve laboratory capacity, goes unmatched with resources and in-kind support. *Technical accompaniment* is needed in most of the places burdened with drug-resistant tuberculosis epidemics, which are, almost without fail, among the poorest countries in the world.[108] Diagnostics and therapeutics to control drug-resistant disease exist, as do health care models capable of delivering them in resource-poor settings. What's missing is delivery—and on a scale large enough to catch up with resurging epidemics of MDRTB around the world.

What does this example reveal about the use of metrics like the

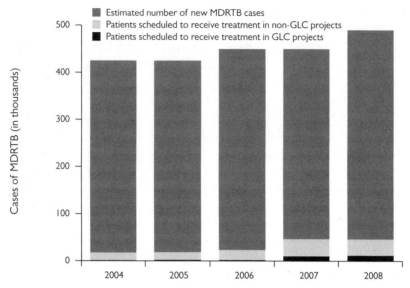

FIGURE 8.6. MDRTB patients receiving treatment versus those in need, 2004–2008. The number of MDRTB patients scheduled to be treated in projects approved by the Green Light Committee (GLC) and others (non-GLC projects) represents only a small portion of the estimated number of patients who require treatment. Source: Salmaan Keshavjee, Kwonjune Seung, et al., "Stemming the Tide of Multidrug-Resistant Tuberculosis: Major Barriers to Addressing the Growing Epidemic," in Institute of Medicine, *Addressing the Threat of Drug-Resistant Tuberculosis: A Realistic Assessment of the Challenge. Workshop Summary* (Washington, D.C.: National Academies Press, 2009), www.iom.edu/~/media/Files/Activity%20Files/Research/DrugForum/IOM_MDRTB_whitepaper_2009_01_14_FINAL_Edited.pdf.

DALY in global health? One lesson is that widespread use of any intervention—even one deemed highly cost-effective and endorsed by global public health authorities—can have unintended, and sometimes harmful, consequences, especially if implementation strategies lack critical feedback loops, such as rigorous monitoring and evaluation. A careful look at the clinical literature on antituberculous drug resistance and at prior experiences combating MDRTB in various countries led some to predict that blanket use of DOTS would trigger drug resistance as occurs with most microbial pathogens. More ongoing monitoring and evaluation might have been able to detect the development of drug resistance earlier and help practitioners contain MDRTB before it spread so widely.

This example also reveals the challenge inherent in attempts to reduce the biosocial complexity associated with a disease like MDRTB into quantifiable attributes (DALYs, cost of intervention, and so on) that fit into a chosen decision-making framework—in this case, cost-effectiveness analysis. As noted, DOTS was advocated by global public health authorities in large part because it was considered highly cost-effective. The 1993 *World Development Report* argued that short-course chemotherapy was characterized by "extremely favorable cost-effectiveness," which warranted government intervention, including subsidies.[109] The WHO also highlighted the cost-effectiveness of DOTS, which it strongly supported across the developing world.[110] But by scrupulously following DOTS protocols, which used first-line drugs as empiric retreatment regimens for patients not cured with the first regime, Peru's National Tuberculosis Program—regarded by the WHO as a paragon of TB control[111]—unwittingly fueled epidemics of drug-resistant disease.

How did a model national program fail to recognize and respond to epidemics of MDRTB within its borders? Max Weber's insights about bureaucracy, which we considered in chapter 2, suggest one answer. This case exemplifies the double-edged sword of bureaucratic rationality. The targeted, algorithmic nature of DOTS was key to its cost-effectiveness and rapid implementation; it helped transform Peru's national program into one of the best tuberculosis-control programs in the world. By providing clear guidelines and benchmarks, the protocol improved the quality and efficiency of TB treatment, and in doing so boosted clinical reach and staff morale. But it also hamstrung practitioners, keeping them from responding nimbly when drug-resistant disease ensued. The rationalization of the clinical encounter into a set of procedures restricted the agency of health workers to address cases that diverged from the norm. Individuals who acquired MDRTB were blamed as problem patients. True to Weber's insights, bureaucratic rationality improved efficiency but also created rigidity—an "iron cage" of rationality—that blinded practitioners to the emergence of drug-resistant tuberculosis.

It also blinded international public health policymakers to the risk of drug resistance. MDRTB treatment appeared in the WHO's Stop TB strategy for the first time in 2006.[112] Perhaps the reported cost-effectiveness of DOTS played a part in leading public health authorities to underestimate the growing threat of drug-resistant tuberculosis. As chapter 4 described, cutting costs was often deemed paramount during the age of structural adjustment programs. The slow reaction to MDRTB epidemics also reflects the difficulty of enacting policy change in a large, bureaucratic organization. The "iron cage" arguably becomes more constraining the larger and more bureaucratic the organization is; and the WHO and other international health bodies are, by necessity, large and bureaucratic.

CONCLUSION

Quantitative instruments like the DALY and cost-effectiveness analysis are essential tools for global health policymakers, practitioners, and researchers. Accurately measuring disease burden can reveal neglected health issues, such as global mental health and tuberculosis control, and help rationalize resource allocation by targeting areas of greatest need. But there are also tensions and trade-offs inherent in developing such instruments.

Despite its algorithm's clear rationale, the DALY necessarily embeds certain values, such as productivity maximization, that must be taken into consideration if it is to be deployed effectively and equitably as a tool for setting health priorities. Many important dimensions of the illness experience—distress, demoralization, stigma, collateral suffering, to name just a few—remain unmeasured by the DALY. Even calculating an accurate DALY-defined burden of disease is problematic, given the many social barriers to care-seeking and adequate case ascertainment in resource-poor regions of the world. Because the validity of tools like the DALY is premised on an accurate case count, imputed data must be considered with some skepticism. The DALY is a welcome addition to the global health practitioner's toolbox, but it cannot be the only tool used. The limitations and embedded assumptions of the DALY and other quantitative instruments should, when possible, inform the interpretation of the data they generate, which should be used alongside other types of data, especially that drawn from the resocializing disciplines, to paint a more comprehensive—and accurate—portrait of the global burden of disease.

Furthermore, by simplifying the profound biosocial complexity associated with global health, such instruments—if used uncritically—can lead to unintended, and sometimes harmful, consequences. The regnant paradigm of cost-effectiveness analysis among policymakers has, among other things, undergirded the anemic response to multidrug-resistant tuberculosis epidemics around the globe. Critical feedback loops linking policymaking and service delivery to rigorous monitoring and evaluation, biosocial research, advocacy, and training can help enhance and leverage quantitative instruments to advance global health equity.

SUGGESTED READINGS

Acland, Sarah. "Mental Health Services in Primary Care: The Case of Nepal." In *World Mental Health Casebook: Social and Mental Health Programs in Low-Income Countries,* edited by Alex Cohen, Arthur Kleinman, and Benedetto Saraceno, 121–153. New York: Kluwer Academic/Plenum, 2002.

Anand, Sudhir, and Kara Hanson. "Disability-Adjusted Life Years: A Critical Review." *Journal of Health Economics* 16, no. 6 (1997): 685–702.

Desjarlais, Robert, Leon Eisenberg, Byron Good, and Arthur Kleinman, eds. *World Mental Health: Problems and Priorities in Low-Income Countries.* New York: Oxford University Press, 1996.

Dye, Christopher, Brian G. Williams, Marcos A. Espinal, and Mario C. Raviglione. "Erasing the World's Slow Stain: Strategies to Beat Multidrug-Resistant Tuberculosis." *Science* 295, no. 5562 (March 15, 2002): 2042–2046.

Good, Byron J. *Medicine, Rationality, and Experience: An Anthropological Perspective.* New York: Cambridge University Press, 1994.

Horwitz, Allan V., and Jerome C. Wakefield. *The Loss of Sadness: How Psychiatry Transformed Normal Sorrow into Depressive Disorder.* New York: Oxford University Press, 2007.

Jamison, Dean T., Joel G. Breman, Anthony R. Measham, George Alleyne, Mariam Claeson, David B. Evans, Prabhat Jha, Anne Mills, and Philip Musgrove, eds. *Disease Control Priorities in Developing Countries.* 2nd ed. New York: World Bank and Oxford University Press, 2006.

Ji, Jianlin, Arthur Kleinman, and Anne Becker. "Suicide in Contemporary China: A Review of China's Distinctive Suicide Demographics in Their Sociocultural Context." *Harvard Review of Psychiatry* 9, no. 1 (2001): 1–12.

Keshavjee, Salmaan, Irina Y. Gelmanova, Alexander D. Pasechnikov, Sergey P. Mishustin, Yevgeny G. Andreev, Askar Yedilbayev, Jennifer J. Furin, Joia S. Mukherjee, Michael L. Rich, Edward A. Nardell, Paul E. Farmer, Jim Y. Kim, and Sonya S. Shin. "Treating Multidrug-Resistant Tuberculosis in Tomsk, Russia." *Annals of the New York Academy of Sciences* 1136 (2008): 1–11.

Keshavjee, Salmaan, and Paul Farmer. "Tuberculosis, Drug Resistance, and the History of Modern Medicine." *New England Journal of Medicine* 367 (2012): 931–936.

Kleinman, Arthur. "A Critique of Objectivity in International Health." In *Writing at the Margin: Discourse between Anthropology and Medicine,* by Arthur Kleinman, 68–92. Berkeley: University of California Press, 1995.

———. *Rethinking Psychiatry: From Cultural Category to Personal Experience.* New York: Free Press, 1988.

Murray, Christopher J.L. "Quantifying the Burden of Disease: The Technical Basis for Disability-Adjusted Life Years." *Bulletin of the World Health Organization* 72, no. 3 (1994): 429–445.

Murray, Christopher J.L., and Alan D. Lopez, eds. *The Global Burden of Disease: A Comprehensive Assessment of Mortality and Disability from Diseases, Injuries, and Risk Factors in 1990 and Projected to 2020.* Vol. 1, Global Burden of Disease and Injury Series. Cambridge, Mass.: Harvard University Press, 1996.

Pablos-Méndez, Ariel, Mario C. Raviglione, Adalbert Laszlo, Nancy Binkin, Hans L. Rieder, Flavia Bustreo, David L. Cohn, Catherina S.B. Lambregts-van Weezenbeek, Sang Jae Kim, Pierre Chaulet, and Paul Nunn (for the World Health Organization–International Union against Tuberculosis and Lung Disease Working Group on Anti-Tuberculosis Drug Resistance Surveillance). "Global Surveillance for Antituberculosis Drug Resistance, 1994–1997." *New England Journal of Medicine* 338, no. 23 (1998): 1641–1649.

Patel, Vikram, Ricardo Araya, Sudipto Chatterjee, Dan Chisholm, Alex Cohen, Mary De Silva, Clemens Hosman, Hugh McGuire, Graciela Rojas, and Mark van Ommeren. "Treatment and Prevention of Mental Disorders in Low-Income and Middle-Income Countries." *Lancet* 370, no. 9591 (2007): 991–1005.

Patel, Vikram, and Arthur Kleinman. "Poverty and Common Mental Disorders in Developing Countries." *Bulletin of the World Health Organization* 81, no. 8 (2003): 609–615.

Patel, Vikram, Benedetto Saraceno, and Arthur Kleinman. "Beyond Evidence: The Moral Case for International Mental Health." *American Journal of Psychiatry* 163, no. 8 (2006): 1312–1315.

Prince, Martin, Vikram Patel, Shekhar Saxena, Mario Maj, Joanna Maselko, Michael R. Phillips, and Atif Rahman. "No Health without Mental Health." *Lancet* 370, no. 9590 (2007): 859–877.

Sen, Amartya. "Missing Women: Social Inequality Outweighs Women's Survival Advantage in Asia and North Africa." *British Medical Journal* 304, no. 6827 (1992): 587–588.

9

Values and Global Health

ARJUN SURI, JONATHAN WEIGEL, LUKE MESSAC, MARGUERITE THORP
BASILICO, MATTHEW BASILICO, BRIDGET HANNA, SALMAAN KESHAVJEE,
ARTHUR KLEINMAN

Beyond great complexity, lies even greater simplicity.

—Father Gustavo Gutiérrez

Global health—the gloss used in this book to describe a complex series of problems, institutions, and aspirations of fairly recent provenance— has been described as "one of the great moral movements of our time."[1] This may make intuitive sense to some readers: there is almost always a moral dimension involved in the decision to do global health work. Great and growing global inequity, the burden of poverty both absolute and relative, millions of preventable deaths every year—these unsettling features of today's world lead many students toward global development and health work because it seems like the only decent thing to do. What are the roots of this moral feeling? By examining moral motivation, might we improve global health practice even as we learn about topics as diverse as modern social movements and pandemics of infectious disease?

This chapter tries to answer these questions by investigating several moral frameworks that are at times invoked in global health scholarship. One goal of the chapter is to trace the genealogy of moral thinking about global health issues. Does every human being deserve good health? Who is responsible for making sure that the ill and disabled receive the care they need within a given country and around the world? These are old questions without easy answers. The idea of human rights, including the right to health care, for example, has a freighted history that informs the nascent field of global health.

Another goal of the chapter is to identify and interrogate moral frameworks that have motivated practitioners, researchers, policymakers, and teachers to take up global health work. Each approach described here can lead toward considered engagement in the movement for global health equity. The framework of human rights occupies the most space because it is perhaps the most widely used approach in the field today. But it does not encompass all motivations, and we do not intend to place it above other approaches or to put forward a hierarchy of values in global health.

A great many individuals dedicated to social justice and global health equity are no doubt motivated by forceful and abiding moral commitments that do not fall into the categories we outline, commitments that cannot be intellectualized beyond a deep-rooted belief that the dignity of every human life demands consideration. Cuban family doctors who specialize in high-quality primary care and prevention services, American managers in emergency relief organizations providing logistical support to operations locally and globally, or BRAC's *shebikas* (described in chapter 7) who provide home-based tuberculosis care in rural Bangladesh might not stop to plumb the moral roots of their work on the front lines of global health efforts. Activists in countries rich and poor may not spend time contemplating the theoretical groundwork of the right to health care, even though they might deploy human rights language to advocate policy change. This chapter in no way seeks to discount the validity of intuitive moral motivation. We hope, rather, that by examining some of the moral frameworks that have led others to global health work, students and practitioners may come to better understand the wellsprings of their own interest.

Another reason to unpack motivation and morals, as Arthur Kleinman and Bridget Hanna argue, is that global health work is extremely difficult. It requires a hard look at preventable suffering and death, global inequalities of disturbing proportions, and many other failures of modernity; these problems lack simple solutions. "What gives strength and fortitude to those who do the difficult work of global health practice on the ground where they may deal with loneliness, privation, illness and other personal trials?" ask Kleinman and Hanna. They answer that "it is a moral practice that draws on deep wells within us."[2] Critical self-reflection—honestly examining one's values, motivations, accomplishments, failures—can help practitioners face the anguish and moral crisis that are often inherent in global health work without resorting to cynicism or despair. Kleinman elaborates:

Learning to picture the world, the patient, and his or her physician as divided and harbouring hidden values is the intellectual complement to the practical interpersonal skills of kindness, respect, compassion, and communicative competence that put together with technical competence contribute what it should mean to be a physician. Skills at critical self-reflection on the complexity and irony of what really matters in living can also enrich life, because this *paideia* and cultivation of sensibility alerts us to the rest of life beyond medicine, where uncertainty, danger, and balancing happiness and disappointment are just as thoroughly caught up with our divided selves and hidden values as they are in the clinic.[3]

Developing such sensibilities takes lifelong engagement that lies beyond the task of this book or any other. Nonetheless, we hope that the subsequent discussion may help students and practitioners of global health begin to develop habits of critical self-reflection in preparation for the challenges ahead.

MORAL FRAMEWORKS AND GLOBAL HEALTH

Utilitarianism

"The greatest good for the greatest number" is a maxim—sometimes called the "greatest happiness principle"—of utilitarianism. Nineteenth-century British utilitarian philosophers such as Jeremy Bentham and John Stuart Mill tried to recast moral philosophy in terms of human happiness: actions were deemed good if they maximized utility (defined as happiness, pleasure, or well-being) for as many people as possible.[4] When facing a moral decision, a utilitarian would tally up the hypothetical good and bad caused to others by different actions and decide the best course based on this calculus. This approach can inspire progressive reform: nineteenth-century British utilitarians included early defenders of women's rights, welfare, inclusive democracy, and penal reform.[5] "At its best," writes one political philosopher, "utilitarianism is a strong weapon against prejudice and superstition, providing a standard and a procedure that challenge those who claim authority over us in the name of morality."[6] But when the many are enfranchised, utilitarian policies risk stepping on the rights of minorities in favor of majority interests. At its worst, then, utilitarianism might lead to a tyranny of the majority. Another problem is how to measure utility: if pleasure were the highest good, why not simply hook people up to machines that pump opiates into their blood?[7]

Despite the pitfalls of utilitarian thinking in its extremes, there is an enduring logic to the goal of maximizing well-being that stimulates much of the global health discourse. It shines a light on the inequities in health outcomes and access to services around the world, for example. What do we make of the fact that an estimated 10 million people, almost all of them in poor countries, die each year from diseases for which treatments are readily available in rich countries?[8] Are we to accept reports of more than one thousand billionaires who can afford luxuries like private Boeing 787 Dreamliners that cost $200 million, when the same amount of money could buy a year of first-line treatment for 1.9 million AIDS patients?[9] Can we justify mundane amenities like a bottle of water that costs $1.50, when more than a billion people live on less than that per day?[10] A utilitarian would find these disparities repugnant: a more equitable distribution of medical care and spending would allow more people around the world to lead full lives in good health for the same cost. This sort of utilitarian calculus moves us toward equity.

One example of the uses of utilitarianism in the health and development discourse is the work of Peter Singer, a philosopher who makes a simple, forceful case for global redistribution and poverty reduction. His argument has four premises:

Suffering and death from lack of food, shelter, and medical care are bad.

If it is within our power to prevent something bad from happening, without sacrificing anything nearly as important, it is wrong not to do so.

By donating to aid agencies, you can prevent suffering and death from lack of food, shelter, and medical care, without sacrificing anything nearly as important.

Therefore, if you do not donate to aid agencies, you are doing something wrong.[11]

Singer makes this argument concrete with an example. He thinks most people would agree that individuals have a duty to save a child drowning in a knee-deep pond—an action that is possible "without sacrificing anything nearly as important" as the child's life. If we agree, then why not support aid agencies that seek to save the lives of children in resource-poor settings around the globe? A similar example pits owning valuable possessions against saving a life: imagine watching a runaway train speed toward a child playing on the tracks, when you have the ability to divert the train so that instead of hitting the child it would wreck your expensive Bugatti automobile. Would you do it? What if the car represents your retirement savings? Singer reports that almost all his students agree that they would divert the train.

He extends this duty to helping poor people who suffer from easily preventable diseases and malnutrition. This argument suggests that, in an age of instantaneous communication and global resource flows, distance is morally arbitrary: that is, not mailing a $5 check to save a starving child in Bengal is just as monstrous as walking by a drowning child.[12] After all, if you're willing to sacrifice the Bugatti and your retirement savings to save a child, why not send a $5 check? "When we spend our surplus on concerts or fashionable shoes, on fine dining and good wines, or on holidays in faraway lands," Singer argues, "we are doing something wrong."[13] Singer's examples are provocative—even Calvinistic—and many believe he goes too far.[14] Nonetheless, his utilitarian moral logic points the way to equity.

Singer's initial premises are not watertight. The third, the efficacy of foreign assistance, is a contentious topic that has spawned a growing literature on failed aid (explored in chapter 10).[15] But such critiques concern the nuts and bolts of aid delivery, not the moral force of the argument. If effective aid delivery models exist—and it is a thesis of this book that they do, at least in the health sector—then Singer's challenge remains intact. His argument also contains other tensions endemic to utilitarianism. For one, he emphasizes targeting "the poorest" and those "most in need," focusing on South Asia because it has "the largest number of people living in extreme poverty."[16] Although defensible, this approach can lead to a slippery slope of helping everyone live a slightly less miserable life, without letting anyone live well.[17] In other words, utilitarianism leads to the rationing of care—a freighted proposition politically (especially during the 2009–2010 U.S. debates on health care reform) and morally (what is the value of life?), but also, Singer argues, one that every American tolerates under the current health care system every day, whether or not they know it, as the U.S. system rations care according to ability to pay.[18]

Although a fair critique, this hypothetical model of extreme equality describes a radically different world than the one we live in. Global income inequality is greater today than it was during the entire twentieth century: the richest 1 percent control 43 percent of the world's wealth; the richest 10 percent own 83 percent; and the poorest 50 percent own 2 percent.[19] We have to look back to the Gilded Age to find

such staggering disparities. Instead of focusing on extreme hypotheti-
cals—of interest to philosophers, but perhaps less helpful in the context
of global health—a more honest and relevant interpretation of utilitarianism leads to moderate (though life-saving) redistribution. If the rich
sacrificed certain luxury items and instead contributed to medical care
for the poor, millions of lives could be spared. The income shortfall of
the 2.5 billion people living in severe poverty (less than $2 per day) is
less than 1 percent of the annual gross national product of countries
in the Organisation for Economic Co-operation and Development.[20] In
other words, for a 1 percent drop in the standard of living among the
rich, the world's poorest could live on at least $2 per day—a humble
goal, but not an unwelcome step toward equity.

Utilitarianism can take us in different directions, however. The concept of cost-effectiveness, like much economic theory and many of its
tools, is predicated on utilitarianism. Interventions are compared to
see which ones mitigate the most death and disability (measured in
disability-adjusted life years, or DALYs) per dollar spent. The goal of
cost-effectiveness analysis is maximizing the impact of global health
outlays, or, in other words, doing the greatest good for the greatest
number. But cost-effectiveness thinking can be a double-edged sword:
it maximizes utility *after assuming scarce resources*. This assumption—the often misleading first principle of cost-effectiveness—can
yield determinations that simply reflect and reproduce global inequalities rather than allocating resources based on the hierarchy of needs.
The poor get cheap care, if they are lucky enough to have access to care
at all. In other words, the logic of cost-effectiveness can also lead to the
pitfalls of "appropriate technology." While selecting and distributing
"appropriate" equipment based on local capacity and economic feasibility are important, some resources, such as diagnostics manufactured
in industrialized countries, are then deemed "inappropriate" for use in
the health programs of developing countries. Long-term, substantial
investments required to strengthen health systems might be written off
because they are too expensive.

But if a life is saved or an injury prevented, doesn't that in itself
mean the intervention was "effective"? How can we compare the effectiveness of targeted, short-term interventions to that of a strengthened
health system? After the past decade demonstrated that global health
funding is eminently variable (see chapters 5 and 11), how might we
reimagine the assumption of scarce resources? The problems of cost-
effectiveness mirror those of utilitarianism: both "cost" and "effective-

ness" are slippery to measure (just like utility), and there is a risk that initial assumptions and definitions are unwittingly predicated on the inequitable status quo.

Liberal Cosmopolitanism

Cosmopolitanism is a blanket term for theories based on "the idea that all human beings, regardless of their political affiliation, do (or at least can) belong to a single community, and that this community should be cultivated."[21] One liberal cosmopolitan philosopher who has developed a normative theory of global justice is Thomas Pogge.[22] A student of the philosopher John Rawls, Pogge extends the duties of Rawlsian political liberalism in the context of global poverty and ill health. In his 1971 work *A Theory of Justice,* Rawls formulates a famous thought experiment in which we are told to imagine an "original position" in which individuals are behind a "veil of ignorance" and don't yet know the circumstances of the life that awaits them. Will they be born into affluent families or impoverished ones? Will they be male or female? Healthy or disabled? Rawls thinks most would hedge their bets when designing the world on the other side of the veil, opting for an egalitarian society with less risk of being born into poverty or discrimination or uncompensated natural disadvantages.[23] In this society, inequalities would be tolerated only if they benefited the worst-off members of society (via nurturing talent in young people, for example)—a proposition known as the "difference principle," and one that led him to endorse massive redistribution from the rich to the poor. But Rawls restricts the implications of his argument to the nation-state, a decision several recent political philosophers, including Pogge, have questioned.[24] The interconnectedness of states through global trade, communication, and migration—not to mention disease vectors that disregard national boundaries—makes a global systems perspective apposite, in Pogge's view, rather than a state-based one.[25]

Pogge uses Rawls's conception of justice as fairness to critique the global institutional order. The reigning economic and political systems of the day, he asserts, exploit the poor to the advantage of the rich. "I deny that our imposition of the existing global order is not *actively causing poverty, not harming the poor,*" Pogge writes. "[The] existence of an adversarial system can justify prioritizing fellow-members and group interests only if the institutional framework structuring the competition is minimally fair. . . . The existing global institutional order falls short of meeting these conditions, on account of the excessive inequalities in bargaining power and the immense poverty and economic inequality that it avoidably reproduces."[26] A contest can be deemed fair only if the players start on an even playing field and compete by the same rules; but the global playing field is riven by inequities and double standards. Pogge is not cautious on this point, highlighting the "causal role of global institutions in the persistence of severe poverty."[27]

The main culprits, for Pogge, are the institutions of global political economy. While most would agree that it is patently unjust for a national economic elite to forcibly impose its will on the majority, few subject the global economic order to the same moral standard, even though the distribution of wealth and bargaining power is analogous. If the rich were to be confronted with the suggestion that current global economic arrangements are unjust, "most would dismiss it as ridiculous or absurd," Pogge writes.[28] He points to international trade agreements policed by the World Trade Organization: while wealthy countries pressure poor ones to open themselves to trade, the former have tariffs on average four times higher than those of the latter, according to *The Economist*, which estimates that poor countries could export an additional $700 billion of goods if rich countries removed their tariffs.[29] On top of this double standard, OECD countries spend an estimated $300 billion on agro-subsidies annually.[30] Imported Western goods thus have artificially low prices and often undersell those of local farmers in developing countries. One recent example is Haiti's failed rice crop. In March 2010, Bill Clinton issued a public *mea culpa* for exporting cheap rice to Haiti in the 1990s:

> Since 1981, the United States has followed a policy, until the last year or so when we started rethinking it, that we rich countries that produce a lot of food should sell it to poor countries and relieve them of the burden of producing their own food, so, thank goodness, they can leap directly into the industrial era. It has not worked. It may have been good for some of my farmers in Arkansas, but it has not worked. It was a mistake. . . . I have to live every day with the consequences of the lost capacity to produce a rice crop in Haiti to feed those people.[31]

Pogge also points to other forms of injustice embedded in international markets. The arms trade is notoriously blithe about furnishing militant groups of ill repute in countries rich and poor with weapons, munitions, and other military equipment.[32] Additionally, the Agreement on Trade Related Aspects of Intellectual Property Rights (TRIPS) restricts global access to the fruits of science and technology. A number of essential medicines, for instance, have been evaluated by clinical trials in developing countries but later denied to them as patented final products distributed through market mechanisms.[33] Pogge aggregates these examples to support his normative theory of global justice:

> The moral point is obvious in small-scale contexts: suppose you can do something that would gain you $10,000 while foreseeably saving three and killing two persons. It would be clearly impermissible to do this if instead you could do something else that would gain you $5,000 while saving three and killing no persons. The case of introducing *this* WTO agreement rather than a less burdensome alternative is analogous. That most of us do not even see how our governments' choice of the first option can be morally problematic shows that we implicitly think of the global poor as a pool, as one homogeneous mass like coffee cream in the fridge: one may take some out provided that, over time, one takes out no more than one puts in.[34]

Thus the global economic system, according to Pogge, actively perpetuates a fundamentally unjust status quo.

But Pogge's critique does not stop there. By underlining ways in which global institutions, norms, and business practices prop up regimes that rule against the interests of the people they claim to represent, he also finds the global political order rooted in injustice. The international system tends to recognize the rulers of resource-rich countries—no matter how they took power—as the legitimate owners of those resources, able to sell them on international markets and pocket the earnings. It is well known that this "international resource privilege," in Pogge's terminology, often ends up benefiting authoritarian governments.[35] The social contract, in which a government bargains with its citizens for income (via taxation) by ruling in their interests and providing certain services, falls apart when the leaders have self-sufficient means, such as natural resource wealth or foreign aid.[36] In fact, Pogge argues that the international resource privilege actually creates an incentive for civil wars and coups d'état because other contenders for power know that the prize is great and easily transferable. Moreover, the ease with which independent sources of income—oil fields or diamond mines, for example—can be taken over by rivals only increases the likelihood that ruling governments will use violence and repression to consolidate power. They can, after all, buy the "means of repression" on poorly regulated international arms markets.[37]

Ruling governments also benefit from what Pogge calls an "international borrowing privilege": the ability to take out loans from foreign creditors on the country's behalf. Not only does this lending system give regimes of dubious legitimacy easy access to resources with which to strengthen their rule, it holds entire nations (and future governments) accountable for money borrowed by a cadre of political elites. "Any successor government that refuses to honor debts incurred by an ever so corrupt, brutal, undemocratic, unconstitutional, repressive, unpopular predecessor will be severely punished by the banks and governments of other countries; at minimum it will lose its borrowing privilege by being excluded from the international financial markets."[38] Indeed, countries that incur a large national debt can lose access to future credit, aid, and trade partners, even if the money owed was spent by governments acting without or against the will of their people. And, because it is granted to most governments regardless of how they came to power, the borrowing privilege further strengthens incentives for rebel groups seeking to supplant existing regimes. Examples of such "odious debt" are easy to come by—from apartheid South Africa to the fledgling government of South Sudan—though some have suggested mechanisms to give legitimate successors to illegitimate debt creators a fair chance at balancing their budgets.[39]

Pogge mentions other ways in which the status quo perpetuates poverty and conflict in poor countries: global warming, caused principally by the developed West, can have especially deleterious effects on agriculture in poor countries;[40] the drug trade, fueled typically by rich-world demand, foments violence and instability across the developing world (especially in Latin America);[41] natural resources and common goods (like fish in the ocean) the world over are increasingly scarce; the list goes on.[42] Some of these sources of harm are difficult to mitigate or offset; others, like the international resource and borrowing privileges, could be addressed by policy change.

By arguing that the reigning economic and political systems actively harm the poor by perpetuating an unfair and exploitive status quo, Pogge's case for reform rests not on good will or charity but on justice. Few would deny the duty not to harm others—what political philosophers call a "negative duty." Even the most dedicated libertarians admit that active harm to others is a moral breach. Pogge's innovation comes with defining the current global institutional architecture as a cause of active harm to the poor. Poverty and the ill health of people in developing countries are usually interpreted as unfortunate circumstances, not the result of specific institutional arrangements created and sustained by political choice, as Pogge suggests. By highlighting the ways rich populations countenance and profit from institutions that actively harm poor populations, Pogge implicates everyone who benefits from the status quo. And, like Singer, Pogge extends his argument into the domain of individual responsibility. Anyone who participates in these same global systems—by buying bananas grown by monopolistic corporations in Central America or conflict diamonds that prop up murderous regimes in West Africa, or simply by enjoying the current international security guarantee—is also morally reprehensible.[43]

Pogge's approach is in many ways an alternate formulation of what we have termed structural violence. He shows the links between the rich and the poor and how such links can lead to poverty, violence, and ill health. This is, at root, an equity argument: when the injustice embedded in the current international system becomes evident, Pogge reasons, a flow of resources to the developing world no longer appears as charity but as the only decent thing to do. As wealthy individuals learn to perceive that the privileges they enjoy on a daily basis are mediated by the same structures that deny the poor a fair shake, many will be compelled to try to change the system. Solly Benatar, a South African physician-ethicist who has dedicated his career to global health inequities, develops a similar line of reasoning: "because wealthy nations, and by association their citizens, are deeply implicated in the generation and maintenance of forces that perpetuate social injustice and poverty, they need to face their responsibilities to alleviate the lives of those most adversely affected." The missing links, according to Benatar, result from "inadequate moral imagination."[44]

The Capabilities Approach

A third moral framework to be considered in the context of development and global health work is the so-called capabilities approach, developed chiefly by Amartya Sen and Martha Nussbaum (both pictured in figure 9.1). Capabilities are the components of flourishing, categories of human experience that enable well-being among individuals and justice among states and societies. Sen describes "elementary capabilities like being able to avoid such deprivations as starvation, undernourishment, escapable morbidity and premature mortality, as well as the freedoms that are associated with being literate and numerate, enjoying political participation and uncensored speech and so on."[45]

Nussbaum is willing to go further in proposing a list of fundamental human capabilities:

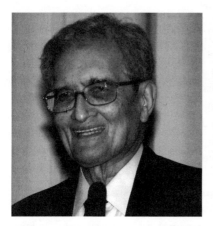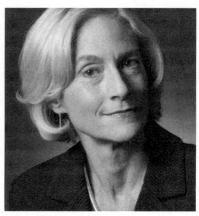

FIGURE 9.1. Economist Amartya Sen and philosopher Martha Nussbaum have helped to integrate a theory of human capabilities into scholarship on global health and development. Sen photograph by Elke Wetzig; Nussbaum photograph by Robin Holland.

1. *Life.* Being able to live to the end of a human life of normal length . . .

2. *Bodily Health.* Being able to have good health. . . . To be adequately nourished; to have adequate shelter . . .

3. *Bodily Integrity.* Being able to move freely from place to place; to be secure against violent assault. . . . Having opportunities for sexual satisfaction . . .

4. *Sense, Imagination, and Thought.* Being able to use the senses, to imagine, think, and reason . . . cultivated by an adequate education . . .

5. *Emotions.* Being able to have attachments to things and people outside ourselves; to love those who love and care for us . . .

6. *Practical Reason.* Being able to form a conception of the good and to engage in critical reflection about the planning of one's life.

7. *Affiliation.*
   a. Being able to live with and toward others, to recognize and show concern for other human beings . . .
   b. Having the social bases of self-respect and nonhumiliation . . .

8. *Other Species.* Being able to live with concern for and in relation to animals, plants, and the world of nature.

9. *Play.* Being able to laugh, to play, to enjoy recreational activities.

10. *Control Over One's Environment.*
    a. Political. Being able to participate effectively in political choices that govern one's life . . .

    b. Material. Being able to hold property . . . and having property on
      equal basis with others . . . [46]

Although Nussbaum considers this list "open-ended," she believes most
would agree that an individual lacking in any of these capabilities cannot be said to be living a good life. When capability deprivations occur,
social reform and policy change are needed.

    The capabilities approach guides us to the source of value in devel-
opment and global health. Sick people do not value medicines per se;
rather, medicines are valued because they remove the burden of illness
and enable the pursuit of other meaningful activities. Sen, therefore,
reimagines development "as a process of expanding the real freedoms
that people enjoy." Instead of measuring development by GNP growth
or rising incomes, which he indicates are useful *means* to expanding
freedom, Sen directs us "to the *ends*" of development, namely the "substantive freedoms—the capabilities—to choose a life one has reason to
value."[47] Framed in this light, development involves removing the barriers to substantive freedoms: barriers such as poverty, discrimination,
state-sponsored violence and repression, lack of access to health care
and education, to name just a few.

    This approach has moral and practical appeal. Nussbaum devel-
ops a normative framework for assessing global justice—an argument
for Aristotelian essentialism, in her terminology.[48] She argues that "a
determinate account of the human being, human functioning, and
human flourishing" can become "the basis for a global ethic and fully
international account of distributive justice."[49] In other words, no society can claim to be just if the components of human flourishing are not
safeguarded for every member.[50] The gap between the existing state of
human functioning and the full realization of human flourishing (exercise of the capabilities) exerts a moral imperative on governments and
societies:

> Human beings are creatures such that, provided with the right educational
> and material support, they can become capable of the major human func-
> tions. When their basic capabilities are deprived of the nourishment that
> would transform them into the higher-level capabilities that figure on my
> list, they are fruitless, cut off, in some way but a shadow of themselves.
> They are like actors who never get to go on the stage or a musical score
> that is never performed. . . . This basic intuition underlies the recommen-
> dation that the Aristotelian view will make for public action: certain basic
> and central human powers have a claim to be developed and will exert that
> claim on others—and especially, as Aristotle held, on government.[51]

What of the 2.5 billion people who live on less than $2 per day? Or disabled individuals who cannot fulfill some of the capabilities Nussbaum identifies? Are these groups not fully human?[52] If nothing is done to compensate such capability deprivations, then yes, Nussbaum would answer; they are like actors barred from the stage. This may seem callous, but Nussbaum intends to set the bar high, to hold everyone accountable when individuals are unable to enjoy what she identifies as basic components of a good human life. She highlights capability violations around the globe as a motivation for social and political change. She also admits that her list of capabilities is not meant to be exhaustive, but a "thick vague theory of the good."[53]

What does this perspective offer over its alternatives? For one, it picks up inequalities that other frameworks overlook. For example, liberal perspectives, including those of Rawls and Pogge, focus primarily on wealth disparities, which can occlude other important disparities. African Americans are richer in aggregate than most people in the developing world, but their life expectancies are substantially lower than those of other Americans.[54] Similarly, although Western European countries have some of the highest rates of income per capita in the world, unemployment rates tend to hang around 10 percent; joblessness, Sen argues, can cause "far-reaching debilitating effects on individual freedom, initiative, and skills."[55] By looking to the end (for instance, living a full life, having a meaningful vocation) instead of the means (for instance, making money), we come to a different and perhaps more complete picture of development. In the words of Aristotle (whom Sen quotes), "wealth is evidently not the good we are seeking; for it is merely useful and for the sake of something else."[56]

Furthermore, the capabilities approach limns structural barriers to freedom, health, fair employment, equality of opportunity. "Women in many nations have a nominal right of political participation without having this right in the sense of a capability," Nussbaum observes. "For example, they may be threatened with violence should they leave the home."[57] Poverty might keep individuals from accessing health services because they have no means of transport to a hospital or because the opportunity cost of leaving their family is too high.[58] The capabilities approach is designed to illuminate the forces that constrain agency in resource-poor settings—the forces that human rights approaches can miss by considering the processes of freedoms (such as the right to vote or the right to education) instead of the exercise of those freedoms (such as the social determinants of voting, the political economy of going to school). In Nussbaum's words, "choice is not mere spontaneity, flourishing independently of material and social conditions."[59]

Considering capabilities can also adjust for the diversity of human needs and preferences. Exclusive focus on equality of aggregate income fails to account for variable needs among individuals: the elderly, for example, need far fewer calories than the young but have greater need for sensory supports like eyeglasses and hearing aids; the chronically ill require more medical care than the healthy.[60] Although Rawls made efforts to tailor his proposals around need variability, at some level the liberal starting point of equality of opportunity struggles to keep pace with the multiplicity of needs fundamental to human agency. Some argue that Rawls's *Theory of Justice* excludes certain social wants that may be what are most at stake for the poor, the disabled, and otherwise vulnerable.[61] By looking to equalize the exercise of human freedoms, the capability approach controls for some of the heterogeneity of human experience.

In fact, it leaves room for individuals to define the good life in their own way so long as certain baseline conditions have been met. Utilitarianism encounters the problem that self-reported preferences, one indicator of happiness or utility, are flexible and changing. Sen notes one such paradox: as countries provide more medical care, self-reported morbidity often increases.[62] Objective health indicators, such as child mortality and maternal mortality, might signal improvements, while at the same time subjective reports signal less satisfaction with the health system paired with increasing demands for better care. This is a product of adaptive preferences: the poor get used to lousy medical care—they become socialized for scarcity—while the rich demand ever more. How might we square this puzzle? The capabilities approach would have us outline the lineaments of good health care and then require that every human receive those provisions. It would not rule out additional health care spending for the wealthy, but it would demand access to basic health services among the poor.

As the next section notes, considering health care as a human right also affords a critique of utilitarianism. The difference, again, is that the capabilities approach demands the fulfilled experience of good health, whereas the human rights framework demands the availability of care. The capabilities approach is therefore a more interventionist position, one that, its critics fear, may lead to standards cooked up in elite universities and think tanks being imposed upon deprived populations around the world.[63] It has also been called utopian in its aspirations.[64] But this may be said of all moral theories interrogating the status quo.

Sen and Nussbaum are not just interested in developing a more accurate metric to expand knowledge about development; they also want to enhance the strategies and tools used to promote development.[65] In Sen's words, the "expansion of freedom is viewed as both (1) the *primary end* and (2) the *principal means* of development."[66] One example of the policy implications of the capabilities approach flows from a striking observation about growth in life expectancy in Britain. During the two world wars, life expectancy increased at a faster rate than during the intervals before, between, or after the wars.[67] Sen uses this counterintuitive empirical finding to demonstrate the role of public service provision in decreasing preventable mortality. In particular, although total food supply dropped, food rationing became more equitable during the wars, which reduced the number of hunger-related deaths. Health care also became more widely available during the wars: the vulnerability of the population led the British government to provide more services for its citizens. Such efforts culminated in the founding of the National Health Service in 1948.

Empirical discoveries such as this, guided by a focus on capabilities (in this case, on the ability to live a full life), provide important data for policymakers. These examples, Sen argues, suggest boosting state-led food rationing and health care services for the poor and vulnerable. He finds similar results in certain developing countries: the Indian state of Kerala experienced a drastic reduction in premature mortality rates, which correlated closely with the expansion of public-sector health care services among poor populations.[68] Studies have attributed rising life expectancies in Costa Rica, Sri Lanka, and China (before economic reform) in part to public-sector health care initiatives directed to the poor.[69] But Sen does not stretch these conclusions. He differentiates between countries with "growth-mediated" and "support-led" paths toward increasing life expectancy. For a country to see significant health improvements based on economic growth alone, Sen suggests that "the growth process [must be] wide-based and economically broad" and be oriented toward increasing employment.[70] Brazil and South Africa, for example, saw their economies grow and premature mortality rates decline in the last few decades without significant expansions in public service provision. Life expectancy—a fundamentally *biosocial* phenomenon—is mediated by multiple biological and social factors that vary across space and time.[71]

Rather than championing one over the other, Sen underscores the links between the "growth-mediated" and "support-led" paths: "It so happens that the enhancement of human capabilities also tends to go with an expansion of productivities and earning power."[72] The argument that so-called human development enhances economic growth has a long and complicated history, but it has begun winning favor again in recent years.[73] Whether or not we accept a causal link between expanded capabilities and growth, few would deny that these goals are mutually reinforcing. Sudhir Anand and Martin Ravallion published a landmark paper in 1993, for example, which tries to parse the effects of GNP per capita on life expectancy.[74] They find a positive correlation that is explained in large part by two factors: income increases among the poor and government expenditures in the health sector. This study affirms a virtuous cycle between "support-led" and "growth-mediated" human development, so long as wealth trickles down to the poor.

Nussbaum introduces another example of how the capabilities approach might enhance the work of global health and development practitioners. Martha Chen's 1983 book *A Quiet Revolution* describes a female literacy project in rural Bangladesh at a time of rapid social change.[75] At first, the project followed recommendations from the United Nations Educational, Scientific, and Cultural Organization (UNESCO) and launched a campaign to distribute free reading aid materials among women. Nussbaum describes this first phase of the program as having a "liberal" approach: provided with the necessary inputs for an education, women could seize the opportunity to educate themselves and advance their social standing.[76] Its initial results, Chen reports, were mediocre: literacy rates did not increase substantially, and participation remained low.[77] The program later shifted toward discussion-based seminars that brought rural women together in common spaces. Chen notes that this approach was more successful in boosting female literacy, and it also seemed to help stimulate microenterprises run by women. Nussbaum uses this story to illustrate the capability approach in practice: the first phase stopped at literacy—a mere *means* to other social goods, in her language—whereas the second phase focused on the *end* of female literacy, namely education and empowerment.[78]

However far we are willing to take such examples, the capabilities approach brings with it a moral imperative to promote equity. No society can claim to be just, according to the capabilities framework, unless every individual in that society is able to exercise the components of a good human life. This claim anticipates the moral strength of human rights theories introduced in the next section.

But the scope of capabilities goes further than does that of human rights, and so too, perhaps, does the risk of unintended consequences when this perspective is adopted by global health and development practitioners. Indeed, Nussbaum's theories encounter some of the pitfalls of essentialism, including disregard for local knowledge and custom. She condemns female genital alteration without hesitation, for instance, because it risks the capability of bodily health (for example, the risk of hemorrhage), constrains female sexual freedom, and violates human dignity.[79] There is force to each of these arguments, but Nussbaum, in the view of some, gives short shrift to the historical and deeply politicized context in which genital alteration has been normalized in some settings. Perhaps because the practice has long been reviled by many—including European colonists—it has acquired a defensive local meaning in parts of Africa.[80] Some Kikuyu women in Kenya, for example, have defended genital alteration as having distinctive cultural value; it became enmeshed with postcolonial Kenyan nationalism. Although the practice is repugnant to outsiders, do they have the right to tell Kikuyu women what is best for them? Yet it is true that female genital cutting often leads to fistulas, painful scars that tear more readily in childbirth, and other serious health consequences.[81] Given the complex class and gender dynamics in Kenya and the politicized nature of this issue, to what extent can Kikuyu women who defend genital alteration be autonomous and free from coercion or pressure by local interests? How might considerations of the health sequelae of this practice figure in local and translocal discussions of it? How will such practices be viewed across time as well as in very different local moral worlds? These questions have no easy answers and exemplify the biosocially complex challenges encountered by global health and development practitioners.

How, one might ask, are capabilities different from human rights? One approach promotes the capability of bodily health, which *requires* medical care and shelter, while the other promotes a right to health care and shelter. How do these theories diverge, and what are the implications for global health and development practice? Both human rights and capabilities frameworks define a set of fundamental components of moral experience. The difference is that human rights theories demand that certain processes of freedom be safeguarded (that everyone has *access* to health care, that they have the *ability* to vote), whereas the capabilities approach looks to the fulfilled experiences that those rights defend (that everyone *enjoys* decent health, that they have *control* over the governance of their life). In other words, human rights concern the means of attaining human well-being; capabilities concern its ends. Both frameworks provide compelling reasons—instrumental and moral—to engage in global health and development work, though at times their prescriptions can lead in different directions.

HUMAN RIGHTS

The belief that health is a human right offers a powerful rationale for global health equity: everyone should have access to decent health services by virtue of being human. This section explores the theory, history, and practice of human rights and its link to global health. By exploring the interplay between theory and practice, we examine how human rights frameworks might serve as tools for understanding and advancing global health equity.

A Short History of Human Rights

In Western political philosophy, human rights theories typically describe a set of entitlements with which people have been naturally endowed. While similar notions exist in older and non-Western traditions, European philosophers of the seventeenth and eighteenth centuries, including John Locke, Jean-Jacques Rousseau, and Thomas Paine, developed the notion that autonomous, rational individuals (men, in most cases, and often only wealthy men) deserved certain freedoms and abilities.[82] These philosophers perceived the coercive power of the state as a grave threat to individual liberty and well-being. The concept of rights, therefore, was linked to the freedom of certain individuals from state control; rights represented boundaries around the individual that the state should not transgress.[83]

Related documents such as revolutionary France's Declaration of the Rights of Man and of the Citizen (1789) and the U.S. Bill of Rights (1791) enshrined these ideals in Western thought and practice. The effort to safeguard individual liberties from external coercion is the intellectual forebear of what are today termed "civil and political rights," which include the right to privacy, property, free speech, and assembly.[84] The idea of "social and economic rights," which include the right to food, water, health care, education, and employment, emerged

as a distinct, though related, concept—at least in the Western canon—
amid the wave of social reforms in Europe and the United States in
the nineteenth and early twentieth centuries.[85] These two categories of
rights roughly correspond to Isaiah Berlin's distinction between "negative liberties," such as freedom from coercion, and "positive liberties,"
the state's obligations to provide public services that are essential to
freedom and agency.[86]

The division between civil/political and social/economic rights is of
relatively recent provenance; eighteenth-century rights theorists often
considered them together. Many of the pioneers of the civil and political rights tradition, including Rousseau, Paine, Adam Smith, and John
Stuart Mill, also argued for significant social and economic protections.
Adam Smith's *Wealth of Nations* (1776) calls for publicly financed education;[87] the second part of Paine's *Rights of Man* (1791) espouses a
welfare state;[88] Mill's *Principles of Political Economy* (1848) suggests
state-provided education, health care, and a basic standard of living.[89]
One goal of this chapter is to illustrate the genealogy of this distinction
between civil and political rights on the one hand, and social and economic rights on the other.

In many ways, the Second World War ushered in another strain
of human rights discourse.[90] For example, political theorist Hannah
Arendt found conventional human rights theory anemic in the face
of the failures of the twentieth-century sovereign state system, just as
antislavery activists regarded theorizing as anemic in the face of the
"peculiar institution" and as women's suffrage leaders regarded such
frameworks as focusing on the rights of man but not all. Arendt argued
that rights exist independently and should not be dependent on governments' ability or willingness to uphold them, she argued, pointing to the rise of totalitarian states like Hitler's Germany and Stalin's
Russia, both of which persecuted and murdered millions of people living within their borders. Did stateless people not deserve rights? "The
conception of human rights," Arendt wrote, "based upon the assumed
existence of a human being as such, broke down at the very moment
when those who professed to believe in it were for the first time confronted with people who had indeed lost all other qualities and specific relationships—except that they were still human. The world found
nothing sacred in the abstract nakedness of being human."[91] To move
past this dependency on state citizenship, Arendt asserted that every
human has a "right to have rights," an essential right to the modes of
action that define the human condition.[92] The capacity for meaningful

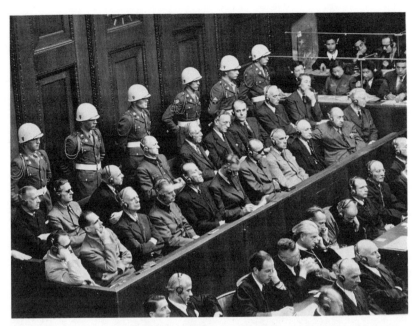

FIGURE 9.2. The 1945–1946 Nuremberg War Crimes Trials exposed to the world the atrocities of the Holocaust. These historic trials were an antecedent to the Universal Declaration of Human Rights. Courtesy United States Holocaust Memorial Museum. (The views or opinions expressed in this text, and the context in which the images are used, do not necessarily reflect the views or policy of, nor imply approval or endorsement by, the United States Holocaust Memorial Museum.)

action—exercised in a public sphere, expressed by language, and medi-ated by interacting with other free individuals[93]—that every human brings into the world at birth is the normative foundation for the right to have rights, according to Arendt.[94] In other words, we need a new conception of human rights to preserve space for agency and original action—a space that was denied to millions of people during the atroci-ties of the twentieth century.

The Holocaust sparked international efforts to prevent similar crimes in the future. Starting in 1945, the International Military Tribunal held the Nuremberg War Crime Trials (see figure 9.2), pros-ecuting most notably the prominent military and political leaders of Nazi Germany. In 1948, the United Nations General Assembly adopted the Universal Declaration of Human Rights, which outlines a broad set of basic entitlements as the birthright of every human being. These rights range from freedom from torture to the right of political assem-

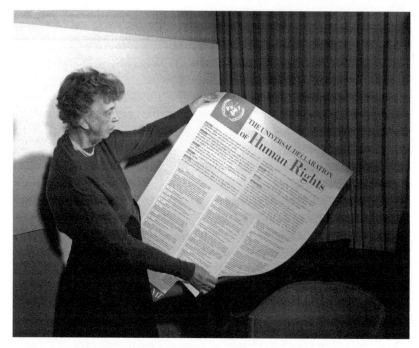

FIGURE 9.3. Former First Lady Eleanor Roosevelt was one of the greatest champions of the Universal Declaration of Human Rights, which was adopted by the UN General Assembly in 1948. Courtesy Franklin and Eleanor Roosevelt Institute.

bly and free primary education to "the right to a standard of living adequate for the health and well-being of himself and of his family including . . . medical care and necessary social services." In other words, the Universal Declaration makes little distinction between civil and political rights versus social and economic rights; it sought to transcend political legacies in order to "promote social progress and better standards of life in larger freedom." Rights were deemed universal in secular terms: we read of "the inherent dignity" of all persons and "the equal and inalienable rights of all members of the human family."[95] Former First Lady of the United States Eleanor Roosevelt (pictured in figure 9.3) chaired the committee that drafted the Universal Declaration of Human Rights. The document passed the UN General Assembly without a single dissenting vote.[96]

Such consensus, however, was short-lived. Cold War divisions found their way into the human rights discourse: the United States government and its allies promoted political and civil rights as inalienable freedoms, while the Soviet bloc polities promoted social and economic rights as a duty of the state.[97] Two separate human rights manifestos—the International Covenant on Economic, Social, and Cultural Rights and the International Covenant on Civil and Political Rights— were written to defend the competing ideologies.[98] The two covenants were initially conceived as a single Bill of Rights to accompany the Universal Declaration. In fact, some had hoped that the Universal Declaration itself would contain binding provisions. But largely as a result of Cold War tensions, it remained a statement of principles; the legal implications of the Universal Declaration were left to the dueling covenants.[99] And the schism ran deep: the United States still has neither signed the Covenant on Economic, Social, and Cultural Rights nor endorsed the right to health care for its own citizens, much less for the rest of the world.[100]

These divisions have stalled progress toward the realization of human rights around the globe. Many human rights organizations, for example, have been slow to embrace social and economic rights. In the 1980s, Amnesty International did not "ignore the importance of [social and economic] rights," but chose to "concentrate our resources on civil and political rights . . . because we recognize that we can only achieve concrete results within set limits."[101] When Amnesty International expanded its focus to include social and economic rights fifteen years later, it was widely rebuked. *The Economist,* for example, argued that "few rights are truly universal, and letting them multiply weakens them"; it warned against the "woollier cause of social reform."[102] In 2001, Michael Ignatieff made a similar argument about the "minimalism" mandated by any universal conception of human rights. If a human rights regime is to be acceptable everywhere, he argues, it must advocate only for "the minimum conditions [necessary] for any kind of life at all."[103]

Perhaps social and economic rights could be taken too far. But is it so difficult to imagine a set of basic entitlements common across different contexts, similar to the list of capabilities proposed by Nussbaum? It may be possible to avoid triviality and identify a minimum basket of entitlements that would be essential regardless of culture. Many would agree that basic primary health care services should be available to everyone in order to avoid easily preventable suffering and death.[104] Basic shelter, clothing, food, water, and health care are the components not of life in a particular culture or community but of life itself. Moreover, many social and economic rights initiatives are synergistic. "Education, health, nutrition, and water and sanitation complement each other," writes Navanethem Pillay, the U.N. High Commissioner for Human Rights, "with investment in any one contributing to better outcomes in the others."[105] In other words, comprehensive efforts to safeguard basic rights can launch virtuous cycles of human development.[106]

Other critics note the difficulty of enforcing social and economic rights as legal claims. Human Rights Watch, an NGO that operates internationally, tends to avoid tackling violations of social and economic rights because such cases lack a clear perpetrator and remedy.[107] This is another common critique of social and economic rights: violations are seldom discrete events with an easily identifiable perpetrator and remedy, making legal action difficult, costly, and perhaps infeasible.[108]

We do, however, have examples of violations of social and economic rights that have proven justiciable. The verdict in *The Government of the Republic of South Africa vs. Irene Grootboom* found the South African government guilty of not upholding the right to housing—enshrined in the country's constitution—after it evicted residents of a shantytown without constructing alternative housing for them.[109] Nonetheless, it has proven difficult to use legal activism to remedy abuses of social and economic rights, especially when they occur in settings of widespread privation and in a world, as Thomas Pogge notes, in which the fruits of development are spread so unevenly. Scholars continue to investigate how to make rights claims more substantial.[110] While some conceive of rights deriving from legislation, as "children of law,"[111] others consider them the moral grounding of legislation, as "parents of law."[112] In practice, they are both: the relationship between rights and laws is dynamic and reciprocal. Advocates fight for legislation that will give teeth to the moral claims of human rights, while citizens demand the fulfillment of their rights by referring to the authority of laws.

Realizing the moral claims embedded in human rights of course requires more than legislation. Rights abuses are embedded in history, political and economic arrangements, and local custom; they inhere in structures of violence that perpetuate poverty and inequalities of ownership and bargaining power, uneven access to education and health care and food, discrimination, stigma, corruption, and political instability. Rights abuses are local and translocal and, therefore,

TABLE 9.1   THE CLOSE RELATIONSHIP OF CIVIL AND POLITICAL RIGHTS TO
SOCIAL AND ECONOMIC RIGHTS: EXAMPLES FROM INTERNATIONAL COVENANTS

International Covenant on Civil and Political Rights (ICCPR)		International Covenant on Economic, Social, and Cultural Rights (ICESCR)
Self-determination (Article 1)	<— appears in both treaties —>	Self-determination (Article 1)
Freedom of religion (Article 18)	<— similar in both treaties —>	Right to take part in cultural life (Article 15)
Right to peaceful assembly (Article 21) Freedom of association (Article 22)	—> implies —>	Right to form unions (Article 15)
Right to life (Article 6)	—> implies —>	Right to health (Article 12)
Freedom of speech (Article 19) Right to political participation (Article 25)	<— enhances <—	Right to education (Article 13)

"symptoms of deeper pathologies of power."[113] All human rights initiatives—whether civil and political or social and economic—must begin by discerning how large-scale social forces become embodied as de facto constraints on personal agency among the destitute and disenfranchised.[114] Fulfilling human rights claims, at least in the context of global health and development, would in most cases require broad-based social change.

As we come to understand the power relations that mediate human rights abuses, divisions between civil and political rights and social and economic rights begin to fade, just as do some of the distinctions between a capabilities approach and rights frameworks. How can a woman fulfill her civic duties when she can barely put food on the table for her family? How can a man find outlets for self-realization and cultivation of individuality when he works two jobs and cares for many children? As importantly, how can a government hope to promote rights to housing or health care when its asset and budgets are minuscule? Safeguarding each class of rights—whose boundaries are often fluid (as table 9.1 illustrates)—is a necessary but insufficient minimum condition of a good human life. Efforts that approach human rights holistically are likely to be more ethical and humane and also more effective and efficient, owing to the many links and synergies among rights of different designation.

Health as a Human Right

The right to health further blurs the divisions in the human rights discourse. The Universal Declaration of Human Rights ushered in a bold, holistic definition of health: "everyone has the right to a standard of living adequate for the health and well-being of himself and his family, including food, clothing, housing, and medical care and necessary social services, and the right to security in the event of unemployment, sickness, disability, widowhood, old age or other lack of livelihood in circumstances beyond his control." The International Covenant on Economic, Social, and Cultural Rights provides more concrete objectives for achieving the right to health and well-being:

a. To ensure the right of access to health facilities, goods and services on a non-discriminatory basis, especially for vulnerable or marginalized groups;
b. To ensure access to the minimum essential food which is nutritionally adequate and safe, to ensure freedom from hunger to everyone;
c. To ensure access to basic shelter, housing and sanitation, and an adequate supply of safe and potable water;
d. To provide essential drugs, as from time to time defined under the WHO Action Programme on Essential Drugs;
e. To ensure equitable distribution of all health facilities, goods and services;
f. To adopt and implement a national public health strategy and plan of action, on the basis of epidemiological evidence, addressing the health concerns of the whole population; the strategy and plan of action shall be devised, and periodically reviewed, on the basis of a participatory and transparent process; they shall include methods, such as right to health indicators and benchmarks, by which progress can be closely monitored; the process by which the strategy and plan of action are devised, as well as their content, shall give particular attention to all vulnerable or marginalized groups.[115]

Like the Universal Declaration, the ICESCR embraces a broad conception of health that encompasses social determinants such as nutrition, access to care, and basic living conditions as well as political factors such as nondiscrimination and participatory processes. As Rachel Hammonds and Gorik Ooms argue, expanding health services is necessary but not sufficient for realizing the right to health.[116] Guaranteeing this far-reaching conception of health to all people would require political reform, economic redistribution, and massive social change in countries rich and poor alike. It would, in short, require the realization of other human rights—social, economic, civil, and political. In the words of the late Jonathan Mann, former director of the World Health Organization's Global Program on AIDS, "re-thinking of the taxonomy of health calls for re-consideration of the conceptual framework of human rights."[117] But should health or access to health care be considered a human right?

The alternative, which has long been the predominant paradigm in many parts of the world and in the global health and development discourse, is that health is a commodity that can be most efficiently allocated by the market according to consumers' willingness to pay. As chapter 4 details, the gradual unraveling of the 1978 Alma-Ata consensus supporting "health for all"—an affirmation of the right to health care—and the rise of selective primary health care and structural adjustment programs meant that market-based, not rights-based, approaches to health reform became the norm among international policymakers in the 1980s and 1990s. Health care, many then assumed, could be delivered more efficiently and even more equitably by private markets.[118] In fact, the World Bank and the International Monetary Fund, the architects of the structural adjustment era, have tended to eschew human rights language altogether. Of twenty-one World Bank Poverty Reduction Strategy Papers published in the past few decades, none mention health as a human right.[119] The World Bank's website couches the AIDS epidemic as a "development problem that threatens human welfare, socio-economic advances, productivity, social cohesion, and even national security," but does not describe it as a human rights issue.[120] Scholars have pointed to a similar avoidance of human rights frameworks among most international institutions established in the decade after World War II.[121]

Alfredo Sfeir-Younis, a senior advisor at the World Bank, defends a "gradualist" approach to human rights: growth and economic development will foster human rights gains over time. "Without wealth creation," he argues, "it would be impossible to see human rights being realized."[122] It is no doubt true that growth can in many cases enhance human rights efforts. As chapter 7 noted, there are many synergies between economic development and health system strengthening. But does a gradualist approach justify cutting back on health services in the short term in an effort to generate growth (as structural adjustment programs often recommended)? What if growth proves elusive? In reality, structural adjustment had mixed results both for growth and for the health sector. In some cases, structural adjustment programs likely undermined access to health services.[123] With these lessons in mind, is it prudent to wait for human rights to follow economic development?[124]

Despite the patchy record of market-based approaches in the history of international health, the commodity paradigm continues to animate much of the global health discourse. One example is cost-effectiveness analysis: interventions are deemed cost-effective based on estimated health impacts and the *willingness to pay* of patients, providers, insurance companies, or other public and private funders. Because it rations care according to whether health care consumers will pay for it, cost-effectiveness analysis is predicated on a conception of health as a commodity. Like other market-based health care models we have considered, cost-effectiveness analysis tends to work better in rich areas than it does in poor ones, where a lack of purchasing power breeds market failures. A rights-based approach rations care according to the hierarchy of needs. "An acceptable long-run goal," writes health economist Guy Carrin, "is the equal utilization of health care among those patients who have a similar need for treatment in the event of a given illness."[125]

The global response to the AIDS pandemic highlights the divergence between the commodity and rights paradigms in global health. If antiretroviral drugs were allocated by the market alone, they would remain expensive and available only to the wealthy. But, as chapter 5 describes, a coalition of practitioners, researchers, policymakers, activists, and public figures reimagined access to AIDS treatment as a human right and fought to realize this vision around the globe. Decades of dogged negotiations and advocacy helped to reduce the price of first-line therapy from more than $10,000 per person per year in the late 1990s to about $80 per person per year in 2007, but the cost of these medications remains an important barrier to access to second-line treatments, pediatric formulations, and other supportive technologies.[126] It is a thesis of this book that almost all global health problems demand reimagining: notions of equity and human rights serve to undermine socialization for scarcity and commodity-based health care as first principles of global health.

Reimagining health as a human right, and implementing an ambitious equity agenda capable of realizing that vision, could strengthen other development priorities, too. Some evidence supports the opposite of the gradualist approach outlined by Alfredo Sfeir-Younis: attending to human rights, especially the right to health, can in certain cases bolster economic development.[127] The World Bank in fact made this argument in its landmark 1993 *World Development Report*, subtitled *Investing in Health*. The argument is simple. Initial inequalities in the distribution of basic resources for human development, including physical and human capital, have been shown to have a negative effect on growth; these effects are almost twice as great for the poor.[128] On a micro level, "poverty traps," a concept we explore in chapter 10, prevent people from accumulating sufficient resources to invest—a foundation of economic growth—because they are stuck in a hand-to-mouth struggle for survival.[129] But a growing body of evidence suggests that such traps can be broken by strengthening health and education systems and by safeguarding other basic human rights.[130] Healthy, educated individuals are more likely to find reliable jobs with decent pay; they can then save, invest, and begin to lift their families out of poverty. Complementary investments in human rights work, when pursued together, can help break the cycle of poverty and disease and lay the groundwork for economic development.

Decent health is also, by most standards, a prerequisite to being an active citizen. Philosophers have long described social and economic preconditions of freedom and autonomy. John Rawls built on this tradition, arguing that adequate health care is necessary to safeguard both political and socioeconomic rights. "Primary goods" (including health care) are, Rawls writes, "[needed for] free and equal persons living a complete life: they are not things it is simply rational to want or desire or to prefer or even to crave."[131] Health care fulfills a "necessary condition of the decency of a society's political institutions and its legal order." Examples are not hard to come by: a man bedridden from late-stage AIDS will have a hard time exercising his political right to cast a ballot in an election; a woman given a sack of grain to vote for a particular political party is unlikely to practice democratic self-determination if her children are hungry.

In sum, human rights frameworks can help us reimagine global health. Rights language can expand and situate narrow conceptions of health and development within the large-scale social forces that so often dictate who is struck with disease and who is shielded from harm.[132] A broad human rights approach starts a conversation about the conditions required to live a full life in good health, rather than returning to tired and sometimes bitter debates over limited resources, cost-effectiveness, appropriate technology, and other expressions of socialization for scarcity. In the words of Wendell Berry, "Rats and roaches live by competition under the laws of supply and demand; it is the privilege of human beings to live under the laws of justice and mercy."[133]

Critique and Praxis

Implementing a bold, rights-based health agenda in a world riven by poverty and inequality encounters a great many challenges, and human rights frameworks are not without their critics. Some cite the "abstract universalism" of human rights and contend that it fails to consider local needs, interests, and political environments. Anthropologist Harri Englund, for example, documents how the human rights discourse has been applied as a one-size-fits-all solution to more complex problems in Malawi.[134] James Ferguson makes a similar argument about the development apparatus in Lesotho, describing how outsiders often cling to dated narratives about a generalized Africa instead of understanding local complexities.[135] The idea of "civil society," to which many human rights theorists look to hold states accountable, is undermined wherever the term comes to refer to local elites with little regard for the human rights claims of the poor majority.[136]

Other critics find human rights too narrow, or too individualistic, to promote genuine human flourishing. Most human rights theory, based on political liberalism, focuses on protecting *individuals,* separate from society.[137] But philosopher Michael Sandel, building on a long tradition in Western philosophy, believes that this mischaracterizes human nature: humans are social beings, he points out; many of our needs are contingent on and embedded in the communities to which we belong.[138] This critique reflects Karl Marx's conception of *species-being:* according to Marx, human flourishing is predicated on membership in communities, on work that benefits something larger than individual needs.[139] Marxists thereby fault human rights approaches for failing to serve as a platform for broad-based social change capable of enabling the realization of our species-being.[140]

Such critiques are echoed in mainstream debates about human rights. For example, Lee Kuan Yew, former prime minister of Singapore, rejected the Western premise that individuals have inalienable rights that trump the needs of society. "The expansion of the right of the individual to behave or misbehave as he pleases has come at the expense of orderly society," said Lee; the main objective in East Asia, he argued, is "a well-ordered society so that everybody can have maximum enjoyment of his freedoms."[141] "Asian values," Lee suggested, run counter to Western individualism. Others, before and since, and with very different political views, have made similar critiques of the individualistic nature of regnant human rights theory.[142]

Amartya Sen, among many others, has objected to Lee's claims. Populations in East Asia, Sen argues, deserve the same protections as those in Europe and around the world, especially in authoritarian states, such as the one Lee headed, in which the rights of individuals may be more easily trampled.[143] Moreover, seeking to define a homogeneous set of values for any society, not to mention categories as broad as "Western" and "Asian," obscures the diversity and richness of local moral experience. It should suffice to note that Marx's concept of the species-being, not to mention other longstanding traditions in Western political thought, also elevates society as a key locus of human flourishing.[144]

The tension between universal claims of human rights and local moral worlds runs throughout these critiques and must be taken seriously. One means of addressing this tension comes from the discipline of anthropology. (Indeed, many of the critics noted earlier are anthropologists.)[145] Anthropology unites ethnography—thick description of local moral worlds—with critical analysis of large-scale social forces and dominant discourses (including dominant frameworks such as human rights). As global health practitioners seek to discern the causes and consequences of poverty and ill health in a local context, these tools of anthropology can help harness the moral force of such frameworks while adapting programs and interventions to local diversity.

But translating human rights theory into practice brings its own set of challenges. For one, there is no coherent human rights movement; rather, there are many heterogeneous human rights movements, some of which do little for their intended beneficiaries.[146] In his essay "Why More Africans Don't Use Human Rights Language," lawyer and human rights advocate Chidi Odinkalu makes a striking observation: Africans rarely use human rights language, while Western charities, NGOs, and aid agencies use it ad nauseam.[147] To explain this phenomenon, Odinkalu writes that most of these human rights organizations have tended to restrict themselves to civil and political rights initiatives, failing to address (or even acknowledge) widespread violations of social and economic rights—illiteracy, poor health, homelessness, unemployment—in the settings where they work, thus alienating themselves from African movements for social justice and survival. Even those organizations that do pledge to address social and economic rights often fail to

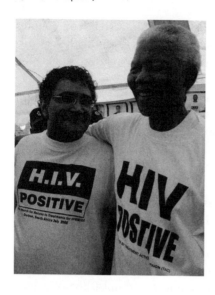

FIGURE 9.4. Zackie Achmat, a founder of the Treatment Action Campaign, and former South African president Nelson Mandela promote expanded access to AIDS treatment. Photograph Anna Zieminski/Agence France-Presse. Courtesy Getty Images.

deliver. Nelson Mandela noted this gap between human rights rhetoric and practice in his address to the UN General Assembly in 1998:

> The unavailability of food, jobs, water and shelter, education, health care and a healthy environment is not a preordained result of the forces of nature or the product of a curse of the deities. . . . [It is the] consequence of decisions which men and women take or refuse to take, all of whom will not hesitate to pledge their devoted support for the Universal Declaration of Human Rights.[148]

With these critiques in mind, how can organizations effectively implement rights-based agendas?[149]

As the case of *The Government of the Republic of South Africa vs. Irene Grootboom* demonstrated, laws provide one means of enforcing human rights claims. One organization that has used legal activism to promote a rights-based approach to health care reform is the Treatment Action Campaign, an AIDS activist group founded in South Africa in 1998 by Zackie Achmat (pictured in figure 9.4, with Mandela) and Mark Heywood. When the administration of South African president Thabo Mbeki suggested treating AIDS with plant-based remedies instead of antiretroviral therapy, TAC launched a grassroots campaign to insist on the right to effective treatment. In fact, the South African constitution guarantees every citizen the right to health care, including AIDS treatment. TAC first sued the government in 2001, winning treatment rights for pregnant women, including prenatal care and prevention of mother-to-child HIV transmission. After further legal battles led by TAC, which were bolstered by growing international consensus about the urgency of treating AIDS in poor countries, the South African government committed to providing universal access to antiretroviral therapy in August 2003. But with 5.2 million South Africans living with HIV (the largest such population in the world) and less than half of those needing treatment receiving it as of 2009, TAC has a long road ahead.[150] The June 2010 cover of the organization's magazine, *Equal Treatment*, says it all: "The struggle for treatment continues."

Legal activism is not the only way to make human rights efforts substantial. The work of Partners In Health and Zanmi Lasante in Haiti, described in chapter 6, is illustrative of a different type of rights-based approach in practice. The strategy of these organizations has, from the beginning, been rooted in the belief that the world's poorest communities deserve world-class standards of medical care. Their mission, in other words, was to realize the human right to health, and their model—to this day—embodies that mission. First, Partners In Health and Zanmi Lasante seek to avoid punitive user fees and other "cost-sharing" devices that shift the burden of payment to those least able to pay. Instead of delivering only cheap interventions approved by gurus of cost-effectiveness, the organizations offer a preferential option for the poor by providing the highest possible quality of care. Second, Partners In Health and its partner organizations seek to overcome the social barriers to accessing care, such as transportation costs and food insecurity. Their Program on Social and Economic Rights provides complementary services that range from education to safe housing to clean water (see, for example, figure 9.5). These wraparound services help address some of the social and economic determinants of ill health. Finally, Partners In Health is committed to working in public-sector health systems because only governments can enshrine health as a human right and then implement programs to safeguard this right for its citizens on a national scale.

In sum, a human rights approach identifies minimum standards of existence that should be available to all human beings. It can serve as a useful tool for holding state and nonstate providers accountable for safeguarding such rights and thus help mobilize social and political change in the direction of justice and equity.[151] The moral force of human rights logic derives from the conviction that global inequities in health care, education, employment, access to credit, freedom of

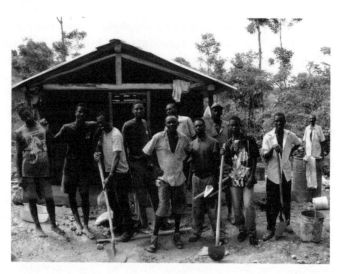

FIGURE 9.5. In Haiti, the Program on Social and Economic Rights established by Partners In Health and Zanmi Lasante improves homes like this one to help address some of the economic determinants of ill health among the population served.

speech, political self-determination, and many other components of human flourishing are not "woolly" problems; they are violations of basic human dignity. By providing a common vocabulary of basic needs that applies to the rich and the poor, the well and the unwell, human rights approaches can help translate unstable emotions like pity, compassion, and solidarity into meaningful action to help remediate global inequities.[152] It is the role of civil society—including the students and practitioners reading this book—to hold governments, near and far, and other institutions charged with protecting the vulnerable accountable when markets fail to do so.[153]

RELIGIOUS VALUES AND GLOBAL HEALTH

While dedication to human rights—social and economic rights in particular—impels some to devote their lives to the fight for global health equity, another set of motivations with deep historical roots and numerous adherents in the history of global health can be described as religious in character.[154] Here, the term "religious" refers not so much to institutionalized religion or religious doctrine as to an inchoate personal religiosity that recognizes the sacredness of relationships to others, our sensibility to care for the afflicted and marginalized, and our desire to do good in the world. William James saw these fundamental human sentiments as the psychophysiology of religious inspiration.[155] This kind of religiosity helps many individuals working in global health to sustain themselves in the face of injustice and inequities of daunting scope and scale as well as the day-to-day adversity, privation, loneliness, and failure that such work entails. The role of religious values in global health work—indeed, in all forms of moral practice—is not always conscious, yet such values can fortify one's aspirations. A deep personal faith often animates the impulse to give care and to protect others, especially the poor and otherwise marginal; it can help us reimagine the human condition as something better, more just, more beautiful.

But the religious underpinnings of global health work remain undertheorized by scholars and unvoiced by many practitioners. Leading thinkers from the Enlightenment to the early twenty-first century—including many religious thinkers—have sought to frame human rights claims within secular philosophical and legal traditions. The culture of biomedicine also obfuscates religious motivations of moral action because cosmological claims are regarded as neither scientific nor rational.

Histories of humanitarianism, long the province of missionaries, sometimes also excerpt religious motivations. The origin of global health is instead understood as the union of the science of medicine and humanitarian assistance. Religious values did not fade from the subjectivities of global health practitioners and policymakers with the late twentieth-century crescendo of secular human rights language. On the contrary, they are a continuing source of inspiration for many who choose this work. This failure to recognize the importance of religiosity in global health obscures rich religious and spiritual traditions that furnish many practitioners with abiding commitments to the long march toward global health equity.

Chapter 3 discussed some of the links between Christianity and state power—and imperial power—during the colonial and postcolonial eras. This legacy may in part explain why global health practitioners today might choose to elide their own religiosity in personal narratives. Even Albert Schweitzer, a theologian and physician, framed his own work as reparation for atrocities perpetrated in the name of God during the colonial period:

For every person who committed an atrocity in Jesus' name, someone must step in to help in Jesus' name; for every person who robbed, someone must bring a replacement; for everyone who cursed, someone must bless. . . . When you speak about missions, let this be your message: We must make atonement for all the terrible crimes we read of in the newspapers. We must make atonement for the still worse ones, which we do not read about in the papers, crimes that are shrouded in the silence of the jungle night.[156]

Any honest account of religion and global health begins with this mixed legacy. Perhaps as a result, many individuals mentioned in these pages have tended to cloak the religious roots of their commitment to global health in secular language. This section draws out some of those connections in order to explore the ways in which religion can be a productive moral force.

Indeed, the movement for global health equity, if it can be called a movement, bears certain resemblances to the late nineteenth-century moral movements that followed the "Second Great Awakening" in American Christianity.[157] Examples include the medical missionary movement, the Boy Scouts and Girl Scouts of America, the Young Men's Christian Association, the Young Women's Christian Association, the Red Cross movement, and the first efforts in what we now call global health. The quintessential organization of nonsectarian medical aid during conflicts, the Red Cross, was founded in 1863 in Switzerland by Henri Dunant, a businessman shocked by the bloody battlefield of Solferino in Italy during the Second Italian War for Independence. The Red Cross symbol originated from the Swiss flag, a reversal of its white cross on a red field. Although the cross on the Swiss flag was derived from the Christian symbol, the Red Cross chose this design primarily because of its resonance with the neutral state of Switzerland.[158] But the red cross may have also had particular religious connotations for its founder, who was raised in the Calvinist tradition and who established the Swiss branch of the Young Men's Christian Association in his youth.[159]

The first generations of medical missionaries in China from the mid- to late nineteenth century drew their inspiration from religion, though they quickly determined, in their words and actions, that they had to save bodies before they could save souls. They built medical schools and universities in China aimed at dealing with the great health and social scourges of the time. John D. Rockefeller funded the faculty of Peking Union Medical College, still China's premier medical research

Clara Barton and the American Red Cross

The biography of Clara Barton, famed nurse, abolitionist, and founder of the American Red Cross, demonstrates a commitment to both secular and religious values. Barton trained as a schoolteacher, but she grew up providing nursing care for her family. She first engaged in humanitarian work in the early days of the American Civil War. Within the war's first weeks, she organized a group of volunteers who distributed supplies and cared for wounded soldiers, and she was eventually put in charge of hospitals providing care for the wounded. Barton later continued her nursing and advocacy work in the United States, lecturing on her experiences during the Civil War and becoming involved in women's suffrage and abolitionist circles. In 1869, she went to Europe to recover from an illness, but soon plunged into humanitarian work with the Red Cross during the Franco-Prussian War. After returning to the United States, she founded an American chapter of the Red Cross in 1881. As many Americans doubted that the country would ever see domestic combat again, Barton responded by refocusing the organization on disaster relief and by expanding its reach beyond U.S. shores.[1]

Her letters reveal that Barton drew motivation from religious values, even as she harbored reservations about institutional religion. She wrote in 1899:

> I do not know if I can claim a home in any Church, as I have never been a member of any, but my father heard Hosea Ballou preach the dedication sermon in the old Universalist Church in the town of Oxford, Worcester Co., Mass., and that church was *his* home . . . and that church was my Sunday abiding place. The cool shadows of the afternoon and the long, dark grass of the old burying place alongside are its memories, and I hope that the work of every day of my life had more or less to do with its principles.[2]

In 1904, sending a small cash donation to the Oxford church, she is more explicit:

> There are few people there [in Oxford] who have memories of harder church work or better church love in the old faith than I. In the later years of my life, I have done other things, worked along other lines than subscribing money to churches, although I have in other ways contributed my share, and it seems to me, dear sister, that with a little thought, the old church could get more through me than I could possibly give in a little personal contribution of a few dollars.[3]

Barton's work, while connected to experiences in the Oxford church, was transformed into a commitment to universal, transnational service for people in crisis. Her experience illustrates how religious values can quietly but forcefully shape the work of individuals engaged in humanitarian assistance and global health.

institute, because of a religious conviction that he should help in a country then known as "the sick man of Asia."[160] The founding of Yale-in-China Medical School in Hunan by Edward H. Hume also reflected missionary commitments that broadened out to help the sick poor in rural areas.[161]

Two international public health leaders we encountered in chapter 4 also came, in different ways, out of the medical missionary movement. Halfdan Mahler, director-general of the World Health Organization and charismatic leader of the primary health care movement in the 1970s, began his career in India as a medical missionary.[162] His father was, in fact, a Baptist minister, and Mahler himself has called social justice a "holy phrase."[163] James Grant, head of UNICEF, which launched the "child survival revolution," was born into a family of medical missionaries. Grant's grandfather had been a medical missionary, and his father also did medical missionary work.[164] His father headed the Department of Hygiene and Public Health at the Peking Union Medical College in China—where Grant himself was raised—and worked to develop low-cost medical training models that became the blueprint for the celebrated "barefoot doctors" program (see chapter 4).[165]

More recently, radical strands of theology have impelled new innovations in global health. Liberation theology, a tradition developed largely by Catholic clergy ministering to impoverished congregations in Latin America and Africa, informed the early work of Partners In Health, including that of three of the authors of this volume. Brazilian liberation theologian Leonardo Boff's claim that "the church's option is a preferential option for the poor, against their poverty" has guided the organization's strategy since the early 1980s.[166] The poor face the heaviest burden of disability and disease, which, after all, themselves make a preferential option for the poor. Liberation theology draws attention to the large-scale social forces that pattern risk among populations rich and poor;[167] it thus offers an implicit critique of, and complement to, human rights theory, which has often obscured the structural roots of violence, poverty, disease, and inequality.[168]

Just as physicians and international relief workers have found spiritual sustenance and new theoretical lenses in religious values and teachings, so, too, have policymakers. U.S. president George W. Bush, whose administration ushered in one of the most ambitious health initiatives in history, the President's Emergency Plan for AIDS Relief, frequently framed his global health agenda in religious terms. In a February 2008 interview during a six-nation tour of Africa, Bush described PEPFAR as "a mission of mercy."[169] In his memoir, Bush points to evangelical pastor Franklin Graham, son of Billy Graham and founder of the nonprofit humanitarian aid organization Samaritan's Purse, as a major influence in his decision to devote significant American resources to the worldwide fight against AIDS.[170] Other leaders in global health policy, from former Senate majority leader Bill Frist (a veteran medical missionary) to Episcopalian congressman Jim Leach (whose legislative work on third world debt relief and AIDS treatment was aided by Episcopal bishop Frank Griswold), openly describe the role of religious values in motivating their work.[171] During his tenure as president of the World Bank, from 1995 to 2005, James Wolfensohn, an Australian Jew, regularly organized dialogues to solicit the perspectives and expertise of religious leaders and organizations working in impoverished communities.[172] The Jubilee 2000 debt relief movement had roots in churches in the United Kingdom that drew inspiration from the nineteenth-century abolitionist movement.[173]

Many of the efforts of medical missionaries, especially those who focus on building or rebuilding medical infrastructure or on training health workers in addition to providing direct services, have had long-term impact on health systems across the developing world. Lutheran medical missions from Scandinavia remain important components of East African medical systems, even as Scandinavian aid agencies build on this long tradition to fund major health initiatives in Africa.[174] The Christian Medical College and Hospital in Vellore, India, has trained generations of practitioners and provided care for the poor since its founding in 1900.[175] The World Health Organization estimates that between 30 and 70 percent of health care infrastructure in Africa was established and is operated by faith-based organizations.[176]

These claims about the importance of religious values in global health are not confined to Judeo-Christian traditions. Buddhist philanthropies have played a major role in many responses to natural disasters in Asia, for example.[177] Other faiths—Islam, Hinduism, Confucianism, to name just a few—have long traditions of helping the poor, tending the sick, and providing care in the broadest sense of the term.[178] The impulse to do global health work, to engage in and seek to mitigate the suffering of others, comes not just from theology and scripture; it is also buried deep within the process of fashioning moral individuals—a process that each of these traditions can guide and strengthen.

The progenitors and leaders of global health have drawn on religion

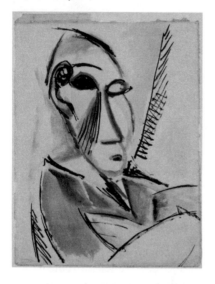

FIGURE 9.6. *Head of the Medical Student (Study for Les Demoiselles d'Avignon),* by Pablo Picasso, June 1907. Digital image © The Museum of Modern Art/Licensed by Scala/Art Resource, N.Y. Gouache and watercolor on paper, 23¾ x 18½ in. Courtesy Museum of Modern Art, New York.

in different ways. Some, like Schweitzer, have openly reflected on scripture and philosophy; others, like Mahler and Grant, have exhibited a religiosity that is buried in their early development as moral individuals. At the level of psychobiology, the visceral sense of religiosity, the embodiment of the religious experience, can shape the choices people make and the ideals to which they aspire. For many global health practitioners, moral motivation stems from lived values, of which they themselves may be unaware. Such values may find expression, for example, in the inherent priority of caregiving—perhaps the most fundamental impulse at the root of the decision to do global health work. Thai Buddhism, for example, has encouraged some extraordinary examples of palliative end-of-life care.[179] Similarly, the Chinese tradition of Confucianism and neo-Confucianism stresses the importance of caregiving: the deeper you cultivate the self in Confucianism, the more you find the universal context of caring for others, rather than the self as partisan.[180]

What is the role of religious values, or other types of values, in the physiology of caregiving? As Kleinman discusses at length elsewhere, the image of a divided self offers one way to conceptualize the dynamic subjective processes that result from the clash of the impulse to care for others and the impulse to pursue selfish interests.[181] The divided self has been depicted in art, including Picasso's *Head of the Medical Student* (reproduced here as figure 9.6).[182]

The figure in this image has one eye opened—to the suffering and pain of others and the need for caregiving—and one eye closed, to protect self-interest and help cultivate habits of critical self-reflection necessary for personal flourishing and prosocial action. The embodied feeling of a religious and ethical impulse shapes how individuals act under this divided condition, which is an ineluctable part of global health work. Without that feeling—that passion—perhaps few would be motivated to engage in work as trying and complex as that demanded to advance global health equity.

We do not intend to overstate the role of religious faith in global health, or to suggest that its legacy warrants uncritical approbation. Beyond their link with colonial medicine, religious values have influenced contentious recent policies, such as PEPFAR's ban on funding groups that provide health care services to commercial sex workers—who are at high risk of HIV infection, not to mention poverty and social marginalization—and its nominal policy that at least one-third of prevention funding be spent on "abstinence-only" education.[183] We are also not claiming that adherence to religious faith is the sole—or even the primary—motivation of any of the figures mentioned in these pages. We simply seek to point out that the religious impulse, religious values, and religious institutions remain an important part of the landscape of global health.

CONCLUSION

This chapter has introduced a necessarily incomplete series of moral frameworks with relevance to global health. It has sought to illustrate the importance of developing habits of critical self-reflection in such a biosocially complex and personally demanding line of work. Most readers will not find their own moral questions, challenges, and aspirations adequately addressed by the frameworks discussed here. But it is our hope that exploring some of the values and theories that have motivated other global health practitioners of all stripes will help readers better understand their own interests in and commitments to the movement for global health equity. Above all, we hope this chapter might serve as a springboard into deeper consideration of the moral roots of engagement in this work that will fortify and sustain future generations of practitioners, policymakers, researchers, advocates, and teachers on the front lines of global health.

SUGGESTED READING

Barry, Brian. *Why Social Justice Matters.* London: Polity Press, 2005.

Cranston, Maurice. "Human Rights: Real and Supposed." In *Political Theory and the Rights of Man,* edited by David Daiches Raphael, 43–51. Bloomington: Indiana University Press, 1967.

Englund, Harri. *Prisoners of Freedom: Human Rights and the African Poor.* Berkeley: University of California Press, 2006.

Farmer, Paul. *Pathologies of Power: Health, Human Rights, and the New War on the Poor.* Berkeley: University of California Press, 2003.

Gutiérrez, Gustavo. *A Theology of Liberation: History, Politics, and Salvation.* Maryknoll, N.Y.: Orbis Books, 1973.

Kleinman, Arthur, and Bridget Hanna. "Religious Values and Global Health." In *Ecologies of Human Flourishing,* edited by Donald K. Swearer and Susan Lloyd McGarry, Center for the Study of World Religions, 73–90. Cambridge, Mass.: Harvard University Press, 2011.

Nussbaum, Martha. "Human Functioning and Social Justice: In Defense of Aristotelian Essentialism." *Political Theory* 20, no. 2 (1992): 202–246.

Pogge, Thomas. *World Poverty and Human Rights.* 2nd ed. Cambridge: Polity Press, 2008.

Sen, Amartya. *Development as Freedom.* New York: Anchor Books, 2000.

———. *The Idea of Justice.* London: Allen Lane, 2009.

Singer, Peter. *The Life You Can Save: Acting Now to End World Poverty.* New York: Random House, 2009.

Taking Stock of Foreign Aid

JONATHAN WEIGEL, MATTHEW BASILICO, PAUL FARMER

In the early 2000s, foreign aid outlays for global health and development projects increased at an unprecedented rate. Within a decade,
development assistance for health nearly tripled, from $8.42 billion
in 1997 to $21.79 billion in 2007 (see figure 10.1).[1] AIDS funding
increased twenty-five-fold in less than two decades, from $200 million
in 1990—with almost none of it supporting treatment at that time—to
$5.1 billion in 2007.[2] Moreover, total development assistance (includ-
ing, but not limited to, health) more than doubled between 2000 and
2010, as figure 10.2 illustrates.

In light of such outlays, the past two decades have given rise to a
lively debate over the efficacy of aid. Has foreign assistance improved
the lot of its intended beneficiaries? Although some doubt the utility of aid per se, substantial evidence demonstrates that development
assistance for health—when delivered strategically—can help to raise
the standard of care and improve health outcomes, even in some of
the world's poorest settings. We also have working models of effective global health delivery, as chapters 6 and 7 describe. The guiding
question of this chapter, therefore, transitions from "does aid work?"
to "*how* does aid work?" Are there principles of effective aid delivery?

Two names that often frame the public discussion are Jeffrey Sachs,
an economist at Columbia University, and William Easterly, a former
World Bank economist currently at New York University. In his book
The End of Poverty: Economic Possibilities for Our Time (2005),

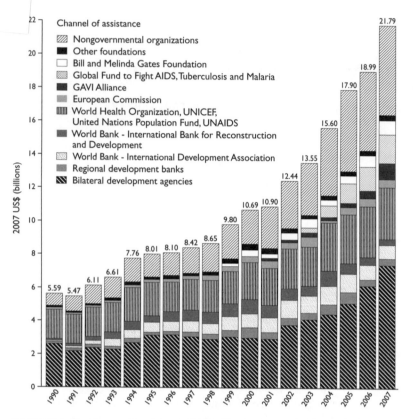

FIGURE 10.1. Development assistance for health, 1990–2007, by channel of assistance. Source: Nirmala Ravishankar, Paul Gubbins, Rebecca J. Cooley, Katherine Leach-Kemon, Catherine M. Michaud, Dean T. Jamison, and Christopher J. L. Murray, "Financing of Global Health: Tracking Development Assistance for Health from 1990 to 2007," *Lancet* 373, no. 9681 (2009): 2115.

Sachs estimates that $135 to $195 billion in foreign aid could help end extreme poverty by 2015.[3] Although this may seem like a large sum, Sachs points out that it amounts to only 0.54 percent of the rich world's gross national product—less than the 0.7 percent target proposed by the UN Millennium Project. (The Millennium Development Goals advanced by this project are introduced in chapter 11.) Sachs's argument rests on the theory of poverty traps.[4] Many poor families, he contends, are unable to reach the first rung of the development ladder because they spend all of their income on basic survival and are therefore unable to begin saving and investing in productivity enhancements (such as better farming technologies or higher-yield seeds), education,

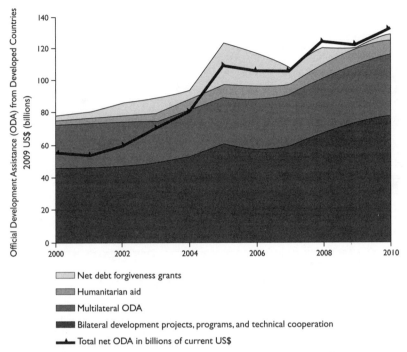

FIGURE 10.2. Official development assistance from developed countries, 2000–2010. Source: United Nations, *Millennium Development Goals Report 2011,* www.un.org/millenniumgoals/11_MDG%20Report_EN.pdf, p. 58.

health care, and other preconditions of escaping poverty.[5] Three development scholars sum up the logic of the poverty trap: "you can't pull yourself up by your bootstraps if you have no boots."[6] Foreign aid, according to Sachs, could help supply the missing resources between the poor and the first rung of development.

In addition to poverty traps, another factor Sachs stresses is the differential burden or blessing of geography: a country that struggles with a large disease burden because it has a tropical climate, or a country that faces high transportation costs because it is mountainous, landlocked, or without navigable rivers, encounters significant barriers to economic activity and growth. With adequate investment, countries can overcome such barriers; Switzerland's prosperity offers one example. But many cash-strapped developing countries may be unable to make the necessary investments without foreign assistance.[7] Pointing to poverty traps and geography as roots of economic stagnation challenges the common perception that the principal roadblock to develop-

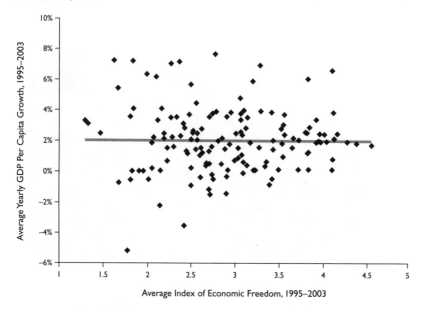

FIGURE 10.3. Growth and governance are not strongly correlated, according to Jeffrey Sachs, who argues that corruption is not a significant determinant of poor growth. (The Index of Economic Freedom is a proposed measure of governance: higher values refer to better governance.) Source: Jeffrey D. Sachs, *The End of Poverty: Economic Possibilities for Our Time* (New York: Penguin, 2005), 320, figure 1. © 2005 by Jeffrey D. Sachs. Used by permission of The Penguin Press, a division of Penguin Group (USA) Inc. Data from Marc A. Miles, Edwin J. Feulner Jr., and Mary Anastasia O'Grady, *2004 Index of Economic Freedom: Establishing the Link between Economic Freedom and Prosperity* (Washington, D.C.: Heritage Foundation and *Wall Street Journal*, 2004).

ment in poor countries in Africa and elsewhere is corrupt or incompetent governance.[8] Although Sachs agrees that corruption can stymie development, he argues that the link between governance and growth is often overstated, as figure 10.3 highlights. Ultimately, Sachs is optimistic, but cautiously so: aid can help reduce poverty, he argues, only if it is overhauled into an efficient, transparent, and accountable system that effectively channels resources to the people who need them most.[9]

In his 2006 work *The White Man's Burden: Why the West's Efforts to Aid the Rest Have Done So Much Ill and So Little Good,* Easterly rebukes Sachs's optimism about aid. Easterly writes the history of foreign assistance as a sequence of failed grand schemes. Using cross-sectional statistics to compare and analyze aid delivery programs, Easterly argues that not only has aid failed to promote growth (see fig-

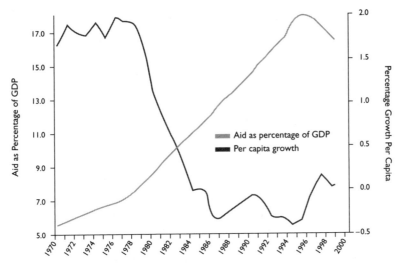

FIGURE 10.4. Aid and growth in Africa (ten-year moving averages), 1970–1999.
Source: William Easterly, *The White Man's Burden: Why the West's Efforts to Aid the Rest Have Done So Much Ill and So Little Good* (New York: Penguin, 2006), 46, figure 2. © 2006 by William Easterly. Used by permission of The Penguin Press, a division of Penguin Group (USA) Inc.

ure 10.4), but it has bred dependency and corruption in poor countries. For example, he claims that Paul Biya, the president of Cameroon since 1982, siphons off 41 percent of the foreign aid his country receives.[10] Easterly also highlights how much aid money is consumed by operating costs: in some cases, aid agencies spend more money on overhead such as salaries and transport costs than they spend on aid projects.[11]

According to Easterly, the underlying problem with aid is that its initiatives are hatched by "planners" in the United States and Western Europe—aid officials seeking to impose top-down solutions to poverty and other problems of development. But such blanket cures will not trigger economic growth and social developments, he argues. Growth and progress are instead attributable to the work of "searchers," individuals in poor countries who start businesses or find creative solutions to reducing poverty and solving social problems. Muhammad Yunus pioneering microcredit in Bangladesh and commercial sex workers in Calcutta's red-light district educating fellow workers about condom use and the dangers of AIDS are two of his examples. Easterly's argument is that markets work, but not when planned from the top down; democracy also works, he adds, but it too must emerge from the bottom up to avoid capture by dictators and predatory elites. "The dynamism of the poor at the bottom," he writes, "has much more potential than plans at the top."[12] Easterly's conclusions offer few easy takeaways for foreign aid agencies, but the overall message is that they must shift their focus from increasing overall sums of aid to scrutinizing how (if at all) aid can spur growth. He thinks this means bypassing governments and allowing resources to flow directly to the private sector.[13]

Amartya Sen has critiqued Easterly's approach, commenting that his claims are often overstated and ignore the heterogeneous effects of foreign aid:

> To arrive at his negative view of economic aid, Easterly draws on large-scale cross-sectional statistical analysis as well as on case studies of particular plans and programs. Such intercountry comparisons have become fashionable as a way of isolating solid connections between causes and effects, but they are seriously compromised by the difficulty of comparing diverse experiences: countries can differ significantly in variables other than those that are brought under cross-sectional scrutiny. Many such studies are also impaired by difficulties in identifying what is causing what. For example, a country's economic distress may induce donors to give it more aid—which may, in terms of associative statistics, suggest a connection between aid and bad economic performance. But using such a correlation to prove the bad effects of aid turns the causal connection on its head. Easterly tries to avoid such pitfalls, but the statistical associations on which he draws for his comprehensive pessimism about the effects of aid do not offer a definitive causal picture.[14]

Despite the limitations of his methodology, however, it must be acknowledged that Easterly's emphasis on critically examining the effects of foreign aid is a welcome demand of an industry that has long escaped rigorous scrutiny.[15]

The Sachs-Easterly debate is often boiled down to simple optimism and pessimism about aid. But polarizing the debate by asking the question "does foreign aid work?" misses the point, which is to interrogate facile claims about causality concerning health and well-being for those left behind by development. Sachs and Easterly both put forward thoughtful and mixed diagnoses explaining the failures of foreign aid. In fact, they both encourage the question we posed at the start: "*how* does foreign aid work?"

This question has been taken up by a number of scholars and practitioners seeking to examine and improve the machinery of foreign aid.[16] One example is the Abdul Latif Jameel Poverty Action Lab (J-PAL) at the Massachusetts Institute of Technology. Led by Esther Duflo and

Abhijit Banerjee, who co-wrote *Poor Economics: A Radical Rethinking of the Way to Fight Global Poverty,* the development economists at J-PAL and its many partner organizations have pioneered the use of randomized controlled trials in development economics.[17] By implementing a development intervention as a "treatment" and comparing it to a "control" in a comparable population that does not receive the intervention, RCTs enable economists to measure the specific effects of that intervention.

For example, an RCT conducted in Kenya by economists Michael Kremer, Edward Miguel, and colleagues found that children who were given deworming medications stayed in school longer and had 20 percent higher earnings as young adults than those who did not receive such medications. The study estimated a lifetime income increase of $3,269 from deworming.[18] By comparing Kenyan schools that provided deworming drugs with similar ones that did not, the RCT isolated the specific (and profound, in this case) effect of the intervention under scrutiny. Duflo, Banerjee, and a growing number of other development economists have launched thousands of RCTs across the developing world to evaluate interventions pertaining to health, education, agriculture, microfinance, family planning, and other facets of development. Their work has added nuance and rigor to our understanding of the mechanics of implementing development programs, financed by foreign aid or national governments.

RCTs, despite their well-known limitations in medical research,[19] offer one useful if imperfect tool for development researchers and policymakers. But they raise troubling questions in development work, too. In a number of cases, global health and development interventions have already been proven effective and deliverable in resource-poor settings. People with life-threatening diseases like HIV or cancer or cholera need treatment, which, as chapter 6 illustrates, can be delivered anywhere in the world. How do we deliver it better? How do we create a science of delivery? Today, more than ever before, there is a growing armamentarium of proven interventions for health and education and other components of development. Once we know what works, the question becomes more focused: how do we bring effective delivery models to scale? Or, more broadly, how can we build systems that will provide quality care in the long term—independent of foreign aid flows—and trigger virtuous social cycles and suitable economic development?

THE ACCOMPANIMENT APPROACH AND AID REFORM

One approach to this challenge has been discussed and supported by examples and case studies throughout this book: *accompaniment*. The accompaniment approach means supporting developing country partners—public and private—until they have the capacity to deliver services and improve livelihoods in the long term. It entails patience, flexibility, and commitment to doing whatever it takes to help the poor and their allies in the public and private sectors to build effective systems for economic development and health care delivery. Above all, it acknowledges (and seeks to redress) unequal development and the effects of large-scale social forces linked to history and geography.

In addition to informing service delivery for specific projects, accompaniment offers a strategy for foreign assistance in general, including global health initiatives. Foreign contractors and international NGOs could find ways of accompanying their intended beneficiaries on development projects of all kinds. Sometimes this might mean providing budgetary support for beleaguered and underfunded government health and education authorities, or investing in local firms, or procuring goods and services locally.[20] There is no one-size-fits-all package. As we know, all social action risks unanticipated consequences. So too does inaction. Accompaniment offers a means of preparing for the unforeseen: by adapting to the local context and by following the lead of local partners, the accompaniment approach enables aid groups to tackle challenges nimbly.

What, exactly, is accompaniment? We start by distilling the accompaniment approach into eight principles:[21]

FAVOR INSTITUTIONS THAT THE POOR IDENTIFY AS REPRESENTING THEIR INTERESTS

Accompaniment starts with listening, to determine which institutions the intended beneficiaries believe to be acting in their interests. The poor endure the local context and have learned from it; they have watched past aid projects succeed or fail. They often know what development opportunities exist and what combination of institutions—public and private, local and international—will be most likely to deliver aid effectively. Accompaniment hinges on finding good partners, and the poor are necessary consultants for that task.

FUND PUBLIC INSTITUTIONS TO DO THEIR JOB

One unintended and harmful consequence of foreign assistance—noted by Paul Collier and others[22]—is that funding NGOs can effectively drain the public sector of resources and skilled personnel. For example, of the $2.4 billion in humanitarian aid disbursed in Haiti after the January 2010 earthquake, less than 1 percent went to the Haitian government.[23] Although at times—and a devastating quake in a setting of poverty may be one of those times—governments are not the only partners for development work, they should be protagonists in such efforts whenever possible. Large-scale implementation usually requires partnering with national and local governments; sustainable development also usually requires working in the public sector, which will still be there long after aid workers have packed their bags. Donors concerned with corruption or lack of capacity on the part of recipient governments often unwittingly fuel a self-fulfilling prophecy. The best way to build capacity and combat corruption is to support the development of systems of accountability and transparency (see the discussion of Haiti's General Hospital later in this chapter)—that is, by practicing accompaniment.

MAKE JOB CREATION A BENCHMARK OF SUCCESS

Donors for all sectors of development—health, education, environment, energy, infrastructure, trade, finance—and all those engaged in global health equity should prioritize local job creation and transfer of capacity to local partners. Beyond helping individuals and families achieve autonomy and basic well-being, jobs confer dignity, self-worth, and opportunities to pursue professional development. Job creation can also stimulate local economies and strengthen the national tax base—two cornerstones of a robust public-sector health system.

BUY AND HIRE LOCALLY

Most foreign aid projects procure goods, services, and personnel outside beneficiary countries, which misses an opportunity to stimulate local development and can even weaken local economies (by importing goods and services at artificially low prices). A year and a half after the Haiti earthquake, only 2 percent of reconstruction contracts had been awarded to Haitian firms.[24] But buying and hiring locally can help create jobs, develop local markets, boost tax revenues, and stimulate entrepreneurship. Some commodities can also be sourced locally. For example, so-called ready-to-use therapeutic foods (especially important for maternal and child health, as chapter 11 describes) can be manufactured in resource-poor settings using produce from local farmers.

CO-INVEST WITH GOVERNMENTS TO BUILD STRONG CIVIL SERVICES

Workforce development in the public sector proceeds best with platforms of transparent hiring and firing, including performance reviews, continuing training programs for civil servants, and the ability to assess workforce needs. This applies as much to a health workforce as to any other. But instead of strengthening civil services, aid programs often erect parallel (or competing) structures and provide technical assistance (usually an expert or two from donor nations) without helping to develop robust training programs that can build in-country capacity. In 2002, the cost of 700 international advisors to the Cambodian government was $50–$70 million, just shy of the wage bill for the country's entire 160,000-strong civil service.[25] An accompaniment approach seeks to shore up and modernize existing human resource systems.

WORK WITH GOVERNMENTS TO PROVIDE CASH TO THE POOREST

A growing body of evidence suggests that cash transfers can be a useful, complementary tool to reduce poverty, boost demand for goods and services, and thus stimulate local economies. In South Africa, for example, cash transfers have been highlighted in helping to reduce the poverty gap.[26] Mexico's conditional cash transfer program—which requires that, among other things, families bring their children to a clinic for a basic package of health interventions—has been credited with improving child health.[27] Cash transfer programs are no panacea and can accomplish little without decent institutions and service-delivery platforms. But they can help empower "searchers," to use Easterly's term, and complement the toolkit for development assistance and global health equity.

SUPPORT REGULATION OF INTERNATIONAL NONSTATE SERVICE PROVIDERS

The status quo in foreign assistance often involves contracting with nongovernmental organizations—local and international—instead of the governments of recipient countries. Thousands of NGOs are operating in Haiti, a country of 10 million. A majority of NGOs (in Haiti and elsewhere) do valuable work, but without coordination and regulation, they run the risk of being duplicative, inequitable, and unaccountable to the communities they serve. We add up to less than the sum of our parts. Cash-strapped ministries of health—and the public clinics and hospitals they run—cannot compete with better-funded NGOs, leading to an internal brain drain that is at times as pernicious as the global one. Harmonizing foreign aid efforts increases their likelihood of helping to generate meaningful, lasting change for their intended beneficiaries.

APPLY EVIDENCE-BASED STANDARDS OF CARE THAT OFFER THE BEST OUTCOMES

Rich and poor settings are almost always separated by different standards of health care. Budgets and funding streams, rather than strategy to increase value and quality of services, too often drive implementation, which usually means paltry health care services are available in poor places. But the accompaniment approach, premised on equity, demands raising the standard of care in resource-poor settings to a level that would be acceptable in affluent settings.

What does accompaniment mean in practice? We can look, for example, at the efforts of the American Red Cross to strengthen the largest public-sector hospital in Port-au-Prince. After a disaster, the Red Cross typically spends a large proportion of its resources working with NGOs. But after the January 2010 earthquake, the General Hospital in Port-au-Prince, which itself sustained major damage, was swamped with patients seeking care for crush injuries and other associated complications. Even before the earthquake, it had faced one of the highest caseloads in the country, and its employees received lower salaries than competing private hospitals and NGO outfits.[28] In an effort to help the beleaguered staff at the General Hospital, the Red Cross agreed to spend $3.8 million on a salary support program. Starting this program was no easy task: the hospital lacked modern bookkeeping and adequate computing systems to keep track of staff work hours, as American accountability norms require. Installing or upgrading computer systems was not what the Red Cross had signed up for, but in this particular time and place, accompaniment demanded the patience to overcome snags as they arose and an investment in solving the root problems—in this case, an underdeveloped "infrastructure of transparency."[29]

This approach is premised on the idea that the hard work and open-ended commitment of accompaniment are worthwhile because a stronger and more durable health system will provide better care for all maladies, despite the ebb and flow of foreign aid through programs such as the President's Emergency Plan for AIDS Relief and the Global Fund to Fight AIDS, Tuberculosis and Malaria. Though a contingency plan was developed a few months later, the 2011 decision that the Global Fund would be unable to approve new projects until 2014 was a reminder not only of the importance of health system strengthening but of the need for long-term assistance guided by these basic principles of accompaniment.[30]

Beyond Red Cross support of a crumbling public hospital, there are many other examples of foreign aid projects that follow an accompaniment approach: nonstate health providers who coordinate their efforts with local ministries of health; international groups that purchase food and supplies in-country from local farmers instead of importing them; donors who prioritize job creation or contract local initiatives alongside foreign ones.[31] One initiative seeking to systematize and disseminate information about such programs is the Global Health Delivery

Project, described in chapter 7.[32] Led by a small team at Harvard, GHD develops case studies of health programs in resource-poor settings around the world in an effort to help build a science of global health delivery.[33] But such initiatives are still the exception, not the norm, in the business of foreign assistance. The accompaniment approach thus entails significant reform—new rules of the road[34]—of the machinery of foreign aid.

Even proponents of increased aid, such as Jeffrey Sachs, argue for fundamental changes to the existing systems of foreign assistance. "If we are to get agreement by the rich world's taxpayers to put more aid through the system," he writes, "we first have to show that the plumbing will carry the aid from the rich countries right down to where the poorest countries need it most—in the villages, slums, ports, and other critical targets."[35] As Easterly and others highlight, the majority of foreign assistance is fragmented, nontransparent, and diluted by high overhead costs; and it often comes with strings attached that suit the interests of donors more than those of the intended beneficiaries.[36] In short, most aid programs are nowhere near as effective as they could be.

The accompaniment approach can help guide foreign aid practitioners in designing projects that are adaptable to diverse local settings, durable over the long term, and therefore more likely to move closer to a broadly shared vision of ending extreme poverty. It also outlines an answer to Easterly's call for aid programs that work from the bottom up: accompaniment starts (and ends) with listening to the problems and priorities described by the intended beneficiaries. Chapter 7 outlines a framework for delivering health care in poor settings; the accompaniment approach is a strategy for implementing that framework effectively. And the accompaniment approach can be leveraged in most types of development work. Unlike traditional aid modalities, accompaniment is a long-term pledge to walk with the poor, to help strengthen and improve existing public and private efforts to promote health and equitable development—replace them with a parallel aid architecture.

MORE (GOOD) AID

Guided by models of effective aid delivery, including the accompaniment approaches, development assistance could be strengthened and expanded to meet these goals. Although aid outlays have increased in the past few decades, they remain small compared to the basic deficits in most poor countries. The authors of this book—along with many policymakers, scholars, and practitioners, not to mention intended beneficiaries—believe that, overall, available evidence suggests the utility of increasing foreign assistance, even as its machinery needs reform. These approaches can be informed and complemented by social justice efforts, both "grassroots" and large-scale, to promote equitable and just development. In particular, aid for global health projects, when delivered according to principles such as those outlined in this volume, has been proven effective in saving lives and mitigating suffering around the globe.

Estimates of the gap between aid provided and aid needed typically range from $40 billion to $52 billion per year.[37] Sachs estimates that an additional $40 billion per year in foreign aid could provide primary health care for the billion poorest people on the planet (who live on less than $1 per day). That is 40 percent of what the United States alone has spent each year on the war in Afghanistan, and less than 5 percent of the 2008–2009 bank bailouts.[38]

For many, even those casting a gimlet eye on foreign aid, health projects occupy a privileged position in the spectrum of development assistance. In a 2009 survey conducted by the Kaiser Family Foundation in the United States, 52 percent of respondents thought the government was spending too much on foreign aid. When asked about "efforts to improve health for people in developing countries," however, this number dropped to 23 percent; when asked about efforts to fight AIDS, it dropped to 16 percent. Thirty-nine percent supported maintaining U.S. government spending on global health, and 26 percent favored increasing spending.[39]

There is also reason to believe that many more Americans would support expanding U.S. global health programs if they understood how little the government currently spends relative to other budget items and relative to the contributions of other high-income countries. A 2010 study found that many Americans thought foreign aid constituted up to 25 percent of the federal budget and suggested reducing it to 10 percent (see figure 10.5);[40] another study found that 69 percent of Americans thought the United States gave a greater percentage of its gross national income than other high-income countries did.[41] But in 2008, aid actually accounted for about 1 percent of the U.S. budget (the equivalent of one-thirteenth of annual defense spending), and the United States in fact spent the lowest percentage of gross national income on foreign aid among all high-income countries: 0.18 percent,

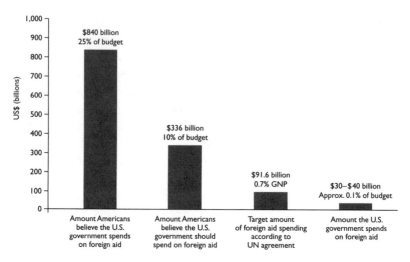

FIGURE 10.5. Perception versus reality regarding U.S. foreign assistance. Source: WorldPublicOpinion.org, "American Public Opinion of Foreign Aid," November 30, 2010, www.worldpublicopinion.org/pipa/pdf/nov10/ForeignAid_Nov10_quaire.pdf.

well below the 0.7 percent target set by a 1970 UN General Assembly resolution.[42] (A number of high-income countries, including Denmark, Sweden, and Norway, have already surpassed the 0.7 percent target, which was reaffirmed by the UN in 2002.) Sachs estimates that the United States could provide primary health care to the "bottom billion" for $40 billion and still remain shy of the UN target, which in any case is much less than the levels of foreign aid that most Americans deem acceptable in opinion polls.[43]

Strategies for closing the gap between perceived and actual global health aid—and between promises and delivery—are explored in the final chapter of this book. Of course, the governments of developing countries are the protagonists in the movement for global health equity, and many have begun devoting more resources to health. In 2001, dozens of African leaders signed the Abuja Declaration, pledging to increase government health spending to 15 percent of total expenditures. Ten years later, median annual government health spending in African Union countries had increased from $10 to $14 per person in real terms; twenty-seven African Union countries spent a larger portion of their budget on health in 2009 than in 2001.[44] In Rwanda, the government's successful National AIDS Control Commission paved the way for increasing government investments throughout the health sector; it is one of the only countries in the developing world close to universal access to AIDS care (see chapter 6). Rwanda—one of two African countries to have reached the Abuja target by 2010, and the only one on track to meet the Millennium Development Goals—has emerged as a model of health system strengthening by channeling tax revenues and more of its foreign assistance from public and NGO sources into a stronger public health system.[45] Other governments in Africa and across the developing world will likely need to increase expenditures on health care if global health programs are to have large-scale and long-lasting impact.

There is only so much, after all, that cash-strapped government ministries can accomplish without support—or accompaniment—from wealthy countries or from a healthy tax base. The budget of one Harvard-affiliated teaching hospital far exceeds that of the government of Haiti. After the 2010 earthquake, some international health NGOs raised more than twice the total budget of the Haitian Ministry of Health.[46] In other words, there remains great need for foreign aid for the work and resources of international NGOs and other partners in equitable development. The accompaniment approach provides one model of how to make foreign assistance more needs-based, adaptable, and sustainable in the long term.

SUGGESTED READING

Acemoglu, Daron, and James A. Robinson. *Why Nations Fail: The Origins of Power, Prosperity, and Poverty.* New York: Crown, 2012.

Banerjee, Abhijit V., and Esther Duflo. *Poor Economics: A Radical Rethinking of the Way to Fight Global Poverty.* New York: PublicAffairs, 2011.

Collier, Paul. *The Bottom Billion: Why the Poorest Countries Are Failing and What Can Be Done about It.* Oxford: Oxford University Press, 2007.

Easterly, William. *The White Man's Burden: Why the West's Efforts to Aid the Rest Have Done So Much Ill and So Little Good.* New York: Penguin, 2006.

Farmer, Paul. "Partners in Help: Assisting the Poor over the Long Term." *Foreign Affairs,* July 29, 2011. www.foreignaffairs.com/articles/68002/paul -farmer/partners-in-help?page=show.

Sachs, Jeffrey D. *The End of Poverty: Economic Possibilities for Our Time.* New York: Penguin, 2005.

Sen, Amartya. "The Man without a Plan," *Foreign Affairs,* March/April 2006. www.foreignaffairs.com/articles/61525/amartya-sen/the-man-without-a -plan?page=show.

United Nations Office of the Special Envoy for Haiti. "Has Aid Changed? Channeling Assistance to Haiti before and after the Earthquake." June 2011. Video presentation, by Katherine Gilbert, www.lessonsfromhaiti.org/press -and-media/videos/presentation-accompany-haiti/; published report, www .lessonsfromhaiti.org/download/Report_Center/has_aid_changed_en.pdf.

11

Global Health Priorities for the Early Twenty-First Century

PAUL FARMER, MATTHEW BASILICO, VANESSA KERRY,
MADELEINE BALLARD, ANNE BECKER, GENE BUKHMAN, OPHELIA DAHL,
ANDY ELLNER, LOUISE IVERS, DAVID JONES, JOHN MEARA,
JOIA MUKHERJEE, AMY SIEVERS, ALYSSA YAMAMOTO

We live in a world that is not only full of dangers and
threats, but also one where the nature of the adversities is
better understood, scientific advances are more firm, and the
economic and social assets that can counter these menaces
are more extensive. Not only do we have more problems to
face but we have more opportunities to deal with them.

—Amartya Sen, 2000 Tokyo International Symposium
on Human Security

The first decade of the twenty-first century has been termed the "golden
age of global health." Stirred by the AIDS pandemic, the world turned
its eyes toward the diseases of the poor and the inequities in health
care. The worldwide AIDS movement catalyzed global health as a field
distinct from international health (and colonial medicine before that)
and added the delivery of longitudinal treatment to a public health
agenda weighted in favor of health promotion and disease prevention.[1]
This was no zero-sum game. Anthony Fauci, director of the National
Institute of Allergy and Infectious Diseases, and colleagues argue that
the global attention directed toward AIDS reinvigorated support for
fighting ancient killers such as malaria and tuberculosis.[2] New transnational funding mechanisms invested billions of dollars in efforts to
prevent and treat leading infectious killers and promote human health
around the globe. The health effects have been dramatic: today, nearly

8 million people with AIDS worldwide have access to antiretroviral therapy, a feat many considered impossible as recently as 2002;[3] efforts to combat malaria and tuberculosis have improved markedly (if unevenly) around the globe;[4] and community-based health delivery has proved capable of raising standards of care and strengthening health systems in poor countries and in poor parts of rich countries alike.[5]

But history reminds us of the risks of complacency concerning global health. The 1978 Alma-Ata Declaration enshrined a bold vision of equity, "health for all by the year 2000." After the success of smallpox eradication in 1979, many hoped that effective health services would reach more and more people around the world. As chapter 4 recounts, such ambitions fell prey to economic troubles in the 1980s; the fiscal austerity measures instituted in many developing countries during the next decades further starved public-sector health systems. Moreover, significant inequities remain today. More than one-third of the world's population (some 2.5 billion people) still lives on less than two dollars per day, and an estimated 18 million people die prematurely from poverty-related causes every year.[6] Too few global health efforts have tackled the heavy burden of cardiovascular disease, cancer, and mental illness in the developing world. The distribution of disease tracks with the availability of health resources: according to the World Health Organization, Africa bears 24 percent of the global burden of disease but has only 3 percent of total health care personnel and 1 percent of the world's financial resources for health, including loans and grants from abroad.[7]

This chapter outlines a number of key global health priorities for the second decade of this century, introducing a series of ongoing conversations that reflect, in broad strokes, the current field of vision. The model of health care delivery and health system strengthening discussed in chapter 7 includes each of these priority areas, and many others. The authors of this volume believe that scaling up these efforts, and the vision of global health equity on which they are based, is the greatest priority in global health. We also believe that health equity is one of the ranking human rights challenge of our times. Building better health systems offers patients and providers and health activists a platform to reduce the burden of disease, address social determinants of health, and build long-term care delivery capacity capable of tackling whatever challenges come along. Short-term, low-cost interventions alone are less likely to move us closer to these goals. Advancing global health equity entails transformational social change—the subject of the final chapter.

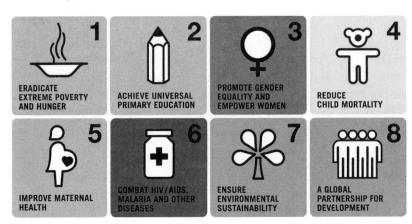

FIGURE 11.1. The eight Millennium Development Goals, supported by countries and development institutions around the world, offer a blueprint for global progress. Source: Millennium Project, "About MDGs: What They Are," www .unmillenniumproject.org/goals/index.htm. Courtesy United Nations.

Given the potential for increasing the effectiveness and quality of aid delivery as discussed in chapters 7 and 10, what are key priorities in global health for the early twenty-first century? The answer to this question necessarily varies across regions and must be based on undemanding local burdens of disease and on bridging gaps in the availability of services. The topics discussed in this chapter are meant to illustrate some key areas of focus; they do not represent an exhaustive list, and many are bound to change from year to year. Almost regardless of what have to be the ranking health problems in a given setting, a *diagonal* approach—responding to specific leading causes of mortality and morbidity in ways that strengthen health systems in general[8]—offers the most compelling strategy for tackling these priorities.

The Millennium Development Goals, formulated at the dawn of the golden age of global health, are a useful place to begin a discussion about global health priorities. In 2000, 192 countries and 23 international organizations pledged support for realizing the eight goals by 2015 (see figure 11.1). All of the MDGs have some bearing on global health; and Goal 4 (reduce child mortality), Goal 5 (improve maternal health), and Goal 6 (combat HIV/AIDS, malaria, and other diseases) are directly relevant to health. Progress on other MDGs, such as eradicating extreme poverty and hunger (Goal 1), promoting gender equality (Goal 3), and ensuring environmental sustainability (Goal 7), is also fundamental to advancing global health equity.

For each goal, specific targets have been set: reducing mortality rates for infants and children under five by two-thirds, for example, and achieving universal access to AIDS treatment.[9] Although few of the Millennium Development Goals will be met by 2015, they have helped generate support, in high-income countries as in many of those in which poverty and disruption make such goals a matter of urgency, for more ambitious agendas in global health and development. The targets and benchmarks of the MDGs have also motivated diverse actors to coordinate their efforts, much as the GOBI-FFF interventions did during the child survival campaign led by the United Nations Children's Fund in the 1980s, which chapter 4 describes in depth.

The next two sections consider Goals 4 and 5 (maternal and child health) and Goal 6 (combating AIDS, TB, and malaria) in more detail.

MATERNAL AND CHILD HEALTH

Millennium Development Goals 4 (reduce child mortality) and 5 (improve maternal health) are often coupled under the rubric of maternal and child health because of the many synergies that exist between these two concerns. A number of clinical processes, such as antenatal care and safe delivery, can improve the health of both mother and child. The same holds for family planning. Every health system needs robust efforts to promote maternal and child health care delivery.

Between 1990 and 2008, the mortality rate for children under five in developing countries dropped by 28 percent.[10] This is an important accomplishment, but the rate of progress falls short of the 4.2 percent average annual reduction needed to reach the MDG target.[11] The great majority of child mortality is attributable to infectious diseases and malnutrition that are treatable or preventable: pneumonia, diarrhea, and malaria accounted for 36 percent of all deaths among children under five worldwide in 2011; more than a third of all child deaths were attributable to malnutrition.[12] Most children who die of infectious pathologies are also malnourished, although their deaths are not always reported as such.[13]

As UNICEF's GOBI-FFF campaign demonstrated, widening access to low-cost interventions like childhood vaccines, oral rehydration therapy, and the promotion of breastfeeding can rapidly reduce mortality and morbidity among children around the world. Over the past dozen years, the Global Alliance for Vaccines and Immunization and its many partners have significantly expanded access to childhood vaccines (see the accompanying box).[14] A decade after its founding in 2000, GAVI had spent nearly $3 billion helping to provide vaccines to more than 250 million children and raising the immunization rate among children in low-income countries to 79 percent—an all-time high, according to the WHO. GAVI estimates that these efforts averted some 5 million child deaths.[15] The organization has been not only effective but also creative: its novel financing strategies—including a "matching fund" that brings together foreign aid organizations, private donors, and recipient country co-funding—are helping to build sustainable immunization programs in countries with low coverage rates.

In addition to childhood immunizations, numerous studies have found that deworming programs offer a range of benefits for child health, including increasing weight gain by 10 percent and reducing school absenteeism by 25 percent. Other studies observe that dewormed children score higher on cognitive exams and earn 21 to 29

The GAVI Alliance

Although the WHO's Expanded Program on Immunization and UNICEF's child survival campaign boosted global childhood immunization rates in the 1980s, vaccine coverage declined in the 1990s.[1] By 2000, some 30 million children in developing countries still had not received some or all of the six basic childhood vaccinations: tuberculosis, diphtheria, tetanus, pertussis (whooping cough), measles, and polio.[2] The GAVI Alliance, a coalition of UN organizations, governments, vaccine manufacturers, researchers, nongovernmental organizations, and philanthropists, took shape in 1999 with a $750 million contribution from the Bill and Melinda Gates Foundation. The Alliance was officially founded in 2000 at the Davos World Economic Forum.

GAVI has four principal goals. First, it seeks to increase vaccination rates in poor countries that have low coverage. Originally focusing on underutilized vaccines against yellow fever, diphtheria, tetanus, pertussis, hepatitis B, and *Haemophilus influenzae* type b (Hib), GAVI, in its second decade, has sought to maintain this coverage while also promoting adoption of new vaccines against meningitis, pneumococcal disease, and rotavirus. It encourages immunization scale-up by providing funds to low- and middle-income countries, offering technical assistance on national immunization strategies, and setting up procurement, monitoring, and evaluation. In some countries, GAVI has supported programs to scale up polio vaccine coverage. The Alliance is now beginning to explore vaccina-

percent more in wages as adults ten years later.[16] Organizations such as the Task Force for Global Health (formerly the Task Force for Child Survival) and Deworm the World, working with many governments in developing countries, have made significant strides in scaling up deworming programs. For example, by 2010, Kenya's national school-based deworming program had treated approximately 3.6 million children at a cost of $0.36 per child.[17] (Other efforts to scale up deworming are examined later in the chapter, in the section on neglected tropical diseases.)

Especially among children, malnutrition and food insecurity underpin much of the risk posed by both acute and chronic infections, from diarrheal diseases to tuberculosis. Among the best treatments for childhood malnutrition are ready-to-use therapeutic foods (RUTFs), fortified and calorie-dense pastes that are easy to package, ship, and store.[18] Médecins Sans Frontières, for example, pioneered use of a vitamin-

---

tion against cervical cancer and rubella as part of a broader focus on women's health.[3]

Second, GAVI seeks to strengthen routine immunization capacity in poor countries by funding training programs, public information campaigns, and "immunization services support" (essentially, reward payments to countries that expand coverage of DTP3 vaccine, which protects against diphtheria, tetanus, and pertussis). The latter program significantly increased DTP3 use in countries with low initial coverage, at an average cost of $14-$20 per child, according to one study. GAVI estimates that 76.5 million children received DTP3 with such support.[4]

Third, GAVI seeks to maintain multiyear, predictable financing for global immunization by marshaling resources from private and public donors and increasing co-investments from developing countries. The 2011 GAVI replenishment cycle raised $4.3 billion, increasing GAVI's total resources to $7.6 billion allocated for use in 2011–2015.[5]

Finally, GAVI uses advance market commitments—securing purchase agreements to incentivize vaccine development and manufacturing[6]—to stimulate research and development of new vaccines and to lower costs of underused vaccines. GAVI's efforts to engage pharmaceutical companies are among its most innovative contributions to global health. For example, GAVI's ability to organize demand helped create reliable markets that spurred development of new rotavirus, pneumococcal, and meningitis vaccines.[7] GAVI's model of delivering available vaccines while also creating incentives to develop new ones balances short- and long-term needs—and at low cost.

enriched peanut paste in Niger, recording a cure rate of up to 90 percent among children who suffered from severe acute malnutrition; similar efforts are under way in Malawi, India, Haiti, and many other countries.[19] In accordance with WHO recommendations, RUTFs are increasingly being used to treat children with severe acute malnutrition, with excellent results.[20]

Some have voiced concern that overuse of RUTFs could create dependency on imported foods and damage local agricultural production, although evidence from one fledgling initiative to produce vitamin-enriched peanut butter in Haiti suggests the contrary.[21] By building processing plants in countries with high rates of malnutrition and by procuring agricultural goods, such as peanuts, from local farmers, RUTF initiatives can create jobs and boost local production capacity—helping to ensure that the availability of such foods does not depend on donor dollars. Such projects exemplify the accompaniment approach outlined in chapter 10.

Maternal mortality remains high across the developing world, and the MDG 5 target of universal access to reproductive health care is still far from being met. More than 350,000 mothers die in childbirth each year, and access to reproductive health services such as family planning, antenatal care, and skilled assistance during delivery follows the fault lines of global purchasing power.[22] Extreme disparities of risk are the rule. The WHO estimates that in 2008, 99 percent of global maternal mortality occurred in developing countries; 65 percent occurred in just eleven countries. That same year, twenty-seven middle- and high-income countries had five or fewer total maternal deaths.[23] Among women living in Niger, the estimated lifetime risk of dying in childbirth is 1 in 7; in middle- and high-income countries, the figure is 1 in 7,300.[24] As of 2008, only nineteen developing countries were on pace to meet the MDG targets.[25]

Recent experiences in a number of countries demonstrate that maternal mortality can be reduced by improving health worker training, enabling referrals to proper facilities, and providing regular antenatal care. For example, in the 1990s, Honduras focused on developing a robust referral system for complicated deliveries, including training traditional birth attendants to determine when mothers should be referred to health facilities able to offer modern obstetrical care. Between 1990 and 1997, maternal mortality rates in Honduras dropped from 182 maternal deaths per 100,000 live births to 108.[26] Other low-cost interventions have also been shown to improve maternal health in resource-poor settings: access to family planning services reduces unintended pregnancies and decreases maternal mortality.

Targeted interventions are a critical short-term answer to the global disparities in maternal health. But improving women's health around the globe means addressing structural forces that affect their access to health care, including the greater burden of farm and household work that women bear, their caregiving responsibilities, and their lower social status. Gender inequity and poverty enjoy a noxious synergy. Food security is a daunting challenge for women living in poverty, especially during pregnancy when nutritional needs increase.[27] A growing literature suggests that integrating maternal health interventions into primary health care delivery may offer a better way to improve health outcomes for mothers over the long term.[28] In Indonesia, rural health outposts and their outreach workers have long provided a range of maternal and child health services, including nutrition, family planning, immunization, and prevention of diarrhea. These community-based primary care initiatives are credited with decreasing fertility rates and improving child survival.[29] In Lesotho, a number of rural health facilities offer HIV testing and family planning services to every woman seen in the clinics, obviating the need for follow-up appointments and increasing the overall efficiency of care delivery.[30]

Addressing maternal and child health comprehensively will require training more health workers; strengthening referral networks between communities, health centers, and hospitals; and ensuring adequate supplies at care centers—all elements of a robust health system. Indeed, no health system can be deemed complete without guaranteeing women access to the full panoply of modern obstetrics, including surgery, blood-banking, antihemorrhagics, and postpartum care. In many regions plagued with high maternal mortality, integrating malaria prophylaxis, HIV testing, micronutrient supplementation for mothers and children, immunizations, and health education into regular antenatal and infant health center visits can also capture synergies between maternal and child health priorities and help to strengthen health systems. HPV vaccines and early diagnosis and treatment of cervical cancer are other inexpensive and straightforward interventions that balance the agenda of women's health.[31]

In 2005, the leaders of hundreds of advocacy, funding, and implementation groups focused on maternal and child health formed the Partnership for Maternal, Newborn, and Child Health to redouble global efforts in support of MDGs 4 and 5. The partnership is principally an advocacy organization seeking to raise global ambitions in maternal and child health. It also helps disseminate evidence about effective interventions and supports ongoing monitoring and evaluation efforts. As ever, it will be necessary to link advocacy and raised ambitions to robust delivery efforts. The challenge for the next decade, as it is for all priorities in global health, will be scaling up targeted interventions in ways that enable health systems to provide quality services for mothers, infants, and children now and in the long term.

THE "BIG THREE": AIDS, TB, MALARIA

Progress has been made on Millennium Development Goal 6—combating HIV/AIDS, malaria, and other diseases—though we are still far from achieving the targets. Estimates of the number of new HIV infections has fallen from a peak of 3.5 million in 1996 to 2.5 million in 2011. Nearly 8 million people with AIDS have access to antiretroviral treatment.[32] (Just a decade ago, this number was close to zero among the poor of Africa, the most affected continent.) Similarly, the number of malaria cases decreased from 244 million in 2005 to 216 million in 2010; deaths from malaria fell from 985,000 in 2000 to 655,000 in 2010.[33] Whereas tuberculosis remains one of the leading infectious killers (after AIDS, diarrheal diseases, and other respiratory infections), its prevalence is falling in all regions except Asia.[34]

Because other chapters have considered elements of these diseases in depth, our focus here is limited to recent developments and to future needs. Several promising developments for treatment and prevention are taking shape: a malaria vaccine candidate and a new combination therapy for tuberculosis are undergoing clinical trials.[35] Evidence has shown that, by suppressing patients' viral loads, antiretroviral treatment is also an important tool for prevention: people living with HIV who are enrolled in antiretroviral treatment are 96 percent less likely to pass the virus to their partners.[36] Other advances such as male circumcision, vaginal microbicide gels, and pre-exposure prophylaxis with antiretrovirals have expanded the arsenal of tools for HIV control. Though none have yet been approved by the U.S. Food and Drug Administration, several HIV vaccine candidates have provided glimmers of hope, including those developed by the Ragon Institute as well as the National Institute of Allergy and Infectious Diseases.[37] Even without a vaccine, decades of experience in settings rich and poor have revealed that the best—perhaps the only—way to control this modern plague is nothing less than fully integrated prevention and treatment, using all the tools currently available.[38]

But major challenges remain. The Joint United Nations Programme on HIV/AIDS estimates that, in 2011, fully 34 million people world-wide were living with HIV, and 1.7 million died from AIDS-related ill-nesses.[39] Universal access to treatment, an unrealized 2010 target of MDG 6, would have averted almost all of these 1.7 million deaths. And in much of the world, the pandemic continues to grow: at current rates, five people are newly infected for every two who start antiretroviral treatment.[40] From 2002 to 2008, international assistance for integrated prevention and care rose sharply. But with the onset of the economic cri-sis in 2008–2009, the upward arc began to flatten. In 2010, for the first time since the early 2000s, funding for global AIDS programs declined; and in 2011, the Global Fund to Fight AIDS, Tuberculosis and Malaria

The Bill and Melinda Gates Foundation

No organization has demonstrated the promise of philanthropy in global health more than the Bill and Melinda Gates Foundation (BMGF). Since 1994, BMGF has committed more than $15 billion to global health research and implementation. A 2008 report found that BMGF funded nearly 18 percent of all research on neglected diseases, behind only the U.S. National Institutes of Health (NIH), which funded almost 42 percent.[1] After the U.S. Congress flattened the NIH budget in 2004, BMGF played an even larger role. In 2006, investor Warren Buffet contributed some $30 billion to BMGF, nearly dou-bling its size. Despite a 20 percent endowment drop during the 2008 financial crisis, BMGF has continued to increase spending every year.

BMGF's global health program outlines its mission as follows: "Our Global Health Program harnesses advances in science and tech-nology to save lives in poor countries. We focus on the health prob-lems that have a major impact in developing countries but get too little attention and funding. Where proven tools exist, we support sustainable ways to improve their delivery. Where they don't, we invest in research and development of new interventions, such as vac-cines, drugs, and diagnostics."[2]

BMGF has mobilized novel partnerships, many of them engag-ing the pharmaceutical industry, to target most of the global health priorities discussed in this chapter, including AIDS, tuberculosis, malaria, neglected tropical diseases, and maternal and child health. It is a major supporter of the Global Fund to Fight AIDS, Tuberculosis

was forced to cancel its upcoming funding cycle, Round 11, citing insufficient donor contributions.[41] Facing these daunting trends, the United Nations announced a global target of 15 million people on treatment by 2015, and President Barack Obama pledged that U.S. global AIDS programs would support 6 million on treatment by the end of 2013.[42] These targets are promising, but they do not necessarily signal robust funding: though U.S. funding has gone back up since 2010, it remains at 2009 levels, while international assistance overall has returned only to 2008 levels.[43] Tens of millions of lives are at stake as we fight an intensifying pandemic with inadequate financial support.

As this book argues throughout, programs targeting HIV, tuberculosis, and malaria can be leveraged to promote broader health system performance over the long term. The targets set by the Millennium Development Goals and other UN resolutions offer useful metrics to

and Malaria; the GAVI Alliance; and the Program for Appropriate Technology in Health (PATH), which works on discovery and development of new technologies in the fight against diseases of poverty. Some of the foundation's principal accomplishments include leading eradication campaigns against polio and malaria, developing a new meningitis vaccine, and increasing access to childhood vaccines. BMGF also supported the International Vaccine Initiative in developing Shanchol, a novel oral cholera vaccine, which is at least as effective as earlier vaccines, at about one-third the cost.[3]

A few critics have questioned whether BMGF's emergence as one of the largest funders for global health may have skewed the research agenda toward its own preferences. Anne-Emanuelle Birn, professor of public health at the University of Toronto, has suggested that BMGF focuses on developing new technologies—seeking "magic bullets" against HIV and malaria, for example—at the expense of scaling up access to existing health interventions.[4] Although technology development is a priority of BMGF, it has also funded large-scale delivery efforts. It is a strong supporter of the Global Fund and the Roll Back Malaria Partnership and in 2007 launched the Malaria Control and Evaluation Partnership in Africa,[5] which cut Zambia's malaria incidence in half. In addition, BMGF was the sole funder of the most ambitious effort to date to take the high road against multidrug-resistant tuberculosis—treating tens of thousands of patients in Peru and Russia, radically decreasing both mortality and transmission.[6] In fact, a close look at BMGF's current investment profile reveals a balance between discovery, development, and delivery.

track priorities and progress in global health. But achieving them in the next decade will require substantial and sustained contributions to integrated and comprehensive health system strengthening efforts around the globe.

NEGLECTED TROPICAL DISEASES

The fight to scale up control strategies against HIV, tuberculosis, and malaria worldwide still struggles to attract adequate funding. Other diseases, including those classified as "neglected tropical diseases," attract even less funding, although they too cause substantial mortal-

---

The Drug Development Pipeline

Discovery and development of new medicines and technologies that target neglected health problems in poor countries are global health priorities. At the same time, safe and effective interventions against many diseases—AIDS, tuberculosis, malaria, and numerous enteric pathogens, to name just a few—already exist and yet remain unavailable to people living in poverty. Thus effective delivery of existing tools must also be a top priority.

Conceptually, the drug development pipeline has three phases. *Discovery* involves research in basic science to identify molecular targets and drug or vaccine candidates. *Translation* (or development) optimizes such candidates into useful vaccines, diagnostics, and medicines by testing to determine whether compounds are effective, stable in human cells, safe in human populations, and deliverable to hospitals, clinics, or patients' homes. *Delivery* is the process of getting vaccines and drugs into the bodies of people who need them.

Figure 11.2 identifies three gaps that can disrupt the flow of technology in the pipeline. The first gap occurs because basic research in biomedical sciences emphasizes diseases that affect patients in the developed world, with its lucrative markets. Diseases that predominantly affect the developing world attract a significantly smaller proportion of basic science researchers' time, in large part because less support is available for this work. For these diseases, then, fewer molecular targets are identified, fewer candidates for therapy or prevention are described, and fewer papers are published. Thus the number of potential candidates for the second phase—translation—is diminished.

The second gap occurs when drug and vaccine candidates are not

ity and morbidity. It is important to understand, however, that framing NTDs in competition with the "big three" or maternal and child health or any of the other key global health priorities is misguided. Most of these areas are complementary; all of them are critical. Building robust health systems readily available to the poor will help to address all of these scourges.

These days, the WHO's Department of the Control of Neglected Tropical Diseases addresses twenty such conditions: Buruli ulcer, Chagas disease, cysticercosis/taeniasis, dengue, dracunculiasis (guinea-worm disease), echinococcosis, foodborne trematode infections, human African trypanosomiasis (sleeping sickness), leishmaniasis, leprosy, lymphatic filariasis, onchocerciasis (river blindness), rabies, schistosomiasis, soil-transmitted helminthiasis (hookworm), trachoma, yaws,

---

pursued because they are deemed unlikely to be safe, effective, and stable—or unlikely to recoup the costs of development. Although estimates of drug development costs are disputed,[1] the pharmaceutical industry reports that average research and development for a new drug costs from $800 million to $1 billion.[2] Upstream in the process, basic science discovery research is conducted by universities and public research institutes as well as corporations. But later stages of development, including human clinical trials, are run primarily by profit-oriented pharmaceutical and biotech companies, which are less likely to pursue technologies that fail to yield high financial returns (even if they bring a high return in, say, lives saved). Thus, many drugs for diseases of the poor stall in the translation phase because they are unlikely to be big sellers in rich-country markets.[3]

The third gap is the implementation, or delivery, bottleneck. Even when medicines are readily available, most health systems in poor countries have underdeveloped infrastructure, too few health workers, and patchy supply chains. More than 10 million deaths could be prevented each year simply by delivering existing interventions to all who need them.[4] This is the *delivery-failure death rate*. Integrated systems of care delivery (see chapter 7) are needed to be sure new interventions—and old ones—reach patients around the globe.[5]

These gaps in the drug development pipeline help explain the lack of essential medicines in many resource-poor settings in high- and low-income countries alike. But the picture—a picture of failure for the 10 million lost—is complete only when we look hard at all three gaps. One of the greatest challenges in global health is building systems of innovation, translation, and care delivery that rapidly move new interventions "from bench to bedside"—to the people who will benefit from them most.[6]

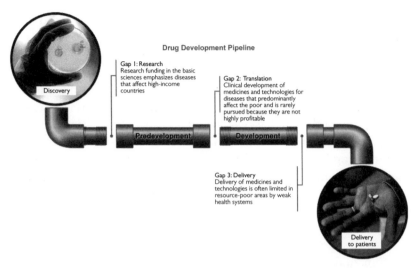

FIGURE 11.2. The drug development pipeline, showing three gaps that slow the discovery and diffusion of new interventions. Source: Adapted from Bernard Pécoul, "New Drugs for Neglected Diseases: From Pipeline to Patients," *PLoS Medicine* 1, no. 1 (2004): e6.

podoconiosis, snakebite, and strongyloidiasis. An estimated 1 billion people—a seventh of the world's population—suffer from one or more NTDs, some of which are deadly and almost all of which are disabling or disfiguring if untreated.[44] Each year, approximately 534,000 of these people, almost all of them living on less than a dollar per day, perish.[45] By thinning workforces and reducing worker productivity, NTDs can also undermine economic development.[46]

Despite the significant global burden of NTDs, they receive little funding for research or delivery of interventions. The WHO estimates that 90 percent of the global disease burden—the diseases of poverty—attracts only 10 percent of health-related research around the world. This disparity has been termed the "90–10 gap." Neglected tropical diseases represent a large share of the 90 percent, along with diseases like malaria and tuberculosis and cholera. When considering only NTDs, the situation is even worse: one study found that only 10 of the 1,556 new drugs registered between 1975 and 2004—fewer than 1 percent—were intended to treat NTDs.[47] In the current system of drug development, driven by estimated market size, a good deal of private investment of drug development goes toward lucrative products like

Viagra and Rogaine instead of new technologies to diagnose and treat diseases that claim millions of lives every year.[48]

Why do diseases that make up a considerable share of the global burden of disease receive so little research or implementation funding? At the root of this neglect is a market failure: there is little financial incentive to invest in new medicines to combat the diseases of the poor, who lack the purchasing power that would allow pharmaceutical companies to recoup the costs of development and delivery. So private-sector research and health care industries instead prioritize the health needs of high-income populations. Put another way, drug development is demand-based, not need-based. Although they are a significant cause of disability-adjusted life years (DALYs) lost worldwide, diseases that predominantly afflict the poor do not constitute markets profitable enough to stimulate private investment.[49]

Without new technology development, sometimes the only available tools for NTD control are ones that are weakly effective, painful, or dangerous. For example, melarsoprol, an arsenic derivative, is still at times used to treat human African trypanosomiasis and Chagas disease.[50] Administered by painful injection, melarsoprol has many serious side effects, deemed lethal in 8 percent of cases.[51] Another drug, eflornithine, is often a better treatment for human African trypanosomiasis, but it is expensive and in short supply in the poor countries with the greatest need. It can also have significant toxicity, including seizure in up to 8 percent of patients.[52] For the NTDs without safe, effective treatments, new drugs and interventions are urgently needed.

For other NTDs, however, safe, effective, and affordable preventatives and therapeutics have been developed (see table 11.1). Control efforts based on mass drug administration—a strategy pioneered in China to control lymphatic filariasis and schistosomiasis in the 1950s[53]—have made strides toward reducing the global NTD burden. Onchocerciasis control provides a telling case. Transmission of onchocerciasis can be reduced by spraying insecticides that kill its blackfly vector, a strategy that formed the basis of the WHO's Onchocerciasis Control Programme, launched in 1974. Onchocerciasis can also be treated with ivermectin, an antiparasitic medicine produced as Mectizan by Merck. Beginning in 1989, Merck joined the onchocerciasis-control effort, donating more than 300 million treatments to date.[54] According to the WHO, the Onchocerciasis Control Programme has prevented blindness in 600,000 people and eliminated the risk of blindness for another 18 million children in the eleven target countries in

TABLE 11.1 MAJOR CHARACTERISTICS OF THE MOST PREVALENT NEGLECTED TROPICAL DISEASES

Disease	Global Disease Burden (DALYs)	Vulnerable Populations	Primary Interventions	Weakness of Current Approaches
1. Hookworm infection	22.1 million	School-age children, women of reproductive age	Single-dose albendazole or mebendazole (1–3 times/year)	Limited access to essential medicines, low efficacy (mebendazole), rapid reinfection, drug resistance
2. Ascariasis	10.5 million	School-age children	Single-dose albendazole or mebendazole (1–3 times/year)	Limited access to essential medicines
3. Trichuriasis	6.4 million	School-age children	Single-dose albendazole or mebendazole (1–3 times/year)	Limited access to essential medicines
4. Lymphatic filariasis	5.8 million	Adolescents, adults	Single-dose ivermectin or diethylcarbamazine (plus albendazole)	Limited access to essential medicines
5. Schistosomiasis	4.5 million	School-age children, women of reproductive age	Single-dose praziquantel	Limited access to essential medicines, potential drug resistance
6. Trachoma	2.3 million	Children, adults (especially women)	Surgery, azithromycin, face washing, environmental control	Limited access to essential medicines and public health interventions
7. Onchocerciasis	0.5 million	Adults	Single-dose ivermectin	Limited access to essential medicines, potential drug resistance
Total	52.1 million			

SOURCE: Adapted from Peter J. Hotez, David H. Molyneux, Alan Fenwick, Jacob Kumaresan, Sonia Ehrlich Sachs, Jeffrey D. Sachs, and Lorenzo Savioli, "Control of Neglected Tropical Diseases," *New England Journal of Medicine* 357, no. 10 (2007): 1019–1020.

West Africa.[55] Although it is an important success story, global onchocerciasis control also highlights the ironies of a demand-based drug development industry and the inequalities that structure it. Mectizan was first discovered and developed to treat a range of canine parasites.[56] Merck's balance sheet losses from donating large amounts of Mectizan to global onchocerciasis control are offset because of the medication's high profitability in canine use in the United States.[57] Pets owned by the affluent can thus serve as a stronger driver of drug development than millions of poor people at risk of a disabling disease.

Nonetheless, Peter Hotez and others have underscored the key role of pharmaceutical companies in coalitions to control NTDs.[58] Merck and GlaxoSmithKline, for example, participate in the Global Alliance to Eliminate Lymphatic Filariasis by donating albendazole and ivermectin. This initiative has nearly eliminated lymphatic filariasis in Egypt, Zanzibar, and Samoa.[59] Additionally, African children carrying multiple parasitic infections, such as hookworm or ascariasis, can be treated effectively with a combination of albendazole (often donated by GlaxoSmithKline) and praziquantel (available in generic formulations).[60] Deworming initiatives are easily deliverable in resource-poor settings (many are integrated with school lunch programs), cost relatively little, and are credited with significantly increasing school attendance and performance.[61] Pfizer donates azithromycin to the International Trachoma Initiative, which has virtually eliminated blinding trachoma in Morocco.[62] The Schistosomiasis Control Initiative has used donations of generic praziquantel from MedPharm to reduce the burden of schistosomiasis among children in eight countries: Burundi, Burkina Faso, Mali, Niger, Rwanda, Tanzania, Uganda, and Zambia.[63] An eradication effort against dracunculiasis has made considerable headway.[64] Eli Lilly's engagement in multidrug-resistant tuberculosis control and Merck's Mectizan donation have broken new ground in linking discovery to development and then to delivery to the poor and otherwise vulnerable.[65] This is one template for addressing all NTDs.

Although there has been progress in controlling several NTDs in a number of countries, these successful examples are dwarfed by the magnitude of need around the globe. Because of synergies in combating multiple NTDs, a number of which are susceptible to the same chemotherapeutic regimes, Peter Hotez and others at the Global Network for Neglected Tropical Diseases have called for integrated preventive chemotherapy for NTDs.[66] In particular, Hotez and colleagues advocate scaled-up delivery of a "rapid-impact package" of albenda-zole or mebendazole, praziquantel, ivermectin or diethylcarbamazine, and azithromycin—all drugs already donated in large quantities to NTD control efforts by branded or generic pharmaceutical companies. This package, readily deliverable by community health workers, is esti-mated to cost $0.40–$0.79 per person per year in sub-Saharan Africa, a nearly 50 percent cost saving relative to existing programs.[67] Fixed-dose combination therapies, such as those developed for malaria, have also shown promise and could be included in this strategy.[68] A five-year global NTD control and elimination program would cost an estimated $1 billion. Furthermore, Hotez and colleagues point out that this rapid-impact package could be integrated with HIV- and malaria-control efforts, or with health system strengthening in general, to capture fur-ther synergies. Although the Bill and Melinda Gates Foundation, the U.S. Agency for International Development, and others have pledged resources for such initiatives, a global strategy for marshaling $1 bil-lion for NTD control does not yet exist.

The rapid-impact package will not, however, reduce the burden of a number of other NTDs, including the three with the highest case-fatality rates: Chagas disease, human African trypanosomiasis, and visceral leishmaniasis. Although some prevention tools, including vec-tor control, exist for these diseases, new drugs and technologies are urgently needed. Novel public-private partnerships for product devel-opment have started to revitalize empty drug pipelines for NTDs. For example, a product of the Drugs for Neglected Diseases Initiative, nifurtimox-eflornithine combination therapy, has demonstrated en-couraging efficacy and safety results in treating human African try-panosomiasis.[69] A number of other NTD drug candidates have been identified, but there is a long way to go before they are developed into safe and effective medicines and delivered to the people who need them. Key to this effort will be integrating these control tools into ongoing efforts to strengthen health systems around the world.

As a final comment, it is worth noting that the moniker "neglected tropical diseases," a legacy of colonial medicine, is, in one sense, mis-leading.[70] As this book has emphasized throughout, the essential truth is that all diseases of the poor are perforce neglected. Many of these pathogens are controlled in affluent countries and neglected in poor ones. Noncommunicable diseases, the subject of the next section, offer another such example.

NONCOMMUNICABLE DISEASES

One epidemiologic model popular in the 1970s held that the principal health threats faced by low-income countries came from infectious or communicable diseases such as pneumonia, vaccine-preventable illnesses, and tuberculosis, while high-income countries faced noncommunicable diseases such as heart disease, cancer, diabetes, and hypertension. When poor countries developed economically, according to the model, they would undergo an "epidemiologic transition" characterized by a decrease in communicable diseases and an increase in noncommunicable diseases. The underlying logic was that, as they developed, low-income countries would build the health systems and public health infrastructure—municipal water systems, modern sanitation, sufficient food production and care delivery mechanisms—necessary to eliminate many infectious diseases, just as parts of the United States and elsewhere in the developed world had done beginning in the late nineteenth century. Until that time, poor people in those areas most often died of communicable diseases before they could get noncommunicable ones.[71]

Like most past models of epidemiologic transitions, this one is fraught with problems. First, many NCDs—from cervical cancer to certain lymphomas to valvular heart disease—have infectious etiologies. Second, recent research has adjusted this model by revealing a *double* burden of disease in low- and middle-income countries: noncommunicable diseases on top of communicable diseases.[72] In fact, NCDs cause more deaths worldwide than infectious diseases do: they are responsible for 60 percent of global mortality, 80 percent of which occurs in developing countries.[73] The NCDs that cause the greatest mortality and morbidity include cardiovascular conditions such as stroke and heart disease, chronic respiratory conditions, type 2 diabetes, and certain cancers; cardiovascular illnesses are the single greatest cause of death in developing countries.[74] Studies using DALYs as a combined measure of morbidity and mortality estimate that mental illnesses are responsible for 14 percent of the global burden of disease; three-quarters of the global burden of mental illness falls in low- and lower-middle-income countries.[75] NCDs also have significant economic costs: one model estimates that the global burden of cardiovascular disease, chronic respiratory disease, cancer, diabetes, and mental health will depress global output by $47 trillion—some 75 percent of global GDP in 2010—over the next twenty years.[76]

What are the noncommunicable diseases of the bottom billion? Some, such as ischemic heart disease, type 1 diabetes, mental illness, and cervical cancer,[77] occur in both poor and affluent settings. Others, such as rheumatic heart disease and malignant hypertension, have been virtually eliminated in high-income countries with the help of modern diagnostics, preventatives, and therapeutics.[78] Though habits and lifestyles are frequently blamed for heart disease, lung disease, cancer, and type 2 diabetes, the burden of NCDs is compounded by endemic environmental conditions, malnutrition, and lack of access to care.[79] People living in settings of poverty are those who bear the brunt of these structural and environmental risk factors. For example, indoor cooking with biomass fuels like charcoal, wood, and animal dung increase the risk of chronic obstructive pulmonary disease. Yet more than 40 percent of households globally—especially in poor, rural areas—use solid fuels daily; in India, some 70 percent use such fuels; in Rwanda, almost all do so.[80] In addition, as noted, a number of NCDs have infectious origins. Peter Hotez and colleagues underscore the links between neglected tropical diseases and noncommunicable diseases: Chagas disease can cause cardiomyopathy; trichuriasis can trigger inflammatory bowel disease; asthma sometimes results from toxocariasis.[81] The boundaries between communicable and noncommunicable diseases are often indistinct.

NCDs afflicting people who live on less than a dollar per day typically follow a specific pattern: the "long tail" of global health equity. Individual NCDs are not always leading causes of morbidity and mortality in low-income countries, but, taken together, they account for a substantial burden of disease. In Rwanda, for example, NCDs account for approximately 17 percent of the disease burden, measured in DALYs (see figure 11.3).[82]

Although many NCDs can be effectively managed with existing medical and public health tools, most initiatives launched during the golden age of global health have not targeted them. Nonetheless, there is a growing body of evidence on the management of NCDs in resource-poor countries. As chapter 7 explains, strengthening health care systems—expanding access to primary care services, training health professionals, and shoring up supply chains, for example—can create delivery platforms to respond more effectively to a wide range of diseases, including NCDs. The WHO now considers key NCD interventions to be pillars of health system strengthening.[83]

Governments in some low-income countries have acted on this in-

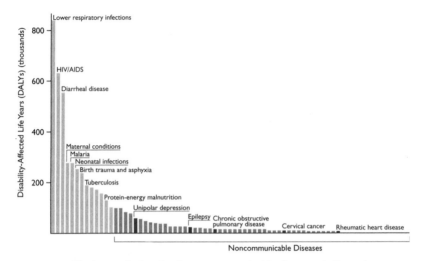

FIGURE 11.3. The long tail of endemic noncommunicable diseases in Rwanda, 2004. Source: Adapted from Gene Bukhman and Alice Kidder, eds., *The Partners In Health Guide to Chronic Care Integration for Endemic Non-Communicable Diseases, Rwanda Edition* (Boston: Partners In Health, 2011), 4, figure 1.1, http://act.pih.org/ncdguide; data from World Health Organization, *The Global Burden of Disease: 2004 Update* (Geneva: World Health Organization, 2008).

sight. In addition to implementing a successful AIDS treatment program that has increased coverage dramatically, Rwanda has also launched an ambitious program to integrate chronic care for NCDs with its efforts to strengthen the national health system.[84] Referral centers with surgical capacity, oncology units, radiology, and other medical specialties can be linked to distinct hospitals and health centers that offer integrated chronic care for NCDs, along with care for AIDS, tuberculosis, and neuropsychiatric disorders. Community health workers can provide chronic care services, such as following up on patients with insulin-dependent diabetes, heart failure, and malignancies. By 2011, the Rwanda Ministry of Health was running three district-level NCD clinics and four integrated chronic care clinics at health centers, which followed some 2,300 patients with chronic diseases.[85] Scaling up Rwanda's model of integrated chronic care elsewhere in the developing world could save millions of lives.

The mistake of pitting one set of pathologies against another is an unwelcome result of the socialization for scarcity. But progress toward one global health priority often strengthens, not weakens, efforts to achieve other priorities. So it is with NCDs. Especially because communicable and noncommunicable diseases can be linked epidemiologically and etiologically, efforts to reduce mortality and morbidity associated with either will be more effective if they are coordinated by building platforms to deliver both chronic and acute care. Julio Frenk has proposed the diagonal approach to combating NCDs (and other leading causes of death).[86] When integrated into primary care delivery, the provision of high-quality services for specific diseases such as hypertension or heart disease can help strengthen health systems in general.

NCDs are gathering attention from global policymakers. At a United Nations high-level meeting on noncommunicable diseases in September 2011, delegates from around the world rallied behind the need to raise the bar in preventing and controlling global NCDs.[87] Although the meeting helped draw attention to the need for concerted action against NCDs, it framed NCDs in terms of four lifestyle risk factors (tobacco use, unhealthful diet, unhealthy alcohol use, physical inactivity) and four diseases (heart diseases, lung diseases, cancer, and diabetes), which mischaracterizes the burden of NCDs among the world's bottom billion. Many of the "best buys" endorsed by the meeting's delegates, such as a polypill, a fixed-dose combination, for vascular diseases, are geared toward the NCDs of high- and middle-income countries.[88] In particular, this definition of noncommunicable disease excludes mental disorders, which make up a substantial percentage of the global burden of disease.[89] Furthermore, the meeting notably lacked firm financial commitments for implementation. Nonetheless, this was only the second disease-focused high-level meeting the UN has ever called; the first, on global AIDS in 2001, helped build momentum toward the Global Fund and PEPFAR. Similar, coordinated, and integrated initiatives are needed to prevent millions of deaths and untold disability caused by NCDs worldwide.

CANCER

One disease process—usually classified as noncommunicable, despite exceptions—warranting closer consideration is cancer. Sometimes considered a problem exclusive to the developed world, cancer is a leading cause of disability and death in low- and middle-income countries, which face 80 percent of the global burden of cancer (measured in DALYs) and yet attract only 5 percent of global resources directed toward cancer care and control.[90] Almost two-thirds of the 7.6 million cancer deaths worldwide occur in such settings.[91] Moreover, as a result of population growth, aging, and reduced mortality associated with infectious diseases, the proportion of the global cancer burden borne by the poor is growing: in 1970, 15 percent of newly reported cancers were in developing countries; in 2008, this figure was 56 percent; and it is expected to rise to 70 percent by 2030.[92]

Although cancer incidence and mortality rates are on the decline in the United States and other wealthy countries—thanks to increased awareness and prevention, prompt detection, and new therapeutics— little progress has been made in cancer care and control in poor countries. The same rhetoric of doubt that was initially heard concerning global AIDS policy crops up in discussions of cancer in poor countries: treatments are too "complex" and "expensive" for poor countries; "scarce resources" would be better spent on more "cost-effective" interventions; prevention and palliation—"comfort care," without narcotics, instead of "heroic measures" like chemotherapy or radiation therapy—are the best bet. In 1993, two researchers affiliated with the U.S. National Cancer Institute put it this way: developing countries "currently lack sufficient economic resources to support the high cost of cancer treatment. . . . Thus, the economic incentive to focus on cancer prevention, which requires less sophisticated and less expensive resources, is particularly compelling in developing countries."[93]

Similar arguments persist today. In 2006, an article summarizing the WHO's "comprehensive approach to cancer control" highlighted the importance of palliation and prevention instead of treatment: "Palliative care . . . should be given high priority in every country. This is especially true in poor countries where . . . the majority of cancer patients will remain uncured in the coming decades."[94] Palliation can significantly improve patients' quality of life and is an important tool in the cancer care arsenal.[95] Pursuing it to the exclusion of available treatments, however, fails to take full advantage of extraordinary recent achievements in cancer care and control.

In the past decade, a growing body of evidence supports the efficacy of treating certain malignancies in resource-poor settings.[96] In fact, many cancers that are prevalent in the developing world are amenable to treatment with off-patent chemotherapeutic regimens—some of them on the WHO's Essential Medicines list—that can be produced by generic pharmaceutical companies at low cost. In Ghana, Cameroon, and Malawi, for example, generic chemotherapy drugs with a 50 percent cure rate for Burkitt's lymphoma are available for less than $50 per patient.[97] Low-cost and effective treatment options are also avail-

TABLE 11.2 CANCERS AMENABLE TO PREVENTION, EARLY DETECTION, AND TREATMENT IN LOW- AND MIDDLE-INCOME COUNTRIES

Preventable cancers by risk factor:
- Tobacco: lung cancer, head and neck cancer, bladder cancer
- Human papillomavirus: cervical cancer, head and neck cancer
- Hepatitis infection: hepatocellular cancer

Cancers that are potentially curable with early detection and treatment, including surgery:
- Cervical cancer
- Breast cancer
- Colorectal cancer

Cancers that are potentially curable with systemic treatment and for which early detection is not crucial:
- Burkitt's lymphoma
- Large-cell lymphoma
- Hodgkin's lymphoma
- Testicular cancer
- Acute lymphoblastic leukemia
- Soft tissue sarcoma
- Osteosarcoma

Cancers that are often well palliated with systemic treatment:
- Kaposi's sarcoma
- Advanced breast cancer
- Ovarian cancer
- Chronic myelogenous leukemia

SOURCE: Paul Farmer, Julio Frenk, Felicia M. Knaul, Lawrence N. Shulman, George Alleyne, Lance Armstrong, Rifat Atun, Douglas Blayney, Lincoln Chen, Richard Feachem, Mary Gospodarowicz, Julie Gralow, Sanjay Gupta, Ana Langer, Julian Lob-Levyt, Claire Neal, Anthony Mbewu, Dina Mired, Peter Piot, K. Srinath Reddy, Jeffrey D. Sachs, Mahmoud Sarhan, and John R. Seffrin, "Expansion of Cancer Care and Control in Countries of Low and Middle Income: A Call to Action," *Lancet* 376, no. 9747 (2010): 1187.

able for cervical, breast, and testicular cancers as well as childhood leukemia.[98] Although some malignancies—including certain pancreatic and lung cancers—remain difficult to treat in affluent and indigent settings alike, there is nonetheless great potential to curb the mortality and morbidity associated with many forms of cancer in low- and middle-income countries using available (and often low-cost) tools (see table 11.2).

Pilot treatment programs in poor countries have realized good outcomes even in the absence of trained oncologists. One program established by Partners In Health, the Dana-Farber Cancer Institute, Harvard Medical School, and Brigham and Women's Hospital has

Intellectual Property and Global Health Equity

A crucial part of achieving global health equity is expanding access to modern medicines and technologies in poor countries. Because intellectual property regimes are one important set of determinants of access to medicines, we take a step back to examine the institution of the patent and its role in the market.

In most countries, national governments grant patents on newly discovered technologies such as medicines. The patent system, which guarantees monopoly rights for a specified period to the person or company that developed the technology, is designed to incentivize innovative and risky research: it allows the patent holder time to recoup the costs of research without market competition. Thus, a patent is by definition an infringement on the free market. Patent systems are primarily regulated by national legal codes, but in an era of increasing globalization, many multinational corporations and governments of developed countries pushed successfully for international governance of intellectual property.[1] In 1994, the World Trade Organization (WTO) established the Agreement on Trade-Related Aspects of Intellectual Property (TRIPS), setting minimum patent law standards for all member states.

One of the most controversial aspects of the agreement was that it restricted access to medical technologies in poor countries. The ethical difficulty in applying a global patenting standard was apparent. Antiretroviral drugs provide useful case studies of the impact of international intellectual property regulations on access to medicines. Because the AIDS pandemic affects patients in both rich and poor countries, pharmaceutical companies, with their eyes on affluent markets, have sufficient incentives to develop new medicines to combat HIV. But the majority of those afflicted live in low-income countries and are unable to pay the same prices as patients in the developed world; many are unable to pay anything at all. In the 1990s, some developing countries began to produce or import lower-cost generic antiretrovirals to answer some of the need. As chapter 5 details, pharmaceutical companies filed lawsuits to stop such generics, arguing that their patents were being violated.

But in fact only a negligible amount of pharmaceutical revenue came from low-income countries.[2] Hence, burdening such countries with patent requirements served only to restrict access to essential medicines while delivering a trickle of income back to corporations. This made little sense in terms of either public health or economics. Furthermore, the patent system in low-income countries was not serving as an incentive for innovation and technology development:

the lack of drug research targeting neglected tropical diseases under-scored the fallacy of that argument.

As pressure mounted, a 2001 WTO conference adopted the Doha Declaration, which acknowledged that governments of low-income countries had the autonomy to determine when the public health ben-efit of broader production of technologies such as new medicines out-weighed the importance of maintaining a patent[3] (a right that the United States has maintained for itself and has exercised on numer-ous occasions).[4] The Doha Declaration helped several countries avoid onerous conditions for importing or producing affordable life-saving medicines.

However, the WTO is not the only body regulating international trade; many trade deals occur outside the organization. In addition, a great deal of biosocial complexity—local as well as transnational—affects access to low-cost generic medicines.

Despite the Doha Declaration, bilateral and multilateral trade agreements continue to restrict generic drug production in many coun-tries. An agreement currently being negotiated between the European Union and India may affect how India issues patents and the ability of Indian companies to ship affordable medicines to other developing countries.[5] The United States has submitted restrictive intellectual property language in the proposed Trans-Pacific Partnership trade agreement, which will eventually include many Pacific Rim countries as signatories, potentially preventing other countries from developing a patent regime and generic production capacity on par with India.[6] Access to new generations of medicines for HIV, cancer, and other diseases continues to be affected by inequities and inefficiencies in global intellectual property policy.

Licensing strategies that allow generic production or tiered pricing in low-income countries have been shown to increase access to essen-tial medicines while not affecting the profitability of the same pat-ented medicines in high-income countries (and therefore not under-mining pharmaceutical companies' incentives to innovate and develop new products).[7] Advocacy for these policies over the past decade has been driven by a wide coalition including the Universities Allied for Essential Medicines, an international organization that is largely student-run. If adopted by international lawmakers, regulators, and pharmaceutical companies—some of which have already found inno-vative ways to make access-minded approaches part of their profit model[8]—such strategies could remove one important obstacle to bringing health technologies old and new to patients whose health depends on them.

provided chemotherapy to patients with cervical, breast, rectal, and squamous head and neck cancers, Kaposi's sarcoma, and Hodgkin's and non-Hodgkin's lymphoma in the rural reaches of Haiti, Rwanda, and Malawi—all settings in which there are no oncologists but plenty of cancer.[99] Outcomes have been good, with few adverse events. Such efforts are much more common in middle-income countries. In Mexico, the government's popular health insurance covers comprehensive treatments for breast and cervical cancer and for a number of pediatric malignancies.[100] Colombia's universal social health insurance has included treatment for cancer since 1993.[101] The King Hussein Cancer Center in Jordan provides treatment for many patients who can't pay for services, including 60 percent of new breast cancer cases.[102] These few examples demonstrate that cancer treatment is feasible in low- and middle-income countries. But each of these programs pales in comparison to the burden of disease; expanding access to cancer care is an urgent priority of the twenty-first century.

Changing incidence and mortality rates associated with many cancers also depends on controlling key risk factors. Smoking is on the rise across the developing world.[103] Awareness of the importance of screening and prompt detection remains low, while economic barriers to seeking care and disease-related stigma are high.[104] Prevention, including vaccination against hepatitis B and HPV as well as anti-tobacco campaigns, must be significantly ramped up to slow the increasing incidence of cancer in the developing world. Rwanda has led the way in taking on cervical cancer: in addition to vigorous screening efforts, the government has already initiated an effort to vaccinate all adolescent girls.[105]

In 2009, the Global Task Force on Expanded Access to Cancer Care and Control in Developing Countries was launched by leaders in global health and cancer care at Dana-Farber Cancer Institute, Harvard Global Equity Initiative, Harvard Medical School, and Harvard School of Public Health. The goal of the task force is to develop, implement, and evaluate strategies to increase access to cancer care and control in concert with partners in the developing world.[106] The group embraces the diagonal approach outlined by Frenk: that is, specific cancers can be treated effectively in ways that also strengthen primary care, prevention, palliation, and other health services. A recalibrated global response that brings together national governments, key funders of research and implementation, international institutions, and NGOs could rapidly scale up this approach—in conjunction with the other priorities outlined in this chapter—in resource-poor settings around the world.

SURGERY

Surgery is an essential tool of modern medicine that remains scarce in many resource-constrained settings. Diseases treatable by surgery—including a number of infections, noncommunicable diseases, malignancies, and conditions afflicting mothers and children—cause substantial mortality and morbidity around the globe. Of the estimated 350,000 to 500,000 mothers who die in childbirth each year, most could be saved with surgical delivery and other means of addressing postpartum hemorrhage.[107] Farming and motor vehicle accidents, peritonitis, long-bone fractures, abscesses, and blindness usually go unattended among the world's poor.[108] Serious cardiac diseases are almost always a death sentence in low-income regions.[109] Millions of people die each year from heart attacks, especially in India, China, and urban centers elsewhere, but very few have access to potentially lifesaving angioplasty or bypass surgery. In sum, the so-called surgical diseases—a category overlapping both communicable and noncommunicable diseases—account for approximately 11 percent of total DALYs worldwide.[110]

Despite the heavy global toll of surgical diseases, there is little access to surgery in most rural areas around the world. Available surgical services are expensive and concentrated in cities.[111] Why does surgery remain scarce? First, the welcome focus on communicable diseases, such as AIDS and malaria and smallpox, has allowed those socialized for scarcity to argue that these pathogens alone are burden enough for health practitioners and weak care delivery platforms. Second, there are almost no surgeons outside urban centers in many poor countries. By some estimates, Africa has less than 1 percent of the surgical workforce of the United States.[112] Third, surgery is often a complex intervention that requires a surgeon, an operating room, anesthesia, autoclaves, sutures, drapes, and other supplies—plus blood-banking capacity and postoperative care. Some surgeries, such as cataract removal, are straightforward, but most demand substantial investment in infrastructure, training, and supplies.

Given these barriers, can high-quality surgical care be delivered in resource-poor settings? A number of examples suggest that integrating surgical services into health facilities is not only possible but yields a high return in terms of morbidity averted and lives saved. A study of efforts by Partners In Health and Zanmi Lasante to provide surgical services in Cange, in rural Haiti, found positive outcomes as well as massive unmet needs. From January 2002 to September 2005, 2,900 surgeries were performed at the hospital in Cange, which provides such services to those unable to pay for them: about half were general surgery, a third obstetric and gynecological, and the rest urologic, plastic, neurologic, ophthalmologic, and cardiothoracic procedures. The distances patients traveled to reach the hospital were striking: half of all patients traveled more than 50 km; a third of patients came from Port-au-Prince (about 80 km from Cange), the capital city, where the great majority of Haiti's operating rooms are located. (Because private and public hospitals in the capital typically charge user fees, Haiti's poorest people lacked and still lack access to surgery.[113]

Many other health providers have also successfully delivered surgical care in settings of poverty. Most focus on specific surgeries or emergency care. The International Federation of Gynecology and Obstetrics, for example, has supported programs providing district-based emergency obstetric services in Uganda, Ethiopia, and Guatemala.[114] International relief organizations such as Médecins Sans Frontières, the Red Cross, and the Red Crescent are adept at providing emergency surgical care after natural disasters and violent conflict; they also perform cesarean deliveries and other obstetrical care, emergency abdominal surgeries, and repair of congenital abnormalities.[115] A 2010 study found that forty-six international organizations working in developing countries reported performing a total of nearly 225,000 surgical procedures each year.[116] After the 2010 Haiti earthquake, relief and rescue teams from around the world provided critical emergency care, including many thousands of surgeries. Partners In Health and Zanmi Lasante reported seeing some three thousand patients and performing 513 emergency surgeries, including wound debridement, fixation of long-bone fractures, and amputations.[117]

Despite these and other examples, surgery remains inaccessible to the great majority of the world's population, and especially to the poorest, who face the largest burden of surgical disease. What is to be done? There is growing consensus about the feasibility (and imperative) of integrating surgical care into health systems across the developing world.[118] Charles Mock and colleagues have suggested a three-tiered prioritization strategy based on disease burden, procedure efficacy, and cost-effectiveness.[119] First-priority conditions include emergencies and common surgical diseases with elective procedures, such as hernia repair, club foot repair, and male circumcision. Plastic surgeons can treat many such conditions, including trauma, burns, and congenital abnormalities, but these specialists are in short supply in developing countries.[120] Trauma response training programs for laypeople have also been shown to be valuable and low cost in resource-constrained settings.[121] Some researchers have suggested that certain surgical procedures can be as cost-effective as other public health interventions.[122]

In addition to vertical surgical interventions, "twinning programs" link a good number of hospitals in the developed world to those in poor nations. But the latter almost always charge user fees and thus rarely provide surgical services to the poorest populations. These programs could be improved by insisting that surgery be available to those in need but unable to pay. Part of this strategy involves investing in new surgical infrastructure and expanding training initiatives in low-income countries. Even district hospitals need multiple operating rooms (at least one for emergencies, usually obstetric, and one for elective cases), blood-banking, anesthesia machines (and staff to use and repair them), a laboratory, and reliable electricity. Training programs could be ramped up alongside efforts to build and rebuild surgical infrastructure and improve systems of health care delivery.

Expanding and improving surgical capacity in resource-constrained settings is synergistic with many other key global health priorities, such as maternal health, noncommunicable diseases, and cancer—not to mention health system strengthening in general. Surgery is, as noted, a pillar of modern obstetrics. We live in a world in which there are too many Caesarian sections performed in some regions and none at all in others. Millennium Development Goal 5, improving maternal health, will be difficult to realize without significant expansion of surgical services for the poorest. Moreover, a number of noncommunicable diseases, including heart disease and certain malignancies, are treatable by surgery. Such synergies reinforce the need for a diagonal approach to expanding surgical care in poor countries. Integrating surgery into health systems would give doctors, nurses, and other health workers in those countries a critical set of tools for responding to many leading causes of mortality and morbidity.

PRIMARY CARE TRANSFORMATION IN THE UNITED STATES

The term "global health" is often used to refer to the health of populations in developing countries. But the United States is on the globe, too. For the past several years, as health care costs have mounted, thorny debates over health care reform have highlighted key problems facing the U.S. health system: millions of uninsured Americans, stark socioeconomic and geographic disparities in health outcomes, provider incentives that promote overuse of unnecessary treatments and procedures, fragmentation of services across venues of care, high rates of preventable medical errors, and an inability to address the complex needs of increasing numbers of patients suffering from multiple chronic diseases.[123] As one bellwether of these systemic problems, the United States, whose infant mortality rate ranked twelfth in the world some fifty years ago, saw its ranking drop to thirty-first in 2008.[124] And yet health care costs are rising unsustainably: currently, the United States spends more than $8,000 per person per year on health care—far more than any other high-income country, many of which have superior health indices—and this figure is increasing.[125] Given that many of the global health challenges considered in this volume stem, in part, from dire poverty and insufficient funding for health care delivery in developing countries, what parallels can be drawn to the crisis of the U.S. health system, which faces problems of a different order?

In fact, some recent efforts to improve health care in the United States suggest that we may be witnessing a convergence in how high-quality care is delivered in countries rich and poor. In the United States, against a century-long backdrop of soaring innovations in medical science,[126] a sobering realization is emerging: new technology alone—novel pharmaceuticals, powerful imaging devices, miraculous surgical procedures—cannot solve the country's health care crisis. Rather, much like initiatives described in chapters 6 and 7, the most promising efforts to transform U.S. health care share several features, most of them linked tightly to delivery. First, they recognize that, by virtue of its broad mandate, primary care offers the most fertile ground for improving access, quality, and efficiency in the overall health system.[127] Second, such efforts seek to reshape care so that it addresses the many social factors that pattern individual and population health and that determine the outcomes of many interventions.[128] Finally, they acknowledge that, in addition to physicians and other professional health workers, community members can contribute significantly to the provision of health care and prevention efforts. Some of these new models of health care delivery in the United States increasingly resemble those pioneered in places like Haiti and Rwanda. Despite radically disparate epidemiologic, political, and financial environments, there are similar paths to be tread in the quest for high-quality, affordable care for all.[129]

The Prevention and Access to Care and Treatment (PACT) program in Boston has utilized a delivery model similar to that used in Haiti and Peru. Its director, Dr. Heidi Behforouz, traveled to Haiti to examine the *accompagnateur* model with the goal of adapting it to an American city with many hospitals but too little in the way of community- and home-based care for chronic disease. In 1997, PACT adopted the accompaniment approach to provide care for AIDS and other chronic diseases for some of the poorest people in Boston. Community health workers were trained (and paid) to provide directly observed therapy in patients' homes, as well as wraparound services such as health education, housing assistance, food support, and psychosocial support.[130] As in Haiti and Peru, PACT has realized positive outcomes—70 percent of its AIDS patients have shown substantial clinical improvement; 35 percent have had shorter hospital stays—with correspondingly decreasing costs. An examination of Medicaid claims from patients enrolled in the PACT program revealed a 16 percent net savings. The PACT model is now being emulated in Miami, New York City, and within the Navajo Nation.[131] But realigning incentives in the U.S. care system has been difficult, and these efforts struggle to find funding for training and compensation of community health workers.

This struggle has not been for lack of proven effectiveness of community- and home-based care for chronic disease, nor even demonstrable cost-effectiveness of pilot efforts. Another example is the Camden Coalition of Healthcare Providers, started in 2002 by Dr. Jeffrey Brenner. Seeking to cut costs while providing better care, the Camden Coalition began by identifying patients for whom the health system was incurring the highest costs. The result was not surprising: poor patients with multiple chronic diseases received most of their care—much of it uncoordinated and costly to the health system—in the emergency room. Health care expenditures for these patients averaged an astonishing $1.2 million per patient per year. The Camden Coalition sought to change the status quo by providing home-based comprehensive care to a small group of high-cost patients, while also attending to social determinants of ill health: lack of access to healthful foods and regular exercise, drug and alcohol abuse, housing contaminated with mold. The results have been dramatic: hospital and emergency room visits decreased by 40 percent, and costs decreased by more than 50 percent.[132] The Camden Coalition's model of home-based care for the sickest patients improved the quality and equity of care, while bringing down overall health expenditures.

Health Leads, another organization started in Boston, has pioneered a different approach for offering wraparound services to poor patients in several American cities. By setting up volunteer-based service centers in hospital waiting rooms, Health Leads enables doctors and nurses to "prescribe" social services like food support and housing improvements, along with medications. Health volunteers, many of them college students, then help patients attend to these social prescriptions. For example, Harlem Hospital Center refers all patients with elevated body mass index to Health Leads, which helps them access healthy foods, gym memberships, and other weight-loss resources. This approach shifts the burden of addressing patients' social needs—something doctors and nurses are not trained to do—to volunteers and community members who are better suited to help with these problems. One study found that Health Leads more than tripled the demand for social work at a partner clinic, helping overstretched primary care doctors counter the social barriers to good health among their patients.[133]

Yet another example of community-based health care delivery in the United States is Atlantic City's Special Care Center, run by Dr. Rushika Fernandopulle since 2007. By recruiting "health coaches" from patients' neighborhoods, the Special Care Center provides home-based care for poor patients, many of whom have chronic diseases. After one year, an evaluation documented impressive outcomes: 63 percent of smokers with lung disease had quit smoking; hypertension in the patient population was largely under control; and many patients' cholesterol levels had decreased. Moreover, hospital admissions and emergency room visits had dropped by 40 percent, surgical procedures by 25 percent, and costs rose by only 4 percent, compared to a 25 percent increase the previous year.[134] Unpublished data from subsequent years reveal further savings, as the model has been expanded.[135]

These and other examples—all of which seek to foster "patient-centered medical homes"[136]—point to a way forward in the United States. Community-based programs that provide home-based care, including psychosocial and wraparound services, to the most marginalized (and often sickest) people in the country can increase access to care, improve quality of care, and simultaneously cut aggregate costs. And we need to mean it when we say "home-based care," since many of these medical homes are not homes at all. Yet the home is the locus of most caregiving. In other words, health care delivery strategies similar to those pioneered in Haiti, Rwanda, and elsewhere in the developing world might offer a means of easing the U.S. health care crisis.[137]

Policymakers have begun taking steps toward reform along these lines. The 2010 Affordable Care Act created the Center for Medicaid and Medicare Innovation, which has $1 billion to invest in novel initiatives capable of improving quality of care while reducing costs, money that could support, expand, and strengthen programs modeled on the sorts of examples offered here. The Affordable Care Act also offers new incentives for primary care providers, which could help rebalance the health system away from specialty care and, in turn, save thousands of lives and millions of dollars. But further policy change is needed to scale up models of effective and affordable health care delivery capable of transforming primary health care in the United States.

Making sure that the field of global health includes the health challenges of the United States and other high- and middle-income countries—and, conversely, making sure that discussions of health care reform in these wealthier settings include lessons from global health—is crucial for advancing equity around the world. Health inequity is a problem everywhere, not just inside the borders of developing countries. In addition, if global health is perceived as a problem of the "other," of interest only to the few who feel motivated to help poor countries, then it is unlikely to gain the depth and breadth of engagement that will be required to address many of the problems we face.

Fully integrating global health into the feedback loop between medical research, service, and training would bolster the primary care transformation in the United States. It has become increasingly clear that the social determinants of health have a decisive impact on the specific burden of disease experienced by communities anywhere in the world.[138] Yet the great majority of the world's medical students and practitioners are not trained to consider these powerful processes beyond superficial "social histories" of individual patients. Resocializing medical education is among the most important priorities for modern medicine in the early twenty-first century, and global health has a critical role to play in this effort. Case studies drawn from resource-poor settings around the world often provide the starkest demonstrations of how social forces become embodied as adverse health outcomes; students and doctors can apply such lessons about the pathophysiology of social determinants of health wherever they happen to practice. Furthermore, keeping global health as "other" forfeits the chance for reverse innovation—using tools designed for the developing world to address problems faced in places of greater abundance. Efforts to improve health anywhere will need to mine best practices developed in all settings and apply them as befits the local setting. Global health research and practice can enhance knowledge of disease and treatment in countless ways, and it should be integrated fully into the training of health care providers everywhere in the world.

TRANSCENDING TRIBALISM AND EXPANDING THE PIE

If there is a theme to the preceding outline of the key challenges in global health today, it is that pronouncing any one disease or health priority "neglected" is misleading. In fact, such neglect is the chief pathology of all systems that distribute goods and services unevenly and unfairly. When global health is understood as a zero-sum game—when practitioners and policymakers are socialized for scarcity—some priority always loses when another wins. Journalist Laurie Garrett notes that too often Western donors favor "diseases and health conditions that enjoy a temporary spotlight," promoting single-disease programs while public health measures receive little attention. She cites the example of pregnant women with HIV/AIDS who are provided with the antiretroviral zidovudine to prevent transmission of the virus to their babies, but who lack access to most modern obstetrics services such as basic surgery, blood-banking, and antihemorrhagics.[139]

But a simple swing in global priorities—from AIDS to maternal and child health, for example—misses the point. AIDS, tuberculosis, malaria, maternal health, childhood diarrheal and pulmonary diseases, neglected tropical diseases, noncommunicable diseases, mental health, cancers, surgical diseases, not to mention clean water, malnutrition, and many other public health priorities—all of these areas demand increased funding and more substantial engagement. The best approach is to respond to ranking causes of mortality and morbidity in ways that strengthen health systems.

If the golden age of global health has taught us anything, it's that we must avoid the theory, dimly articulated, of limited good.[140] This theory is predicated on the assumption of scarce resources—the same pathology that triggered chronic failures of imagination in responding to the AIDS pandemic and many other leading killers around the globe in the last century. But the resource pie is not fixed. There's not a single compelling argument to support the claim that the approaches we have advocated are too expensive or beyond our means. In 1998, most Western leaders and opinion-makers believed that treating AIDS in developing countries was too difficult and too expensive. A coalition of health practitioners, advocacy groups, and policymakers reimagined the possible in the fight against global AIDS, as outlined in chapter 5. In 2000, President Bill Clinton issued Executive Order 13144 supporting the use of a compulsory license for generic production of antiretroviral medications in South Africa and elsewhere. The Global Fund and PEPFAR were launched in the next three years. And there has since been a dramatic rise in development assistance for health, which increased from $5.59 billion in 1990 to $21.79 billion in 2007.[141]

Instead of jockeying for a thin sliver of the resource pie, energies should be spent expanding the pie, capturing synergies and spill-over effects of health and development initiatives, and strengthening health systems until they are capable of delivering high-quality care for all. Resources may be limited but, despite a global recession, they are less limited now than ever before. Times of crisis can in fact motivate greater concern for equity by exposing the vulnerability of the poor. The U.S. government passed Social Security during the Great Depression; Britain established the National Health Service right after World War II; and Mexico launched its landmark universal health insurance program, Seguro Popular, after the 1995 financial meltdown. "History teaches us that many of the most enlightened social protection measures have been crafted precisely at times of economic or political crisis," says Julio Frenk.[142] The second decade of the twenty-first century could be the dusk of the golden age of global health, or it could continue and even accelerate the progress of the last ten years, beyond the imagination of practitioners today. In part this will depend on sustaining a movement for global health equity, the topic of the final chapter.

SUGGESTED READING

Bukhman, Gene, and Alice Kidder, eds. *The Partners In Health Guide to Chronic Care Integration for Endemic Non-Communicable Diseases, Rwanda Edition: Cardiac, Renal, Diabetes, Pulmonary, and Palliative Care.* Boston: Partners In Health, 2011.
Abdallah S. Daar, Peter A. Singer, Deepa Leah Persad, Stig K. Pramming, David R. Matthews, Robert Beaglehole, Alan Bernstein, Leszek K.

Borysiewicz, Stephen Colagiuri, Nirmal Ganguly, Roger I. Glass, Diane T. Finegood, Jeffrey Koplan, Elizabeth G. Nabel, George Sarna, Nizal Sarrafzadegan, Richard Smith, Derek Yach, and John Bell. "Grand Challenges in Chronic Non-Communicable Diseases." *Nature* 450, no. 7169 (November 22, 2007): 494–496.

Farmer, Paul, Julio Frenk, Felicia M. Knaul, Lawrence N. Shulman, George Alleyne, Lance Armstrong, Rifat Atun, Douglas Blayney, Lincoln Chen, Richard Feachem, Mary Gospodarowicz, Julie Gralow, Sanjay Gupta, Ana Langer, Julian Lob-Levyt, Claire Neal, Anthony Mbewu, Dina Mired, Peter Piot, K. Srinath Reddy, Jeffrey D. Sachs, Mahmoud Sarhan, and John R. Seffrin. "Expansion of Cancer Care and Control in Countries of Low and Middle Income: A Call to Action," *Lancet* 376, no. 9747 (2010): 1186–1193.

Frenk, Julio. "Bridging the Divide: Global Lessons from Evidence-Based Health Policy in Mexico." *Lancet* 368, no. 9539 (2006): 954–961.

Hotez, Peter J. *Forgotten People, Forgotten Diseases: The Neglected Tropical Diseases and Their Impact on Global Health and Development.* Washington, D.C.: ASM Press, 2008.

Institute of Medicine. *Unequal Treatment: Confronting Racial and Ethnic Disparities in Health Care.* Edited by Brian D. Smedley, Adrienne Y. Stith, and Alan R. Nelson. Washington, D.C.: National Academies Press, 2002.

Jamison, Dean T., Joel G. Breman, Anthony R. Measham, George Alleyne, Mariam Claeson, David B. Evans, Prabhat Jha, Anne Mills, and Philip Musgrove, eds. *Disease Control Priorities in Developing Countries.* 2nd ed. Washington, D.C.: World Bank, 2006.

Kapczynski, Amy, Samantha Chaifetz, Zachary Katz, and Yochai Benkler. "Addressing Global Health Inequities: An Open Licensing Approach for University Innovations." *Berkeley Technology Law Journal* 20, no. 2 (2005): 1031–1114.

Kremer, Michael, and Rachel Glennerster. *Strong Medicine: Creating Incentives for Pharmaceutical Research on Neglected Diseases.* Princeton, N.J.: Princeton University Press, 2004.

Mock, Charles, Meena Cherian, Catherine Juillard, Peter Donkor, Stephen Bickler, Dean Jamison, and Kelly McQueen. "Developing Priorities for Addressing Surgical Conditions Globally: Furthering the Link between Surgery and Public Health Policy." *World Journal of Surgery* 34, no. 3 (2010): 381–385.

Mukherjee, Joia S., Donna J. Barry, Hind Satti, Maxi Raymonville, Sarah Marsh, and Mary Kay Smith-Fawzi. "Structural Violence: A Barrier to Achieving the Millennium Development Goals for Women." *Journal of Women's Health* 20, no. 4 (2011): 593–597.

Ozgediz, Doruk, Peter Dunbar, Charles Mock, Meena Cherion, Selwyn O. Rogers Jr., Robert Riviello, John G. Meara, Dean Jamison, Sarah B. Macfarlane, Frederick Burkle Jr., and Kelly McQueen. "Bridging the Gap between Public Health and Surgery: Access to Surgical Care in Low- and Middle-Income Countries." *Bulletin of the American College of Surgeons,* 94, no. 5 (2009): 14–20.

Samb, Badara, Tim Evans, Mark Dybul, Rifat Atun, Jean-Paul Moatti, Sania Nishtar, Anna Wright, Francesca Celletti, Justine Hsu, Jim Yong Kim, Ruairi Brugha, Asia Russell, and Carissa Etienne (World Health Organization Maximizing Positive Synergies Collaborative Group). "An Assessment of Interactions between Global Health Initiatives and Country Health Systems." *Lancet* 373, no. 9681 (2009): 2137–2169.

World Health Organization Mental Health Gap Action Programme (mhGAP). *Scaling Up Care for Mental, Neurological, and Substance Use Disorders.* 2008. www.who.int/mental_health/mhgap_final_english.pdf.

A Movement for Global Health Equity?

A Closing Reflection

MATTHEW BASILICO, VANESSA KERRY, LUKE MESSAC, ARJUN SURI, JONATHAN WEIGEL, MARGUERITE THORP BASILICO, JOIA MUKHERJEE, PAUL FARMER

This text has stressed that the limited vision of what is currently deemed possible, whether in the halls of power or in the midst of great privatism, is not immutable—just as resources need not always be "scarce" or technologies static. Prevailing notions of the possible may be expanded by new experience, strong partnerships, and strategic advocacy. We have recounted a number of efforts to reimagine the possible in global health, and this chapter will describe a couple more. Some stories are of visionary policymakers; some are about people living with AIDS and their allies, including students; many involve a wide range of individuals and organizations. These are stories of courage in the face of seemingly insurmountable challenges. While moving from inspiration to action may be risky—fraught with unintended consequences—it can be done by accompanying, over the long term, the intended beneficiaries of the action, while cultivating habits of critical self-reflection. One powerful form of engagement in global health work, discussed in chapter 5 but warrants further analysis, links evidence to advocacy and activism.[1]

ADVOCACY AND ACTIVISM: GRASSROOTS EFFORTS

Advancing global health equity demands broad-based and transnational movements. Meaningful reforms in domestic and foreign policy rarely come about without sustained advocacy efforts. The roots of the abolition of the slave trade in the British Empire in 1807 can be traced to a decades-long grassroots movement spawned by a small group of Quakers and a young Baptist minister.[2] The anti-apartheid movement targeting the South African government during the 1980s and early 1990s mobilized concerned individuals and groups from the slums of Johannesburg to the campuses of American universities. These and other campaigns highlight the ability of informed and dedicated advocates, including students, to bend the arc of history toward justice a little more rapidly.

The past few decades have also furnished examples of effective global health activism focused on increasing access to modern medicine and advancing a broader movement for social and economic rights. Activists, along with health practitioners, researchers, and policymakers, were a key part of the coalition that reimagined the global AIDS effort—and got the rest of the world to do the same. This chapter briefly reconsiders three notable advocacy campaigns in the recent history of global health.

AIDS Coalition to Unleash Power

The U.S. Food and Drug Administration granted federal approval to the first AIDS drug in March 1987. The long-awaited azidothymidine (AZT)—branded as Retrovir—was soon released by pharmaceutical company Burroughs Wellcome with a price tag of $8,000 per patient per year. The most expensive medicine in history, Retrovir was inaccessible to many Americans needing treatment, especially the poor and otherwise vulnerable, not to mention those in other countries. Burroughs Wellcome defended the price by citing high research and development costs as well as plans to continue research. But with 33,000 new U.S. cases of HIV/AIDS reported in 1987 and an additional 250,000 then expected by 1991, many urged price reductions to make the drug more widely available.[3]

People living with HIV/AIDS and their friends, families, caregivers, and allies came together in early 1987 in New York City to form the AIDS Coalition to Unleash Power—ACT UP—an organization that aimed to combat "the government's mismanagement of the AIDS crisis."[4] Only weeks after its founding, activists staged their first demonstration, on March 24, 1987, protesting Burroughs Wellcome's profit model and the drug-approval policies of the FDA, which, they argued, contributed to the limited supply and high price of Retrovir.

In a *New York Times* op-ed released the day before the protest, Gay Men's Health Crisis co-founder and ACT UP founding member Larry Kramer wrote:

> There is no question on the part of anyone fighting AIDS that the FDA constitutes the single most incomprehensible bottleneck in American bureaucratic history—one that is actually prolonging this roll call of death. . . . AIDS sufferers, who have nothing to lose, are more than willing to be guinea pigs. . . . We cannot understand for the life of us, or for what life in us many of us still cling to hungrily, why the FDA withholds them—especially when the victims are so eager to be part of the experimental process.[5]

Given that two-thirds of people with HIV at that time were expected to die within five years,[6] gaining access to new drugs before the FDA had completed its approval process was quite literally a matter of life and death. Of course, many of the drug candidates were simply toxic; Western medicine's long history of ineffective and unsafe therapeutics is the reason for the cautious policies of the FDA.[7] Nonetheless, as Kramer pointed out, there were viable drugs pending approval that could save patients' lives. Shortly after ACT UP's first demonstration, the FDA announced that it would shorten its approval process for HIV drugs (and, later, for other drugs) by two years.[8] With continued pressure, including repeated public protests such as the one shown in figure 12.1, the FDA eventually allowed AIDS patients to participate in clinical trials.[9]

Burroughs Wellcome was another of ACT UP's targets. In 1989, two years later in the course of the epidemic, AZT still cost $8,000 a year and remained the most expensive medicine in history. Activists kept up the pressure. On September 14, 1989, ACT UP members protested the high price of Retrovir on Wall Street, holding banners and chanting, "Sell Wellcome!" at the New York Stock Exchange. Within days, Burroughs Wellcome decreased the price of Retrovir 20 percent, from $8,000 to $6,400.[10]

Such initiatives had effects beyond policy change. Building on grassroots movements to expand access to family planning, given the role of contraceptive barrier methods as an AIDS prevention strategy,[11] AIDS treatment activism helped increase the public's participation in consumer health policy. The AIDS movement spurred citizens to engage with pharmaceutical companies and the FDA to push for the development and approval of treatment options. "AIDS activism has changed activism itself," writes political scientist Patricia Siplon, "partly as a result of

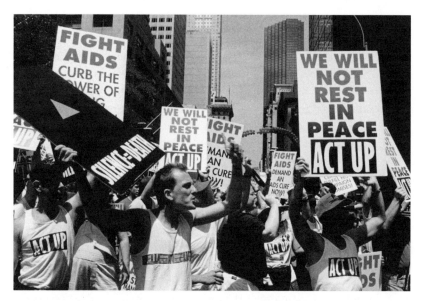

FIGURE 12.1. An ACT UP protest in New York City, June 1993. Courtesy Andrew Holbrooke/Corbis.

some of the special circumstances of the AIDS epidemic. . . . The successes of AIDS activists created a new model featuring direct action, self-empowerment, and self-education first for other health-based groups and ultimately even for activist groups outside the health realm."[12]

ACT UP was the first AIDS activist group "to draw a broad spectrum of people and unite them into a cohesive organization." It was said "to have sparked a new rise in nonviolent, nonpartisan, political advocacy," driven by a diverse group of activists that included people across genders, ages, sexual orientations, and educational and socioeconomic backgrounds, not to mention HIV status, which helped to give it traction. The movement not only utilized civil disobedience tactics to gain attention but also benefited from the work of young, educated activists who learned about the emerging science of HIV in order to better track the research and development of new drugs and treatment programs.[13]

Treatment Action Campaign

The Treatment Action Campaign was initiated in South Africa in December 1998 by a small group of political activists. The two founders, Zackie Achmat and Mark Heywood, were veterans of the anti-apartheid movement and members of the African National Congress. TAC's constitution describes the group's objective: "to challenge by means of litigation, lobbying, advocacy and all forms of legitimate mobilization, any barrier or obstacle, including unfair discrimination, that limits access to treatment for HIV/AIDS in the private or public sector."[14] (Chapter 9 describes TAC's use of legal activism in the fight to secure treatment for AIDS patients.)

When TAC was founded, South Africa's HIV prevalence rate was approaching 25 percent; an estimated six hundred South Africans died of AIDS every day. But while access to antiretroviral treatment remained limited to the wealthy, AIDS claimed little attention in the national political debate. Amid complex cycles of accusation and counteraccusation that surrounded the AIDS epidemic—conspiracy theories, worries of economic ruin, massive loss of life among blacks but not whites, charges that the spread of the virus was evidence of black sexual promiscuity—many of the country's black political leaders were loath to discuss HIV openly.[15]

In poor communities beset by AIDS, TAC members taught infected and affected South Africans about the science of HIV; the group also discussed social and economic rights and the responsibilities of the state in the realization of those rights. While AIDS activism in South Africa had been led primarily by a small, mostly white, group during the 1980s and early 1990s, TAC sought to build a broad-based, racially integrated organization. Membership included young people, faith-based organizations, health care professionals, and labor unions. In 2005, Achmat described the group's membership as 80 percent unemployed, 70 percent women, 70 percent young people between the ages of fourteen and twenty-four, and 90 percent African.[16] TAC also built links with AIDS activists in high-income countries—particularly with ACT UP chapters in the United States—to help develop educational materials to build "treatment literacy" for people living with the virus.

While organizing communities at the grassroots level, TAC engaged its membership in large-scale political advocacy. Using methods ranging from civil disobedience, street demonstrations, lawsuits in constitutional court, data-driven pamphlets, and limited antiretroviral treatment programs for members, TAC sought to keep its members healthy and health literate while pressing the public sector to recognize the right to quality health care.[17] When the Pharmaceutical Manufacturers Association filed a lawsuit to overturn South Africa's Medicines Act in

2000, TAC submitted an amicus curiae brief and organized a march that brought five thousand people to the steps of Pretoria's High Court on the first day of the case. Three years later, when it seemed clear that President Thabo Mbeki would not make treatment access a national priority, TAC led a march of twenty thousand protestors to the South African Parliament to demand a national treatment program. These demonstrations, which highlighted the impact of intellectual property restrictions and government inaction on access to essential medicines, drew international media attention.

TAC built the largest organized activist constituency of people living with AIDS in the developing world. Its protests and litigation helped spur price reductions and public-sector programs that began providing antiretroviral therapy for hundreds of thousands of South Africans.[18] Beyond expanding access to treatment, TAC also tried to reimagine what it meant to live with AIDS in South Africa. In 1998, an openly HIV-positive activist named Gugu Dlamini had been stoned to death by her neighbors in KwaZulu-Natal; less than two years later, thousands of South Africans took to the streets in TAC's t-shirts, which read "HIV POSITIVE."[19]

2004 and 2008 STOP AIDS Campaigns

Two advocacy initiatives in which students played an especially important role occurred during the 2004 and 2008 U.S. presidential campaigns. In 2004, a coalition of AIDS activist groups, including Health GAP, the Global AIDS Alliance, and the Student Global AIDS Campaign (who sponsored the demonstration pictured in figure 12.2), collaborated in an effort to garner a commitment from every major presidential candidate to double the Bush administration's five-year $15 billion plan to combat AIDS in poor countries. The tactic of choice was "bird-dogging": questioners were dispatched to hundreds of town hall events in Iowa, New Hampshire, and other states with early primaries to repeatedly ask candidates to pledge to double AIDS appropriations to $30 billion over five years. The questions came from students, church groups, and people living with AIDS, who coordinated their efforts to ensure representation at as many events as possible. The candidates were often noncommittal at first. But early in the primary season, each of the seven Democratic candidates signed a pledge committing to the proposed funding level if elected. President George W. Bush, who had announced PEPFAR in 2003, did not commit to addi-

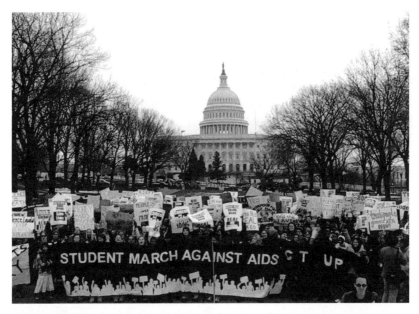

FIGURE 12.2. The Student Global AIDS Campaign organized this 2005 march in Washington, D.C., which drew students from more than one hundred colleges and universities to demand greater support for global health programs. Courtesy Andrew Kohan.

tional funding for global AIDS. In part because he held fewer small-scale question-and-answer events during his reelection campaign, he proved a more difficult target for the activists.

Four years later, activist groups reprised the STOP AIDS campaign, demanding that funding increase to $50 billion over five years. The STOP AIDS 2008 platform also included pledges to train and retain 140,000 new health care workers in poor countries; to repeal the ban on federal funding for syringe exchanges; to expand Medicaid coverage for people in the United States with HIV; and to support trade policies that increased access to generic drugs for important health needs beyond AIDS. Again, candidates responded to voters at pancake breakfasts and barbecues and in hotel lobbies, ice cream parlors, and churches. Once again, each of the Democratic candidates pledged to meet the activists' targets. Then-senator Barack Obama reiterated this pledge at public events and on his campaign website. Although many Republican candidates published platforms on global health and foreign aid, none pledged $50 billion for global AIDS efforts.

Each of these campaigns introduced demands for funding that

reimagined the possible. When the U.S. Congress considered the reauthorization of PEPFAR in the summer of 2008, three of the candidates who had signed the $50 billion pledge—Barack Obama, Hillary Clinton, and Joseph Biden—were members of the U.S. Senate, and one—Biden—was chair of the Committee on Foreign Relations, the body tasked with ushering the reauthorization bill through the Senate. With the presumptive leaders of the Democratic Party bound to this pledge, the Democrat-controlled House and Senate passed a reauthorization bill that included $48 billion over five years to fund the battle against AIDS, tuberculosis, malaria; microbicide development; and health systems strengthening in resource-poor settings. Other elements of the activists' platform, including the repeal of the ban on federal funding for syringe exchange programs, became law in the months following President Obama's inauguration (though the ban on syringe exchange funding has since been reinstated by the Republican-controlled House of Representatives, who inserted such language into the annual federal budget).

There were, of course, many other factors influencing the expansion of PEPFAR: a growing body of evidence from the field that antiretroviral treatment not only was deliverable and effective in resource-poor settings but also boosted prevention and primary care services and health systems in general; increasing acknowledgment of the links between health and economic development; concern about the pandemic's effect on fragile states and the consequences for U.S. national security. Nonetheless, activists played a key part in this story, as they must continue to do in the ongoing movement for global health equity.

THE ADVOCATE'S TOOLKIT: ACTIVIST STRATEGIES FOR GLOBAL HEALTH EQUITY

This chapter argues that supporters of global health equity do not need to hold official positions of power to make a significant impact. Students, health workers, lawyers, people living with HIV, and other grassroots activists have changed global health policy through effective advocacy; their tactics are available to anyone with a passion for equity. Included here are some of the most useful and accessible tools employed by global health activists.

ENGAGE IN CRITICAL SELF-REFLECTION

Effective advocacy begins with thoughtfully considering your own position, sources of inspiration, and potential role in the movement for global health equity. People in all stations of life can find meaningful roles to play;

the challenge is discerning the reaches of your local moral world in the context of the larger movement and preparing (if possible) for unintended consequences of purposive social action.

FIND GOOD PARTNERS

A number of groups, some of them described in this book, are already engaged in building an advocacy movement for global health equity. Such organizations include, for example, Health GAP, the Student Global AIDS Campaign, RESULTS, ACT UP, the ONE Campaign, Oxfam America, the Treatment Action Campaign, Partners In Health, and many others. These groups understand some of the mechanics of policy change; with local chapters across the United States and around the world, they seek to give visibility to key issues and gain political traction. Find a group that fits your interests, or organize your own, and understand that power resides in partnerships. Remember that your partners need to include those most affected by the problems your activism seeks to address.

KNOW THE ISSUES

Effective advocates are well informed about key global health issues and also the local political climate. Determine the issues on which particular political leaders might have leverage—perhaps in congressional committee work or by sponsoring specific pieces of legislation, for example. Always remember that enduring activism needs to be based on careful and accurate analysis of what are complex biosocial issues; such understanding is a chief tool in promoting global health equity. But also remember that these are human problems, and the ability to engage with them is not limited to those with certificates of advanced training.

START A DIALOGUE WITH POLICYMAKERS

Reach out to representatives in local and national government. Get a sense of their position: if they do not support your concerns, find out why. You might have something to learn from them either about the issue or about the mechanics of political change. Think of ways to align their interests with those of the movement for global health equity. If they offer support, ask them to champion efforts or introduce legislation. The authorization of PEPFAR, documented in chapter 5, shows that these issues can have broad appeal across the political spectrum.

HIGHLIGHT KEY ISSUES

If you encounter resistance or aren't granted meetings with political officials, think of creative ways to demonstrate the importance and promote the visibility of global health issues. Tactics such as these have proven effective in building support among members of Congress, state legislators, and local politicians:

- Calling or writing, especially if you can generate great numbers of calls or letters, can draw officials' attention to an issue.

- Bird-dogging can elicit public comments and pledges from political leaders.
- Drafting, circulating, and presenting a petition can demonstrate broad support and can introduce you to new allies.
- Setting up meetings with elected representatives can start a constructive dialogue about the potential for change and any possible obstacles.
- Placing commentary in the media, whether traditional or social media, is another key tool in building public awareness. Op-eds, letters to the editor, blog posts, and posts on Facebook and Twitter can reach a wide audience. Bring printed copies of published writing to events: it shows that you are engaged with the issues and gives others the chance to do the same.

ORGANIZE A PUBLIC DEMONSTRATION

Public displays—for example, a protest, a boycott, a sit-in, a public fast, or performance art—are among the most effective ways to raise the visibility of key issues. Such actions sometimes work best at political events, where officials can be held accountable for their responses. Press coverage and social media can amplify the impact of such events, so reach out to local outlets beforehand.

BUILD A COALITION

A broad base of thoughtful and engaged individuals is the first step in building a movement for global health equity. Reach out to local organizations—religious, community, service-oriented, political, cultural—as well as to students and peers and other informal networks to build a coalition of support for these issues.

BE THE CHANGE

Being humble means listening before speaking out. Listen carefully to others, especially those who disagree with you. Everyone has a valuable perspective worth considering as you seek to improve your own platform and strategy. Don't underestimate one-on-one conversations with peers. Nothing compares to the strength of genuine connection in creating solidarity around a cause.

ADVANCING GLOBAL HEALTH EQUITY

Every storm must begin with a single drop of rain. And so it is with
every worthwhile movement. . . . It begins with an idea that is too
simple to be taken seriously . . . and then comes the storm.
—Marco Caceres

Former U.S. surgeon general Julius Richmond, who taught us a great deal, described three components of policy change: knowledge base, political will, and social strategy.[20] This model is worth adopting in the movement for global health equity. First, as this book emphasizes, policies must be evidence-based; global health practitioners and researchers must continue to build the knowledge base about how to deliver care efficiently and equitably through durable health systems in settings rich and poor. Universities and affiliates, including the students, faculty, and staff, can better contribute to knowledge generation when they are committed to bridging the know-do gap. Second, once we know what works, we need an equity plan. Scaling up evidence-based health care delivery strategies often requires high-level policy change, which demands broad-based political will. One way to build political will—and this brings us to Dr. Richmond's third point—is social strategy: grassroots groups demonstrating support for an issue can spur politicians and other decision-makers to enact large-scale policy change.

For the most ambitious movements, this third component can be the most difficult. To refer back to the writing of Peter Berger and Thomas Luckmann (discussed in chapter 2), the normalization and institutionalization of injustice embeds structures that perpetuate the status quo among dominant political and economic systems—an economy based on transatlantic human trafficking, for example, or a racist political regime. Hence *structural violence*. Breaking free from these structures often hinges on the ingenuity, persistence, and resilience of large-scale social movements. India's fight for independence in the 1940s, the U.S. civil rights movement in the 1960s, the fall of apartheid in the 1990s— each of these twentieth-century milestones drew on vigorous social mobilization.

The global AIDS movement illustrates Dr. Richmond's model. Once it became clear that antiretroviral therapy could be delivered effectively in resource-poor settings—once even a fragment of the knowledge base was established—PEPFAR and the Global Fund funded public and private implementers to increase access to ART around the globe. Millions of lives have been saved. They helped fund the equity plan. Building the political will necessary to launch these ambitious programs—the most ambitious global health initiatives in history—demanded a social strategy capable of bringing together AIDS activists, liberal and conservative U.S. politicians, leading scientists and health practitioners, international policymakers, celebrities, and thought leaders. The history of global health is populated by many other examples. Organizations like the Grameen Bank and BRAC and Village Health Works and Zanmi Lasante have scaled up evidence-based practices by echoing and amplifying voices from the bottom billion and by building alliances with government officials and international policymakers and with patients and families and students and donors. There is great power in partnership.

This volume focuses on the importance of global health as an *academic field,* one drawing on a handful of key disciplines and methodologies. *Reimagining Global Health* reminds readers—and we hope there will be many—that there have been innumerable good-will attempts to improve the health of the poor over the past centuries. But most have had unintended consequences; some have reinforced power structures and ambitions that do not square with equity and a rights-based approach to global health concerns. This scholarly approach can be complemented by tackling policy and implementation efforts. One sketch of a global health advocacy agenda emerges from this volume: increasing aid while improving aid effectiveness, strengthening health systems, and developing and delivering new health technologies, for example. The mainstream international institutions—from the WHO to the World Bank to UNICEF—are now contemplating each of these challenges.

Beyond academia and development agencies bilateral and multilateral, there are many avenues for engagement in the movement for global health equity. Health practitioners willing to tackle the pathologies of poverty by accompanying the destitute sick and those who seek to provide care for them are in short supply. Skilled teachers and pedagogues are necessary to train the next generation of global health practitioners. Researchers employing methodologies from molecular genetics to pharmacokinetics, from epidemiology to econometrics, and from ethnography to history are needed to build robust critical feedback loops and to continue improving the quality of available tools and technologies as well as the efficiency and equity of global health delivery. Practitioners, trainers, and researchers will often be the same people or will work together closely; integrating research, service, and training is the best strategy we know for making global health more than just a collection of problems. Skilled policymakers and informed advocates are urgently required. And activist organizations in both developed and developing countries continue to play a crucial role.

But there is also great need for engaged individuals in diverse fields that this text has not mentioned in sufficient detail. Engineers, such as the recent inventors of a $25 neonatal incubator, can find ways of implementing point-of-care diagnostics and preventatives and therapeutics in remote areas.[21] Business entrepreneurs, such as the founders of Aravind Eye Hospital, a low-cost, tertiary-level ophthalmologic care hospital in south India, can improve the efficiency, scale, and accountability of health care delivery in resource-poor settings. Producers of solar panels, wind turbines, and other clean energy innovations can power hospitals in poor places that often have plenty of sunlight and wind but little affordable energy. Writers like Nicholas Kristof, who has vividly depicted gender disparities and many health challenges around the globe, can help garner public attention and swell the ranks of the movement for global health equity.[22]

Architects and builders can help raise clinics and hospitals that not only promote infection control but also confer dignity upon their patients through elegant design.[23] Painters and sculptors and artists can further enrich such facilities by making them temples not just of healing but also of beauty and color. Musicians, such as Bono and the members of Arcade Fire, can generate support for global health issues among their fans and become thought leaders in the field. Computer scientists can develop effective electronic medical records systems and help deliver them in low-income settings. Scholars can turn their diverse training toward problems that have plagued humanity from time immemorial. This list goes on and on. Just about every skill or occupation can be leveraged in the movement for global health equity.

We hope young people (and more experienced practitioners) who read this book will find ways to become involved in this movement, no matter their level of training or experience. Students are in a privileged position to learn about global health inequities and become engaged, unencumbered by affiliations with institutions who have vested interests in the status quo; they can develop habits of critical self-reflection necessary for smart and effective global health work. This is a potent combination.

The gradients of global health inequality are patterned by large-scale social forces perpetuating poverty, inequality, food and water insecurity, poor education, unsafe housing, and high unemployment. Economic development—growth in GDP, say—can help lift people out of poverty and vulnerability: in most places, increased family income is associated with better access to nutrition, education, and health care. But, as we've learned the hard way, growth is no panacea. Even most high-income countries fail to provide basic protections to all their citizens, especially the poorest.

Joining the movement for global health equity begins by learning about the disparities that prevent billions from living good lives in full health; this is a lifelong pursuit, but one we hope this book has enhanced for its readers. Joining this movement means finding creative ways to leverage one's own skills and interests and to work with others to advance an agenda for social and economic rights. For many, joining the movement will mean accompanying the sick and the poor and sticking with the task until it is deemed completed not by the *accompagnateur* but by those being accompanied. Global health equity is a noble ambition, but it remains only a beginning to the pursuit of a more just, fair society that allows our children, wherever they are born, a decent shot at a decent life.

Declaration of Alma-Ata

International Conference on Primary
Health Care, Alma-Ata, USSR,
September 6–12, 1978

The International Conference on Primary Health Care, meeting in Alma-Ata
this twelfth day of September in the year Nineteen hundred and seventy-eight,
expressing the need for urgent action by all governments, all health and development workers, and the world community to protect and promote the health
of all the people of the world, hereby makes the following

DECLARATION:

I

The Conference strongly reaffirms that health, which is a state of complete
physical, mental and social wellbeing, and not merely the absence of disease or
infirmity, is a fundamental human right and that the attainment of the highest possible level of health is a most important world-wide social goal whose
realization requires the action of many other social and economic sectors in
addition to the health sector.

II

The existing gross inequality in the health status of the people particularly
between developed and developing countries as well as within countries is
politically, socially and economically unacceptable and is, therefore, of common concern to all countries.

III

Economic and social development, based on a New International Economic
Order, is of basic importance to the fullest attainment of health for all and

to the reduction of the gap between the health status of the developing and developed countries. The promotion and protection of the health of the people is essential to sustained economic and social development and contributes to a better quality of life and to world peace.

IV

The people have the right and duty to participate individually and collectively in the planning and implementation of their health care.

V

Governments have a responsibility for the health of their people which can be fulfilled only by the provision of adequate health and social measures. A main social target of governments, international organizations and the whole world community in the coming decades should be the attainment by all peoples of the world by the year 2000 of a level of health that will permit them to lead a socially and economically productive life. Primary health care is the key to attaining this target as part of development in the spirit of social justice.

VI

Primary health care is essential health care based on practical, scientifically sound and socially acceptable methods and technology made universally accessible to individuals and families in the community through their full participation and at a cost that the community and country can afford to maintain at every stage of their development in the spirit of self-reliance and self-determination. It forms an integral part both of the country's health system, of which it is the central function and main focus, and of the overall social and economic development of the community. It is the first level of contact of individuals, the family and community with the national health system bringing health care as close as possible to where people live and work, and constitutes the first element of a continuing health care process.

VII

Primary health care:

1. reflects and evolves from the economic conditions and sociocultural and political characteristics of the country and its communities and is based on the application of the relevant results of social, biomedical and health services research and public health experience;
2. addresses the main health problems in the community, providing promotive, preventive, curative and rehabilitative services accordingly;
3. includes at least: education concerning prevailing health problems and the methods of preventing and controlling them; promotion of food supply and proper nutrition; an adequate supply of safe water and basic

sanitation; maternal and child health care, including family planning; immunization against the major infectious diseases; prevention and control of locally endemic diseases; appropriate treatment of common diseases and injuries; and provision of essential drugs;

4. involves, in addition to the health sector, all related sectors and aspects of national and community development, in particular agriculture, animal husbandry, food, industry, education, housing, public works, communications and other sectors; and demands the coordinated efforts of all those sectors;

5. requires and promotes maximum community and individual self-reliance and participation in the planning, organization, operation and control of primary health care, making fullest use of local, national and other available resources; and to this end develops through appropriate education the ability of communities to participate;

6. should be sustained by integrated, functional and mutually supportive referral systems, leading to the progressive improvement of comprehensive health care for all, and giving priority to those most in need;

7. relies, at local and referral levels, on health workers, including physicians, nurses, midwives, auxiliaries and community workers as applicable, as well as traditional practitioners as needed, suitably trained socially and technically to work as a health team and to respond to the expressed health needs of the community.

VIII

All governments should formulate national policies, strategies and plans of action to launch and sustain primary health care as part of a comprehensive national health system and in coordination with other sectors. To this end, it will be necessary to exercise political will, to mobilize the country's resources and to use available external resources rationally.

IX

All countries should cooperate in a spirit of partnership and service to ensure primary health care for all people since the attainment of health by people in any one country directly concerns and benefits every other country. In this context the joint WHO/UNICEF report on primary health care constitutes a solid basis for the further development and operation of primary health care throughout the world.

X

An acceptable level of health for all the people of the world by the year 2000 can be attained through a fuller and better use of the world's resources, a considerable part of which is now spent on armaments and military conflicts. A genuine policy of independence, peace, détente and disarmament could and should release additional resources that could well be devoted to peaceful aims and in particular to the acceleration of social and economic development of which primary health care, as an essential part, should be allotted its proper share.

The International Conference on Primary Health Care calls for urgent and effective national and international action to develop and implement primary health care throughout the world and particularly in developing countries in a spirit of technical cooperation and in keeping with a New International Economic Order. It urges governments, WHO and UNICEF, and other international organizations, as well as multilateral and bilateral agencies, nongovernmental organizations, funding agencies, all health workers and the whole world community to support national and international commitment to primary health care and to channel increased technical and financial support to it, particularly in developing countries. The Conference calls on all the aforementioned to collaborate in introducing, developing and maintaining primary health care in accordance with the spirit and content of this Declaration.

Notes

Notes for supplementary boxes are found at the end of each chapter's notes section, listed under the title of the box.

PREFACE

1. See, for example, David Brown, "For a Global Generation, Public Health Is a Hot Field," *Washington Post,* September 19, 2008, www.washingtonpost.com/wp-dyn/content/article/2008/09/18/AR2008091804145.html (accessed August 19, 2012); Deirdre Shesgreen, "Riding the Wave of Student Interest in Global Health," *Science Speaks: HIV and TB News,* July 10, 2009, http://sciencespeaksblog.org/2009/07/10/riding-the-wave-of-student-interest-in-global-health/ (accessed November 15, 2012).

2. See, for example, William Foege, "Disease Prevention in the 21st Century," *Global Health Chronicles,* July 12, 2008, http://globalhealthchronicles.org/smallpox/record/view/pid/emory:16nmw (accessed November 15, 2012); William H. Foege, *House on Fire: The Fight to Eliminate Smallpox* (Berkeley: University of California Press, 2011); Paul E. Farmer, Jennifer J. Furin, and Joel T. Katz, "Global Health Equity," *Lancet* 363, no. 9423 (2004): 1832.

3. Jim Yong Kim, Paul Farmer, and Michael Porter, "Redefining Global Health-Care Delivery," *Lancet,* 20 May 2013.

4. See, for example, Barbara Rylko-Bauer and Paul Farmer, "Managed Care or Managed Inequality? A Call for Critiques of Market-Based Medicine," *Medical Anthropology Quarterly* 16, no. 4 (December 2002): 476–502.

5. Richard Horton, personal communication to the author, January 29, 2012.

6. Paul Farmer, "More than Just a Hobby: What Harvard Can Do to Advance Global Health," *Harvard Crimson,* May 26, 2011, www.thecrimson

.com/article/2011/5/26/health-global-training-medical (accessed November 25, 2012). These suggestions are meant to be relevant to any research university or teaching hospital.

7. The landscape of such bilateral efforts may finally be changing, becoming more egalitarian and thus more focused on training needs in resource-poor settings. For example, the Rwandan Ministry of Health, in partnership with the Clinton Foundation and a dozen U.S. universities, has announced a program called Human Resources for Health, which will bring scores of senior medical and nursing faculty to Rwanda to launch training programs intended to build *local* capacity to respond to, say, cancer, noncommunicable diseases, trauma, and complex pathologies too numerous to list. See Clinton Health Access Initiative, "Human Resources for Health," www.clinton foundation.org/main/our-work/by-initiative/clinton-health-access-initiative/ programs/health-systems/human-resources-for-health.html (accessed November 18, 2012).

8. At each level, we've sought to make our teaching materials open-source, so that we might use them not only in Cambridge and Boston but also in any of the settings in which we and our students work. For information on these courses and also on the Master of Medical Sciences in Global Health Delivery (MMSc-GHD) degree that we now offer at Harvard Medical School, see the website http://ghsm.hms.harvard.edu/. We've also developed an online program management guide that synthesizes sundry experiences in providing health care in resource-poor settings around the globe; see www.pih.org/pmg.

9. The syllabus is open-source and can be found at http://ghsm.hms .harvard.edu/education/courses/#ghsm. The course description for 2011 read:

> Social, economic, and political forces powerfully influence who gets sick, what diseases afflict them, which treatments are available, and the outcomes of those treatments. Why else does heart disease persist as the world's leading cause of death, even though the measures needed to prevent it have been known for over fifty years? Why else are outcomes of HIV infection so different in different countries, and why do they vary widely even within the United States?
>
> All physicians encounter such questions in their clinical work, whether they work in Boston, elsewhere in the United States or further afield. These questions cannot be answered by studying molecular biology and pathophysiology alone. Medical education and practice must be grounded in an understanding of social medicine, a field of inquiry that uses the methods of the social sciences and the humanities to analyze disease and medicine.
>
> This course will introduce students to the theory and practice of social medicine to enable them to recognize these forces wherever they work, to understand how they affect their patients, and to develop appropriate responses. Lectures and tutorials will explore (1) the determinants of disease and health inequalities between populations and over time; (2) how social factors influence medical knowledge and health care; and (3) what must be done to combat and prevent health inequalities in local, national, and global contexts. We will emphasize the continuities between local and global, showing how insights gained in one setting can often be applied and adapted in many others.

10. The case studies can be found at http://globalhealthdelivery.org/ library/publications/case-studies/. For a review of these efforts, and the stra-

tegic framework underpinning them, see chapter 7 of this text and also Kim, Farmer, and Porter, "Redefining Global Health-Care Delivery."

11. Disparate claims about the quake's toll are explained in Paul Farmer, *Haiti after the Earthquake* (New York: PublicAffairs, 2011).

12. Some of us tried to take this look back in *Haiti after the Earthquake* (New York: PublicAffairs, 2011).

13. See, for example, *Wòch nan Soley: The Denial of the Right to Water in Haiti,* a 2008 report by the Center for Human Rights and Global Justice and the International Human Rights Clinic at New York University's School of Law, Partners In Health, Zanmi Lasante, and the Robert F. Kennedy Memorial Center for Human Rights, www.pih.org/page/-/reports/Haiti_Report_FINAL.pdf (accessed November 12, 2012).

14. Centers for Disease Control and Prevention, *Acute Watery Diarrhea and Cholera: Haiti Pre-Decision Brief for Public Health Action,* March 2, 2010, http://emergency.cdc.gov/disasters/earthquakes/haiti/waterydiarrhea_pre-decision_brief.asp (accessed November 19, 2012).

15. For further explanation of these claims of causality, see Louise C. Ivers and David A. Walton, "The 'First' Case of Cholera in Haiti: Lessons for Global Health," *American Journal of Tropical Medicine and Hygiene* 86, no. 1 (2012): 36–38; and Jonathan Weigel and Paul Farmer, "Cholera and the Road to Modernity: Lessons from One Latin American Epidemic for Another," *Americas Quarterly* 6, no. 3 (Summer 2012), www.americasquarterly.org/cholera-and-the-road-to-modernity (accessed November 18, 2012).

16. Louise Ivers, Paul Farmer, and William J. Pape, "Oral Cholera Vaccine and Integrated Cholera Control in Haiti," *Lancet* 379 (2012): 2027–2028.

17. Paul Farmer, et al., "Meeting Cholera's Challenge to Haiti and the World: A Joint Statement on Cholera Prevention and Care," PLoS NTD 5, no. 5 (2011): e11145.

18. This point is made effectively in every chapter of João Biehl and Adriana Petryna, *When People Come First: Critical Studies in Global Health* (Princeton, N.J.: Princeton University Press, 2013).

CHAPTER 1

1. See Paul Farmer, "An Anthropology of Structural Violence," *Current Anthropology* 45, no. 3 (2004): 305–326.

2. See, for example, Arthur Kleinman, Veena Das, and Margaret M. Lock, eds., *Social Suffering* (Berkeley: University of California Press, 1997); Arthur Kleinman, *The Illness Narratives: Suffering, Healing, and the Human Condition* (New York: Basic Books, 1988); João Biehl and Adriana Petryna, *When People Come First.*

3. Paul Farmer, "On Suffering and Structural Violence: A View from Below," in *Social Suffering,* ed. Arthur Kleinman, Veena Das, and Margaret Lock (Berkeley: University of California Press, 1997), 261–283; originally published in *Daedalus* 125, no. 1 (1997).

4. Jonathan M. Mann, "Medicine and Public Health, Ethics and Human Rights," *Hastings Center Report* 27, no. 3 (1997): 8.

5. Paul Farmer, "Social Inequalities and Emerging Infectious Diseases," *Emerging Infectious Diseases* 2, no. 4 (1996): 259–269.

6. Kim, Farmer, and Porter, "Redefining Global Health-Care Delivery."

CHAPTER 2

1. Max Weber, "The Nature of Social Action" (1922), in *Max Weber: Selections in Translation*, ed. W.G. Runciman, trans. Eric Matthews (Cambridge: Cambridge University Press, 1978), 7 (emphasis added). At that time, sociology—a field that influenced the foundations of other social sciences—was a blanket term that covered what are now the fields of sociology and sociocultural anthropology.

2. David Ashley and David Michael Orenstein, *Sociological Theory: Classical Statements,* 6th ed. (Boston: Pearson Education, 2005), 241.

3. Anne E. Becker, Rebecca A. Burwell, David B. Herzog, Paul Hamburg, and Stephen E. Gilman, "Eating Behaviours and Attitudes following Prolonged Exposure to Television among Ethnic Fijian Adolescent Girls," *British Journal of Psychiatry* 180 (June 2002): 509–514.

4. See, for example, Randall M. Packard, *The Making of a Tropical Disease: A Short History of Malaria* (Baltimore: Johns Hopkins University Press, 2007), 111–149. See also Peter J. Brown, "Microparasites and Macroparasites," *Cultural Anthropology* 2, no. 1 (February 1987): 155–171.

5. Peter Berger and Thomas Luckmann, *The Social Construction of Reality: A Treatise in the Sociology of Knowledge* (New York: Irvington Publishers, 1966), 3.

6. Ibid., 50. Berger and Luckmann's broad definition of institution refers to anything that has become customary—not solely, though including, large institutional organizations.

7. Ibid., 116.

8. Ibid., 61.

9. American Psychiatric Association, *Diagnostic and Statistical Manual of Mental Disorders: DSM-II* (Washington, D.C.: American Psychiatric Association, 1968), 44; American Psychiatric Association, *Diagnostic and Statistical Manual of Mental Disorders: DSM-III* (Washington, D.C.: American Psychiatric Association, 1980), 281–282. See also Richard Pillard, "From Disorder to Dystonia: *DSM-II* and *DSM-III*," *Journal of Gay and Lesbian Mental Health* 13, no. 2 (2009): 82–86.

10. Allan Young, *The Harmony of Illusions: Inventing Post-Traumatic Stress Disorder* (Princeton, N.J.: Princeton University Press, 1995), 5–6, 89–118.

11. Arthur Kleinman, Leon Eisenberg, and Byron Good, "Culture, Illness, and Care: Clinical Lessons from Anthropologic and Cross-Cultural Research," *Annals of Internal Medicine* 88, no. 2 (February 1978): 251.

12. Leon Eisenberg, "Disease and Illness: Distinctions between Professional and Popular Ideas of Sickness," *Culture, Medicine, and Psychiatry* 1, no. 1 (1977): 9–23.

13. Arthur Kleinman, *Patients and Healers in the Context of Culture: An*

Exploration of the Borderland between Anthropology, Medicine, and Psychiatry (Berkeley: University of California Press, 1980), 25–44.

14. Robert K. Merton, "The Unanticipated Consequences of Purposive Social Action," *American Sociological Review* 1, no. 6 (December 1936): 894–896.

15. Ibid., 901.

16. Fiona Terry, *Condemned to Repeat? The Paradox of Humanitarian Action* (Ithaca, N.Y.: Cornell University Press, 2002), 164–166; Johan Pottier, *Re-Imagining Rwanda: Conflict, Survival, and Disinformation in the Late Twentieth Century* (New York: Cambridge University Press, 2002); Gérard Prunier, *Africa's World War: Congo, the Rwandan Genocide, and the Making of a Continental Catastrophe* (Oxford: Oxford University Press, 2009); Jason Stearns, *Dancing in the Glory of Monsters: The Collapse of the Congo and the Great War of Africa* (New York: PublicAffairs, 2011).

17. Weber developed these "ideal types" in the abstract. He did not believe that these kinds of power existed in their "pure" forms. He viewed power in the world as messy and mixed but believed that by creating these ideal types he could think more scientifically and productively about how the world worked.

18. Max Weber, *The Theory of Social and Economic Organization*, trans. A.M. Henderson and Talcott Parsons (New York: Free Press, 1947), 328.

19. Max Weber, "On Bureaucracy," in *From Max Weber: Essays in Sociology*, by Max Weber, trans. and ed. H.H. Gerth and C. Wright Mills (London: Routledge and Kegan Paul, 1948), 228.

20. Combinations of these types of authority have resulted in some of the worst genocides in history; for example, neither the Holocaust nor the Rwandan genocide would have been possible without well-organized bureaucracies that could efficiently target minority groups.

21. Max Weber, "Politics as a Vocation," in *From Max Weber: Essays in Sociology*, 128.

22. Michel Foucault, *Discipline and Punish: The Birth of the Prison*, trans. Alan Sheridan (London: Allen Lane, 1977), 1.

23. Michel Foucault, *The History of Sexuality*, trans. Robert Hurley (New York: Pantheon Books, 1978), 136.

24. For more on the expansion of these processes into statecraft and social institutions, see Ian Hacking, *The Taming of Chance: Ideas in Context* (Cambridge: Cambridge University Press, 1990).

25. Foucault, *History of Sexuality*, 143.

26. Ibid., 139.

27. Mahmood Mamdani, *When Victims Become Killers: Colonialism, Nativism, and the Genocide in Rwanda* (Princeton, N.J.: Princeton University Press, 2001), 87–102. See also Stephen Kinzer, *A Thousand Hills: Rwanda's Rebirth and the Man Who Dreamed It* (Hoboken, N.J.: Wiley, 2008), 24–29.

28. Bernard S. Cohn, *Colonialism and Its Forms of Knowledge: The British in India* (Princeton, N.J.: Princeton University Press, 1996), 1–20.

29. Veena Das, "Suffering, Legitimacy, and Healing: The Bhopal Case," in *Critical Events: An Anthropological Perspective on Contemporary India*, by Veena Das (New Delhi: Oxford University Press, 1996), 136–174.

30. Adriana Petryna, *Life Exposed: Biological Citizens after Chernobyl* (Princeton, N.J.: Princeton University Press, 2002), 6.

31. Arthur Kleinman, Veena Das, and Margaret M. Lock, eds., *Social Suffering* (Berkeley: University of California Press, 1997), ix (emphasis added).

32. Paul Farmer, *Pathologies of Power: Health, Human Rights, and the New War on the Poor* (Berkeley: University of California Press, 2003), 40.

33. For more on structural violence, see Paul Farmer, "An Anthropology of Structural Violence," *Current Anthropology* 45, no. 3 (2004): 305–326.

CHAPTER 3

1. The history of colonial medicine and international health has become a vibrant arena in postcolonial studies. For a few overviews of the field, see David Arnold, "Introduction: Disease, Medicine, and Empire," in *Imperial Medicine and Indigenous Societies,* ed. David Arnold (Manchester, U.K.: Manchester University Press, 1988), 1–26; Michael Worboys, "Colonial Medicine," in *Medicine in the Twentieth Century,* ed. Roger Cooter and John Pickstone (Amsterdam: Harwood Academic, 2000), 67–80; Warwick Anderson, "Postcolonial Histories of Medicine," in *Locating Medical History: The Stories and Their Meanings,* ed. John Harley Warner and Frank Huisman (Baltimore: Johns Hopkins University Press, 2004), 285–308; and Anne-Emanuelle Birn, Yogun Pillay, and Timothy H. Holtz, "The Historical Origins of Modern International Health," in *Textbook of International Health: Global Health in a Dynamic World,* 3rd ed. (New York: Oxford University Press, 2009), 17–60.

2. These latter distinctions—"developed" and "developing"—are themselves freighted with problematic histories that are explored elsewhere. See, for example, James Ferguson, *Global Shadows: Africa in the Neoliberal World Order* (Durham, N.C.: Duke University Press, 2006).

3. See, for example, Theodore M. Brown, Marcos Cueto, and Elizabeth Fee, "The World Health Organization and the Transition from 'International' to 'Global' Public Health," *American Journal of Public Health* 96, no. 1 (2006): 62–72; and Worboys, "Colonial Medicine."

4. Dorothy Porter, *Health, Civilization, and the State: A History of Public Health from Ancient to Modern Times* (New York: Routledge, 1999), 19.

5. Nikolas Rose, "The Politics of Life Itself," *Theory, Culture, and Society* 18, no. 6 (December 2001): 6.

6. Alfred W. Crosby, *Ecological Imperialism: The Biological Expansion of Europe, 900–1900* (Cambridge: Cambridge University Press, 1993), 7.

7. David Shumway Jones, "Using Smallpox," in *Rationalizing Epidemics: Meanings and Uses of American Indian Mortality since 1600,* by David Shumway Jones (Cambridge, Mass.: Harvard University Press, 2004), 93–117.

8. Maryinez Lyons, *The Colonial Disease: A Social History of Sleeping Sickness in Northern Zaire, 1900–1940* (Cambridge: Cambridge University Press, 1992), 199–219.

9. Arnold, "Introduction: Disease, Medicine, and Empire," 5.

10. Many famines fall into this category, as Mike Davis argues in *Late*

Victorian Holocausts: El Niño, Famines, and the Making of the Third World (London: Verso, 2001).

11. Jones, *Rationalizing Epidemics*, 36, 53.

12. Joyce Chaplin, *Subject Matter: Technology, the Body, and Science on the Anglo-American Frontier, 1500–1676* (Cambridge, Mass.: Harvard University Press, 2001), 8–9.

13. Philip D. Curtin, "The White Man's Grave: Image and Reality, 1780–1850," *Journal of British Studies* 1 (1961): 95.

14. Daniel R. Headrick, *The Tools of Empire: Technology and European Imperialism in the Nineteenth Century* (New York: Oxford University Press, 1981), 74.

15. William B. Cohen, "Malaria and French Imperialism," *Journal of African History* 24 (1983): 23.

16. See Warwick Anderson, *Colonial Pathologies: American Tropical Medicine, Race, and Hygiene in the Philippines* (Durham, N.C.: Duke University Press, 2006).

17. Headrick, *Tools of Empire*, 68.

18. Leo B. Slater, *War and Disease: Biomedical Research on Malaria in the Twentieth Century* (New Brunswick, N.J.: Rutgers University Press, 2009), 17–18.

19. The extraction of quinine did not, however, lead to the ability to synthesize it efficiently until the mid-twentieth century. Until that time, access to quinine remained the subject of bitter imperial rivalries. Indeed, the Japanese occupation of Indonesia in 1942 effectively cut off the Allied forces' access to quinine and was thought to have hindered Allied deployment in the tropical theaters of World War II until synthetic supplies could be adequately secured. See ibid., 109.

20. Arnold, "Introduction: Disease, Medicine, and Empire," 3.

21. Jim Paul, "Medicine and Imperialism in Morocco," *Middle East Research and Information Project [MERIP] Reports* 60 (1977): 7; quoted in Arnold, "Introduction: Disease, Medicine, and Empire," 3, 22.

22. Richard Keller, "Madness and Colonization: Psychiatry in the British and French Empires, 1800–1962," *Journal of Social History* 35, no. 2 (Winter 2001): 297, citing the proceedings of the Congrès des médécins alienistes et neurologistes de France et des pays de langue française, 37th session, Rabat (Paris, 1933), 73–74.

23. Anna Crozier, *Practising Colonial Medicine: The Colonial Medical Service in British East Africa* (London: I. B. Tauris, 2007), 79–91.

24. Worboys, "Colonial Medicine," 75.

25. Philip D. Curtin, "Epidemiology and the Slave Trade," *Political Science Quarterly* 83, no. 2 (1968): 194.

26. For more on the responsibility of the "dressed native" in propagating epidemic disease under colonial rule, see Randall M. Packard, "The 'Healthy Reserve' and the 'Dressed Native': Discourses on Black Health and the Language of Legitimation in South Africa," *American Ethnologist* 16, no. 4 (November 1989): 686–703; and Randall M. Packard, *White Plague, Black*

Labor: Tuberculosis and the Political Economy of Health and Disease in South Africa (Berkeley: University of California Press, 1989).

27. Quoted in David Arnold, *Colonizing the Body: State Medicine and Epidemic Disease in Nineteenth-Century India* (Berkeley: University of California Press, 1993), 189.

28. Institute of Medicine, *America's Vital Interest in Global Health: Protecting Our People, Enhancing Our Economy, and Advancing Our International Interests* (Washington, D.C.: National Academies Press, 1997).

29. John Darwin, *After Tamerlane: The Global History of Empire since 1405* (New York: Bloomsbury Press, 2008).

30. Competing and discrepant claims of causality, then as now, were far too numerous to count. But Pasteur and Koch triggered a revolution within a growing transnational scientific community; see Thomas D. Brock, *Robert Koch: A Life in Medicine and Bacteriology* (Washington, D.C.: American Society for Microbiology, 1999). Nancy Tomes has written about the impact of germ theory on popular notions of etiology in turn-of-the-century middle-class America; see Nancy Tomes, *The Gospel of Germs: Men, Women, and the Microbe in American Life* (Cambridge, Mass.: Harvard University Press, 1998).

31. Brock, *Robert Koch,* 140–169. See also John Aberth, *Plagues in World History* (Plymouth, U.K.: Rowman and Littlefield, 2011), 101–110.

32. Michael Worboys, "The Emergence of Tropical Medicine," in *Perspectives on the Emergence of Scientific Disciplines,* ed. Gérard Lemaine, Roy MacLeod, Michael Mulkay, and Peter Weingart (London: Routledge, 1976), 82–85.

33. Paul Farmer, *Infections and Inequalities: The Modern Plagues* (Berkeley: University of California Press, 1999), 37–58, 76–82.

34. John Farley, *Bilharzia: A History of Imperial Tropical Medicine* (Cambridge: Cambridge University Press, 1991), 20–26.

35. Patrick Manson, Harry Johnston, Jervoise Athelstane Baines, Robert Felkin, and J. W. Wells, "Acclimatization of Europeans in Tropical Lands: Discussion," *Geographical Journal* 12, no. 6 (1898): 599–600.

36. Judith Walzer Leavitt, *Typhoid Mary: Captive to the Public's Health* (Boston: Beacon Press, 1996).

37. Anderson, *Colonial Pathologies,* 44.

38. Warwick Anderson, "Immunities of Empire: Race, Disease, and the New Tropical Medicine, 1900–1920," *Bulletin of the History of Medicine* 70, no. 1 (1996): 110.

39. Warwick Anderson, "'Where Every Prospect Pleases and Only Man Is Vile': Laboratory Medicine as Colonial Discourse," *Critical Inquiry* 18, no. 3 (Spring 1992): 508.

40. Anderson, *Colonial Pathologies,* 59.

41. Ibid.

42. Alison Bashford, "'Is White Australia Possible?' Race, Colonialism, and Tropical Medicine in the Early Twentieth Century," *Ethnic and Racial Studies* 23, no. 2 (2000): 256–257.

43. Jock McCulloch, *Colonial Psychiatry and "The African Mind"* (Cambridge: Cambridge University Press, 1995), 2.

44. Frantz Fanon, "Medicine and Colonialism," in *A Dying Colonialism*, by Frantz Fanon (New York: Grove Press, 1967), 121–147.

45. Robin Wright, "USAID Director Keeps an Eye on Long-Term Recovery," *Washington Post,* January 6, 2005, A17.

46. Worboys, "Colonial Medicine," 68.

47. There are, of course, some notable exceptions to this trend, as discussed in Warwick Anderson's *Colonial Pathologies.*

48. Megan Vaughan, *Curing Their Ills: Colonial Power and African Illness* (Stanford, Calif.: Stanford University Press, 1991), 108.

49. Ibid., 11.

50. Ibid., 57.

51. David Hardiman, "Introduction," in *Healing Bodies, Saving Souls: Medical Missions in Asia and Africa,* ed. David Hardiman (New York: Editions Rodopi B.V., 2006), 24.

52. Ibid., 15.

53. Quoted in ibid., 14.

54. Terence O. Ranger, "Godly Medicine: The Ambiguities of Medical Mission in Southeast Tanzania, 1900–1945," *Social Science and Medicine* 15B (1981): 261–277.

55. Hardiman, *Healing Bodies, Saving Souls,* 25.

56. Vaughan, *Curing Their Ills,* 56.

57. Ibid., 61.

58. Charles M. Good, "Pioneer Medical Missions in Colonial Africa," *Social Science and Medicine* 32, no. 1 (1991): 1–10.

59. Hardiman, *Healing Bodies, Saving Souls,* 13.

60. Vaughan, *Curing Their Ills,* 155.

61. Lyons, *The Colonial Disease,* 62.

62. Porter, *Health, Civilization, and the State,* 79–96.

63. The miasmatic theory was often associated with a broad approach to public health that included sanitation, social reform, and concern with poverty. Ironically, the germ theory, at least initially, sponsored a reductionist focus on germs that weakened broad public health initiatives. See, for example, Barbara Rosenkrantz, *Public Health and the State: Changing Views in Massachusetts* (Cambridge, Mass.: Harvard University Press, 1972).

64. Peter Vinten-Johansen, Howard Brody, Nigel Paneth, Stephen Rachman, and Michael Rip, *Cholera, Chloroform, and the Science of Medicine: A Life of John Snow* (Oxford: Oxford University Press, 2003), 294.

65. See ibid., 8–11.

66. Ibid., 7.

67. Ibid.

68. Ibid., 8.

69. Marcos Cueto, ed., *Missionaries of Science: The Rockefeller Foundation and Latin America* (Bloomington: Indiana University Press, 1994), 11.

70. Ibid., 58–59.

71. Stephen Kinzer, *Overthrow: America's Century of Regime Change from Hawaii to Iraq* (New York: Henry Holt, 2006), 58–59.

72. Ibid., 59.

73. David McBride, *Missions for Science: U.S. Technology and Medicine in America's African World* (New Brunswick, N.J.: Rutgers University Press, 2002), 48–58.

74. The U.S. Army commission used vector control as its primary mode of intervention to restrict the activity of the mosquitoes capable of perpetuating person-to-person transmission of yellow fever and malaria. This measure was chosen from the two competing schools of thought during that period, one that advocated a direct attack on the mosquitoes—the vectors—and another that argued for fighting the malaria parasite within the human hosts. For a more recent example of the prevention-versus-care debate, see chapter 5 of this volume.

75. The convention's geographic delimitation and broad mission differentiated it from the International Sanitary Conferences held in Europe, which had primarily focused on the containment of cholera and the plague.

76. *Transactions of the First General International Sanitary Convention of the American Republics,* held in Washington, D.C., December 2, 3, and 4, 1902, under the auspices of the Governing Board of the International Union of the American Republics (Washington, D.C.: Government Printing Office, 1903).

77. *Transactions of the Second General International Sanitary Convention of the American Republics,* held in Washington, D.C., October 9, 10, 12, 13, and 14, 1905, under the auspices of the Governing Board of the International Union of the American Republics (Washington, D.C.: Government Printing Office, 1906), 94.

78. Ibid., 30.

79. Although yellow fever was successfully eradicated from the region, many other diseases, such as pneumonia and diarrheal diseases, remained unaddressed; see World Health Organization, *Fifty Years of the World Health Organization in the Western Pacific Region, 1948–1998,* Report of the Regional Director to the Regional Committee for the Western Pacific (Geneva: World Health Organization, 1998), 3–8; and Alexandra Minna Stern and Howard Markel, "International Efforts to Control Infectious Diseases, 1851 to the Present," *Journal of the American Medical Association* 292, no. 12 (2004): 1474–1479. This legacy continues today, as resources are dedicated to problem choice diseases—diseases that historically have been prioritized by researchers, funders, and commercial markets—instead of what have now been termed "neglected diseases" (chapter 11 discusses this topic further).

80. Marcos Cueto, *The Value of Health: A History of the Pan American Health Organization* (Washington, D.C.: PAHO, 2007), 29.

81. Stern and Markel, "International Efforts," 1476.

82. PAHO also serves as the Western Hemisphere's branch of the World Health Organization. These institutions are charged with setting global health policies and are influential in steering public and private capital toward certain threats to health—and away from others.

83. Brown, Cueto, and Fee, "The World Health Organization," 64.

84. Anne-Emanuelle Birn and Armando Solórzano, "Public Health Policy Paradoxes: Science and Politics in the Rockefeller Foundation's Hookworm Campaign in Mexico in the 1920s," *Social Science and Medicine* 49, no. 9 (1999): 1197–1213.

85. Ilana Lowy and Patrick Zylberman, "Medicine as a Social Instrument: Rockefeller Foundation, 1913–45," *Studies in History and Philosophy of Science, Part C,* 31, no. 3 (2000): 365–369.

86. Ibid., 369.

87. Cueto, *The Value of Health,* 77–78.

88. Moreover, to properly equip the areas it believed could be moved "forward" with the introduction of Western science, the foundation spent significant resources in Latin American medical schools, advocating for standardized curricula set in the global North—which failed to consider the local context of disease, local beliefs about disease causation, and the structural realities of under-resourced health systems. See, for example, Cueto, *Missionaries of Science,* 126–144.

89. Michael Havinden and David Meredith, *Colonialism and Development: Britain and Its Tropical Colonies, 1850–1960* (London: Routledge, 1993), 209.

90. See Martin Meredith, *The Fate of Africa: A History of Fifty Years of Independence* (New York: PublicAffairs, 2005); Frederick Cooper, *Africa since 1940: The Past of the Present* (Cambridge: Cambridge University Press, 2002), 20, 36–37.

91. Meredith, *The Fate of Africa,* 9.

92. María Josefina Saldaña-Portillo, *The Revolutionary Imagination in the Americas and the Age of Development* (Durham, N.C.: Duke University Press, 2003), 22; Arturo Escobar, *Encountering Development: The Making and Unmaking of the Third World* (Princeton, N.J.: Princeton University Press, 1995), 3–4; Wolfgang Sachs, ed., *The Development Dictionary: A Guide to Knowledge as Power* (Johannesburg: Witwatersrand University Press, 1992), 2–3.

93. Harry S. Truman, "Inaugural Address," delivered in Washington D.C., January 20, 1949, www.presidency.ucsb.edu/ws/index.php?pid=13282 (accessed November 21, 2012).

94. Havinden and Meredith, *Colonialism and Development,* 253.

95. Jeffrey Herbst, *States and Power in Africa: Comparative Lessons in Authority and Control* (Princeton, N.J.: Princeton University Press, 2000), 16.

96. Cooper, *Africa since 1940,* 91–132.

97. Stern and Markel, "International Efforts," 1477.

98. Javed Siddiqi, *World Health and World Politics: The World Health Organization and the U.N. System* (London: Hurst, 1995), 53.

99. Note that cholera vaccinations at this time were less effective than those currently available, but too rarely used. See Aly Tewfik Shousha, "Cholera Epidemic in Egypt (1947): A Preliminary Report," Report to the World Health Organization, *Bulletin of the World Health Organization* 1, no. 2 (1948): 353–381, http://whqlibdoc.who.int/bulletin/1947–1948/Vol1-No2/

bulletin_1948_1(2)_353–381.pdf (accessed November 21, 2012). See also Louise C. Ivers, Paul Farmer, Charles Patrick Almazor, and Fernet Léandre, "Five Complementary Interventions to Slow Cholera: Haiti," *Lancet* 376, no. 9758 (2010): 2048–2051.

100. One can see incarnations of this debate even in contemporary policy circles: a recent endeavor by the Bill and Melinda Gates Foundation and other partners to subsidize antimalarial medication on the private market has drawn applause from parasite-control advocates, but resistance from other experts. Some professionals are concerned about drug resistance developing as medicines are used without the supervision of trained clinicians, and those supporting transformation of socioeconomic conditions believe this technical intervention will be insufficient. (As later chapters detail, this debate has been echoed in policy discussions of many complex ailments requiring prevention and care, including AIDS and tuberculosis as well as malignancies such as cervical cancer.)

101. Edmund Pellegrino, "The Sociocultural Impact of Twentieth-Century Therapeutics," in *The Therapeutic Revolution: Essays in the Social History of American Medicine,* ed. Morris Vogel and Charles Rosenberg (Philadelphia: University of Pennsylvania Press, 1979), 261.

102. Randall M. Packard, *The Making of a Tropical Disease: A Short History of Malaria* (Baltimore: Johns Hopkins University Press, 2007), 156.

103. Socrates Litsios, "Malaria Control, the Cold War, and the Postwar Reorganization of International Assistance," *Medical Anthropology* 17, no. 3 (1997): 255–278.

104. Albert F. Wessen, "Resurgent Malaria and the Social Sciences," *Social Science and Medicine* 22, no. 8 (1986): 3–4.

105. Packard, *The Making of a Tropical Disease,* 160.

106. Frank Fenner, Donald Ainslie Henderson, Isao Arita, Zdeněk Ježek, and Ivan Danilovich Ladnyi, *Smallpox and Its Eradication* (Geneva: World Health Organization, 1988), 493.

107. Meredeth Turshen, *The Politics of Public Health* (New Brunswick, N.J.: Rutgers University Press, 1989), 153–154.

108. Fenner, Henderson, et al., *Smallpox,* 485.

109. Ibid., 494.

110. Paul Greenough, "Intimidation, Coercion, and Resistance in the Final Stages of the South Asian Smallpox Eradication Campaign, 1973–1975," *Social Science and Medicine* 41, no. 5 (1995): 633, 644.

111. This chapter is based on lectures by Jeremy Green and Paul Farmer, Societies of the World 25 at Harvard University. See also Paul Farmer, Peter Drobac, and Zoe Agoos, "Colonial Roots of Global Health," *Harvard College Global Health Review,* September 2009.

112. Fenner et al., *Smallpox and Its Eradication,* 321, 1349.

The McKeown Hypothesis, page 64

1. For work by Thomas McKeown and his colleagues, see Thomas McKeown, R.G. Record, and R.D. Turner, "An Interpretation of the Decline

of Mortality in England and Wales during the Twentieth Century," *Population Studies* 29, no. 3 (1975): 391–422.

2. For commentary on McKeown's work, see John B. McKinlay and Sonja M. McKinlay, "The Questionable Contribution of Medical Measures to the Decline of Mortality in the United States in the Twentieth Century," *Milbank Memorial Fund Quarterly: Health and Society* 55, no. 3 (1977): 407–408. See also James Colgrove, "The McKeown Thesis: A Historical Controversy and Its Enduring Influence," *American Journal of Public Health* 92, no. 5 (2002): 725–729.

CHAPTER 4

1. Eric Hobsbawm, *The Age of Extremes: A History of the World, 1914–1991* (New York: Pantheon Books, 1994).

2. World Health Organization, *World Health Report 2008: Primary Health Care, Now More than Ever* (Geneva: World Health Organization, 2008).

3. Kenneth W. Newell, ed., *Health by the People* (Geneva: World Health Organization, 1975), 70.

4. David Blumenthal and William Hsiao, "Privatization and Its Discontents: The Evolving Chinese Health Care System," *New England Journal of Medicine* 353, no. 11 (2005): 1165.

5. In the last ten years, however, schistosomiasis appears to have been reemerging in parts of China such as the Poyang Lake region in Jiangxi province. See "Hello Again, God of Plague," *Economist,* June 18, 2009, www.economist.com/node/13871961?story_id=E1_TPRSTJGT (accessed September 21, 2012).

6. Blumenthal and Hsiao, "Privatization," 1165. The Cooperative Medical System was an important example of rural health care, which policymakers saw as an alternative to failed Western health programs like the Malaria Eradication Programme. Indeed, the barefoot doctors were often depoliticized and discussed outside the context of the Cultural Revolution. The elimination of diseases is more significant than the program results indicating a change in life expectancy, as even the most basic health data in the People's Republic of China were difficult to come by before the mid-1980s. But the fact that a positive change in life expectancy occurred, regardless of magnitude, is quite exceptional. Against the backdrop of the Great Leap Forward, during which 25–30 million people died of starvation, and the Cultural Revolution, during which 1–2 million died as a result of political violence, this positive shift is even more remarkable.

7. Ibid.; Newell, *Health by the People.*

8. Socrates Litsios, "The Long and Difficult Road to Alma-Ata: A Personal Reflection," *International Journal of Health Services* 32, no. 4 (2002): 713.

9. Ibid., 718–720.

10. Marcos Cueto, "The Origins of Primary Health Care and Selective Primary Health Care," *American Journal of Public Health* 94, no. 11 (2004): 1867–1868.

11. The term "medical elitism" is used in the sense of the following definition: "a fascination with specialists, technically sophisticated achievements, the metropolitan-style medical center." See Ernest W. Boyd, Thomas R. Konrad, and Conrad Seipp, "In and Out of the Mainstream: The Miners' Medical Program, 1946–1978," *Journal of Public Health Policy* 3, no. 4 (1982): 432–444; quoted in "What Is Primary Care?" *Journal of Public Health Policy* 4, no. 2 (1983): 129.

12. U.S. Department of Health, Education, and Welfare, *Healthy People: The Surgeon General's Report on Health Promotion and Disease Prevention,* Public Health Service publication 79-55071 (Washington, D.C.: Government Printing Office, 1979), 124.

13. Lynn M. Morgan, *Community Participation in Health: The Politics of Primary Care in Costa Rica* (Cambridge: Cambridge University Press, 1993), 62.

14. World Health Organization, *Primary Health Care: Report on the International Conference on Primary Health Care,* Alma-Ata, USSR, September 6–12, 1978 (Geneva: World Health Organization, 1978), 78.

15. Cueto, "Origins of Primary Health Care," 1868. See also Paul Ehrlich, *The Population Bomb* (New York: Buccaneer Books, 1968).

16. Julia A. Walsh and Kenneth S. Warren, "Selective Primary Health Care: An Interim Strategy for Disease Control in Developing Countries," *New England Journal of Medicine* 301, no. 18 (1979): 967.

17. Ibid.

18. Cueto, "Origins of Primary Health Care," 1870–1872.

19. Peter Adamson, "The Mad American," in *Jim Grant: UNICEF Visionary,* ed. Richard Jolly (Florence, Italy: UNICEF, 2001), 32.

20. Howard Stein, *Beyond the World Bank Agenda: An Institutional Approach to Development* (Chicago: University of Chicago Press, 2008), 209–213.

21. World Bank, *Health Sector Policy Report* (Washington, D.C.: World Bank, 1975).

22. Frederick Golladay and Bernhard Liese, "Health Problems and Policies in the Developing Countries," World Bank Staff Working Paper no. 412 (Washington, D.C.: International Bank for Reconstruction and Development, 1980); quoted in Stein, *Beyond the World Bank Agenda,* 212.

23. See Paul Isenman, Nicholas Hope, Timothy King, Peter Knight, Akbar Noman, Rupert Pennant-Rea, and Adrian Wood, eds., *World Development Report 1980: Part I, Adjustment and Growth in the 1980s; Part II: Poverty and Human Development* (New York: Oxford University Press, 1980).

24. David de Ferranti, "Paying for Health Services in Developing Countries: An Overview," World Bank Staff Working Paper no. 721 (Washington, D.C.: World Bank, 1985).

25. Stein, *Beyond the World Bank Agenda,* 216.

26. June Goodfield, *A Chance to Live* (New York: Macmillan, 1991), 38.

27. Whether global policymakers' endorsement of scaling back public health systems funding was a prudent course of action in the face of economic troubles is open to debate. When Mexico faced further financial pain in the 1990s, Minister of Health Julio Frenk saw the fragility of the economy as an

opportunity, not as a barrier to effective health spending. Today, Frenk continues to argue that moments of crisis expose the vulnerability of the population and therefore warrant increased commitment to health on the part of the government. Frenk's ideas and actions as Mexico's minister of health are revisited in chapters 7 and 8. See also the recent evaluation of data from several countries, including the United States, in David Stuckler and Sanjay Basu, *The Body Economic: Why Austerity Kills* (New York: Basic Books, 2013).

28. John Gershman and Alec Irwin, "Getting a Grip on the Global Economy," in *Dying for Growth: Global Inequality and the Health of the Poor,* ed. Jim Yong Kim, Joyce V. Millen, Alec Irwin, and John Gershman (Monroe, Maine: Common Courage Press, 2000), 23.

29. Ibid., 20–26; William Easterly, *The Elusive Quest for Growth: Economists' Adventures and Misadventures in the Tropics* (Cambridge, Mass.: MIT Press, 2001), 101.

30. Eliot Berg, *Accelerated Development in Sub-Saharan Africa: An Agenda for Reform* (Washington, D.C.: World Bank, 1981).

31. Brooke G. Schoepf, Claude Schoepf, and Joyce V. Millen, "Theoretical Therapies, Remote Remedies: SAPs and the Political Ecology of Poverty and Health in Africa," in Kim, Millen, et al., *Dying for Growth,* 99–101.

32. Easterly, *Elusive Quest for Growth,* 102.

33. Dani Rodrik, "Goodbye Washington Consensus, Hello Washington Confusion? A Review of the World Bank's Economic Growth in the 1990s: Learning from a Decade of Reform," *Journal of Economic Literature* 44, no. 4 (December 2006): 973.

34. Easterly, *Elusive Quest for Growth,* 102.

35. Ibid.; Gershman and Irwin, "Getting a Grip," 32.

36. Gershman and Irwin, "Getting a Grip," 18–22; Easterly, *Elusive Quest for Growth,* 101–103.

37. World Bank, *World Development Report 1993: Investing in Health* (Oxford: Oxford University Press, 1993), 12.

38. Ibid., 9.

39. David Stuckler, Lawrence King, and Sanjay Basu, "International Monetary Fund Programs and Tuberculosis Outcomes in Post-Communist Countries," *PLoS Medicine* 5, no. 7 (2008): 1085; David Stuckler and Karen Siegel, eds., *Sick Societies: Responding to the Global Challenge of Chronic Disease* (New York: Oxford University Press, 2011), 50.

40. Rob Yates, "Universal Health Care and the Removal of User Fees," *Lancet* 373, no. 9680 (2009): 2078; John S. Akin, Nancy Birdsall, and David M. de Ferranti, *Financing Health Services in Developing Countries,* 1987 World Bank Policy Study (Washington, D.C.: World Bank, 1987).

41. WHO guidelines for the 1987 Bamako Initiative are cited in Barbara McPake, Kara Hanson, and Anne Mills, "Community Financing of Health Care in Africa: An Evaluation of the Bamako Initiative," *Social Science and Medicine* 36, no. 11 (1993): 1383.

42. Gershman and Irwin, "Getting a Grip," 30.

43. Meredeth Turshen, *Privatizing Health Services in Africa* (New Brunswick, N.J.: Rutgers University Press, 1999), 33–50.

44. Barbara McPake, "User Charges for Health Services in Developing Countries: A Review of the Economic Literature," *Social Science and Medicine* 36, no. 11 (1993): 1404.

45. Rob Yates, "International Experiences in Removing User Fees for Health Services—Implications for Mozambique," report prepared for Department for International Development, Health Resource Centre, London, June 2006, 3–13.

46. Jessica Cohen and Pascaline Dupas, "Free Distribution or Cost-Sharing? Evidence from a Randomized Malaria Prevention Experiment," *Quarterly Journal of Economics* 125, no. 1 (2010), www.povertyactionlab.org/publication/free-distribution-or-cost-sharing-evidence-malaria-prevention-experiment-kenya-qje (accessed August 24, 2012).

47. Akin, Birdsall, and de Ferranti, *Financing Health Services in Developing Countries,* 4.

48. Lucy Gilson, Steven Russell, and Kent Buse, "The Political Economy of User Fees with Targeting: Developing Equitable Health Financing Policy," *Journal of International Development* 7, no. 3 (1995): 385.

49. Yates, "International Experiences in Removing User Fees," 15.

50. World Bank, "Cost Sharing: Towards Sustainable Health Care in Sub-Saharan Africa," World Bank Group Findings, Africa Region, no. 63, May 1996.

51. Yates, "International Experiences in Removing User Fees," 7.

52. Giovanni Andrea Cornia, Richard Jolly, and Frances Stewart, eds., *Adjustment with a Human Face: Protecting the Vulnerable and Promoting Growth—A Study by UNICEF* (Oxford: Clarendon Press, 1987).

53. Frances Stewart, "The Many Faces of Adjustment," *World Development* 19, no. 12 (1991): 1851.

54. John Williamson, "What Washington Means by Policy Reform," in *Latin American Adjustment: How Much Has Happened?* ed. John Williamson (Washington, D.C.: Institute for International Economics, 1990), 11.

55. Even Williamson himself acknowledged that policies commonly understood as deriving from the Washington Consensus had strayed far from many of their original intents—including the intent to reduce poverty—and had moved to a more rigid set of neoliberal practices in economic policy. See John Williamson, "What Should the World Bank Think about the Washington Consensus?" *World Bank Research Observer* 15, no. 2 (2000): 252.

56. Easterly, *Elusive Quest for Growth,* 103.

57. Nicholas van der Walle, *African Economies and the Politics of Permanent Crisis, 1979–1999* (New York: Cambridge University Press, 2001).

58. David Stuckler, Sanjay Basu, Anna Gilmore, Rajaie Batniji, Gorik Ooms, Akanksha A. Marphatia, Rachel Hammonds, and Martin McKee, "An Evaluation of the International Monetary Fund's Claims about Public Health," *International Journal of Health Services* 40, no. 2 (2010): 328; Schoepf, Schoepf, and Millen, "Theoretical Therapies, Remote Remedies," 109.

59. Roy Carr-Hill, Kamugisha Joviter Katabaro, Anne Ruhweza Katahoire, Dramane Oula, "The impact of HIV/AIDS on education and institutionalizing preventive education," report to International Institute for Educational Planning/UNESCO (Paris, 2002), 42. Available at http://unesdoc.unesco.org/images/0012/001293/129353e.pdf (accessed 28 May 2013).

60. Rodrik, "Goodbye Washington Consensus," 974.

61. See Daron Acemoglu and James Robinson, *Why Nations Fail: The Origins of Power, Prosperity, and Poverty* (New York: Crown, 2012).

62. Anne O. Krueger, "Meant Well, Tried Little, Failed Much: Policy Reforms in Emerging Market Economies" (paper presented at the Roundtable Lecture at the Economic Honors Society, New York University, New York, March 23, 2004).

63. Richard Cash, preface to *Child Health and Survival: The UNICEF GOBI-FFF Program,* ed. Richard Cash, Gerald T. Keusch, and Joel Lamstein (Wolfeboro, N.H.: Croom Helm, 1987), ix.

64. Gerald T. Keusch, Carla Wilson, and Richard Cash, "Is There Synergy among the Interventions in the GOBI-FFF Programme?" in Cash, Keusch, and Lamstein, *Child Health and Survival,* 109.

65. The term "cold chain" refers to the need for an unbroken system of refrigerated transit and storage for certain health technologies, food items, or commodities.

66. Keusch, Wilson, and Cash, "Is There Synergy among the Interventions in the GOBI-FFF Programme?" 116.

67. UNICEF, *1946–2006: Sixty Years for Children* (New York: United Nations Children's Fund, 2006), 18.

68. Maggie Black, *Children First: The Story of UNICEF Past and Present* (Oxford: Oxford University Press, 1996), 45.

69. Andrea Gerlin, "A Simple Solution," *Time,* October 8, 2006, 40–47.

70. World Health Organization, *World Health Report 2002: Reducing Risks, Promoting Healthy Life* (Geneva: World Health Organization, 2002), 113.

71. Adamson, "The Mad American," 23.

72. Audrey Hepburn's involvement in the GOBI-FFF campaign foreshadowed the many celebrities who would champion public health causes in the following years, especially during the HIV/AIDS epidemic.

73. Richard Jolly, "Introduction: Social Goals and Economic Reality," in *The Progress of Nations 1995,* compiled by United Nations Children's Fund, www.unicef.org/pon95/intro001.html (accessed February 15, 2013).

74. UNICEF, *1946–2006: Sixty Years for Children,* 21.

75. World Health Organization and UNICEF, *Progress Towards Global Immunization Goals: Summary Presentation of Key Indicators,* August 2011, www.who.int/immunization_monitoring/data/SlidesGlobalImmunization.pdf (accessed March 25, 2012).

76. UNICEF, *State of the World's Children 2008* (New York: United Nations Children's Fund, 2007), 1.

77. UNICEF, *1946–2006: Sixty Years for Children,* 17.

78. Jean-Pierre Unger and James R. Killingsworth, "Selective Primary Health Care: A Critical Review of Methods and Results," *Social Science and Medicine* 22, no. 10 (1986): 1003.

79. Morgan, *Community Participation in Health,* 62.

80. UNICEF, *1946–2006: Sixty Years for Children,* 17.

81. Carol Bellamy, "The Time to Sow," in *The Progress of Nations 2000,*

compiled by United Nations Children's Fund, 11, www.unicef.org/ponoo/ponoo_3.pdf (accessed February 15, 2013).

82. UNICEF, *General Progress Report of the Executive Director* (E/ICEF/608) (New York: United Nations Children's Fund, 1971), 1.

83. World Health Organization, *World Health Report 2008*, 3.

84. Walsh and Warren, "Selective Primary Health Care," 967; Theodore M. Brown, Marcos Cueto, and Elizabeth Fee, "The World Health Organization and the Transition from 'International' to 'Global' Public Health," *American Journal of Public Health* 96, no. 1 (2006): 62–72.

85. Gershman and Irwin, "Getting a Grip," 32.

86. Richard Jolly, "Adjustment with a Human Face: A UNICEF Record and Perspective on the 1980s," *World Development* 19, no. 12 (1991): 1809.

87. Ibid.

88. Ibid., 1819.

89. World Bank, *World Development Report 1993*, 4.

90. In low-income countries, government health expenditures were $6 per capita, and total health expenditures were $14 per capita. The World Bank called for increased spending from donors and governments in addition to reallocation of resources.

91. World Bank, *World Development Report 1993*, 10.

92. Ibid., 10.

93. Ibid., 8.

Halfdan Mahler, page 77

1. Marcos Cueto, "The Origins of Primary Health Care and Selective Primary Health Care," *American Journal of Public Health* 94, no. 11 (2004): 1867–1868.

2. Ibid.

3. "Address to the 61st World Health Assembly," Dr. Halfdan Mahler, former director-general of WHO, World Health Organization, 2008, www.who.int/mediacentre/events/2008/wha61/hafdan_mahler_speech/en/index.html (accessed November 12, 2012).

James P. Grant, page 96

1. For an account of Grant's life and career, see Barbara Crosette, "James P. Grant, UNICEF Chief and Aid Expert, Is Dead at 72," *New York Times*, January 30, 1995, www.nytimes.com/1995/01/30/obituaries/james-p-grant-unicef-chief-and-aid-expert-is-dead-at-72.html (accessed November 12, 2012).

Days of Tranquility, El Salvador, 1985, page 99

1. UNICEF, *1946–2006: Sixty Years for Children* (New York: United Nations Children's Fund, 2006), 19.

2. Ibid.

3. UNICEF News Note, "UN Urges 'Days of Tranquility' in Burundi for Vaccination Campaign," June 12, 2002, www.unicef.org/media/media_21527.

html (accessed January 8, 2013); UNICEF News Note, "Nationwide Measles and Polio Vaccination Campaign Launched in Burundi," June 19, 2002, www.unicef.org/media/newsnotes/02nn20measles.htm (accessed August 24, 2012).

4. Thierry Delvigne-Jean, "Pan-African Forum: Immunization as a Way of Building Peace," *UNICEF: Young Child Survival and Development,* October 19, 2004, www.unicef.org/childsurvival/index_23709.html (November 12, 2012).

Trade Liberalization and Food, page 105

1. Adam Drewnowski and Barry M. Popkin, "The Nutrition Transition: New Trends in the Global Diet," *Nutrition Reviews* 55, no. 2 (1997): 31.

2. Pedro Conceição and Ronald U. Mendoza, "Anatomy of the Global Food Crisis," *Third World Quarterly* 30, no. 6 (2009): 1162.

CHAPTER 5

1. Hillary Rodham Clinton, "Remarks on 'Creating an AIDS-Free Generation,'" November 8, 2011, www.state.gov/secretary/rm/2011/11/176810.htm (accessed February 9, 2012).

2. "Development assistance for health" is defined as "all flows for health from public and private institutions whose primary purpose is to provide development assistance to low-income and middle-income countries" (Nirmala Ravishankar, Paul Gubbins, Rebecca J. Cooley, Katherine Leach-Kemon, Catherine M. Michaud, Dean T. Jamison, and Christopher J.L. Murray, "Financing of Global Health: Tracking Development Assistance for Health from 1990 to 2007," *Lancet* 373, no. 9681 [2009]: 2116).

3. Tiaji Salaam-Blyther, *Trends in U.S. Global AIDS Spending: FY 2000–2008* (Washington, D.C.: Congressional Research Service, 2008), 13.

4. Carol Lancaster, *Transforming Foreign Aid: United States Assistance in the 21st Century* (Washington, D.C.: Institute for International Economics, 2000), 46.

5. Steven Radelet, "Bush and Foreign Aid," *Foreign Affairs* 82, no. 5 (2003): 107.

6. Greg Behrman, *The Invisible People: How the U.S. Has Slept through the Global AIDS Pandemic, the Greatest Humanitarian Catastrophe of Our Time* (New York: Free Press, 2004), 27.

7. For a detailed account of how these figures were obtained from congressional legislation, see Salaam-Blyther, *Trends in U.S. Global AIDS Spending.*

8. Office of the U.S. Global AIDS Coordinator, "Treatment Results," in *Sixth Annual Report to Congress on PEPFAR Program Results (2010)* (Washington, D.C.: Government Printing Office, 2010), www.pepfar.gov/press/sixth_annual_report/137133.htm (accessed December 1, 2012). Although the figures in the 2010 report were not questioned, PEPFAR's treatment figures have been subject to dispute in the past. In January 2005, PEPFAR contended that it was supporting antiretroviral treatment for more than thirty-two thousand people in Botswana; health officials in Botswana disputed this claim, pointing out that the United States had yet to fulfill an earlier pledge of $2.5 million.

The Bush administration revised the treatment claim for Botswana down to twenty thousand, although debate persisted about the accuracy of that figure as well. See UN Office for the Coordination of Humanitarian Affairs, *"Lazarus Drug": ARVs in the Treatment Era,* IRIN Web Special, September 2005, www.irinnews.org/pdf/in-depth/ARV-era.pdf (accessed September 2, 2012).

9. Office of the U.S. Global AIDS Coordinator, *Sixth Annual Report to Congress on PEPFAR Program Results (2010).* When this treatment for HIV-positive pregnant women includes a course of three antiretroviral medicines, cesarean sections during childbirth, and the use of formula rather than breast milk, it can reduce rates of mother-to-child transmission of the HIV virus from up to 40 percent to less than 1 percent.

10. See Eran Bendavid, Charles B. Holmes, Jay Bhattacharya, and Grant Miller, "HIV Development Assistance and Adult Mortality in Africa," *Journal of the American Medical Association* 307, no. 19 (2012): 2060–2067. Bendavid and colleagues use a difference-in-difference statistical analysis to determine that age-adjusted mortality in PEPFAR focus countries was lower than in similar AIDS-affected countries that were not PEPFAR focus countries. While the authors determined that all-cause adult mortality declined further in PEPFAR focus countries than in non-focus countries, they were unable to determine whether PEPFAR had an impact on mortality rates related to diseases other than HIV.

11. Bill and Melinda Gates Foundation, "Global Health Program Fact Sheet," 2009, http://docs.gatesfoundation.org/global-health/documents/global-health-fact-sheet-english-version.pdf (accessed February 15, 2013).

12. The Global Fund for AIDS, Tuberculosis and Malaria, "The Global Fund's 2011 Results at a Glance," video, www.youtube.com/watch?v=B20PM p6q3qg (accessed December 1, 2012).

13. International Monetary Fund, "Debt Relief under the Heavily Indebted Poor Countries (HIPC) Initiative," Factsheet, September 30, 2012, www.imf .org/external/np/exr/facts/hipc.htm (accessed January 8, 2013).

14. World Health Organization, *Progress on Global Access to HIV Antiretroviral therapy: A Report on "3 by 5" and Beyond,* March 2006 (Geneva: World Health Organization, 2006), 7.

15. Ibid.

16. Joint United Nations Programme on HIV/AIDS, *2011 UNAIDS World AIDS Day Report: Getting to Zero* (Geneva: UNAIDS, 2011), 5.

17. Ravishankar, Gubbins, et al., "Financing of Global Health," 2115.

18. Peter Berger and Thomas Luckmann, *The Social Construction of Reality: A Treatise in the Sociology of Knowledge* (New York: Irvington Publishers, 1966), 53.

19. José M. Zuniga and Amin Ghaziani, "A World Ravaged by a Disease without HAART," in *A Decade of HAART: The Development and Global Impact of Highly Active Antiretroviral Therapy,* ed. José M. Zuniga, Alan Whiteside, Amin Ghaziani, and John G. Bartlett (New York: Oxford University Press, 2008), 19.

20. Gina Kolata, "Strong Evidence Discovered that AZT Holds Off AIDS," *New York Times,* August 4, 1989, www.nytimes.com/1989/08/04/us/strong-

evidence-discovered-that-azt-holds-off-aids.html?src=pm (accessed February 15, 2013); "AZT's Inhuman Cost," *New York Times,* August 28, 1989, www .nytimes.com/1989/08/28/opinion/azt-s-inhuman-cost.html (accessed January 31, 2013).

21. Given the limits of AZT monotherapy, activists in the United States— many HIV-positive themselves—pushed the U.S. Food and Drug Administration to fast-track the approval process for new antiretrovirals. See Steven Epstein, *Impure Science: AIDS, Activism, and the Politics of Knowledge* (Berkeley: University of California Press, 1996), 270.

22. Centers for Disease Control and Prevention, *AIDS Surveillance: Trends (1985–2010),* "Slide 3: AIDS Diagnoses and Deaths of Adults and Adolescents with AIDS, 1985–2009, United States and 6 U.S. Dependent Areas," www.cdc .gov/hiv/topics/surveillance/resources/slides/trends/slides/2010AIDStrends.pdf (accessed December 1, 2012).

23. Behrman, *The Invisible People,* 125.

24. For a detailed discussion of the U.S. AIDS activist movement, see Patricia D. Siplon, *AIDS and the Policy Struggle in the United States* (Washington, D.C.: Georgetown University Press, 2002).

25. Behrman, *The Invisible People,* 123.

26. David Ho was named *Time* magazine's "Person of the Year" in 1996; see Christine Gorman, Alice Park, and Dick Thompson, "Dr. David Ho: The Disease Detective," *Time,* December 30, 1996. For more information on HAART and Ho's role in its development, see his extended interview filmed for the *Frontline* documentary series *The Age of AIDS,* directed by William Cran and Greg Barker, 2006, www.pbs.org/wgbh/pages/frontline/aids/inter views/ho.html (accessed February 15, 2013).

27. See, for instance, Roy M. Gulick, John W. Mellors, Diane Havlir, Joseph J. Eron, Charles Gonzalez, Deborah McMahon, Douglas D. Richman, Fred T. Valentine, Leslie Jonas, Anne Meibohm, Emilio A. Emini, Jeffrey A. Chodakewitz, Paul Deutsch, Daniel Holder, William A. Schleif, and Jon H. Condra, "Treatment with Indinavir, Zidovudine, and Lamivudine in Adults with Human Immunodeficiency Virus Infection and Prior Antiretroviral Therapy," *New England Journal of Medicine* 337, no. 11 (1997): 734–739; Scott M. Hammer, Kathleen E. Squires, Michael D. Hughes, Janet M. Grimes, Lisa M. Demeter, Judith S. Currier, Joseph J. Eron Jr., Judith E. Feinberg, Henry H. Balfour Jr., Lawrence R. Deyton, Jeffrey A. Chodakewitz, Margaret A. Fischl, John P. Phair, Louise Pedneault, Bach-Yen Nguyen, and Jon C. Cook, "A Controlled Trial of Two Nucleoside Analogues plus Indinavir in Persons with Human Immunodeficiency Virus Infection and CD4 Cell Counts of 200 per Cubic Millimeter or Less," *New England Journal of Medicine* 337, no. 11 (1997): 725–733; Stefano Vella, "Clinical Experience with Saquinavir," *AIDS,* suppl. 2 (1995): S21–S25; Julio S. G. Montaner, Peter Reiss, David Cooper, Stefano Vella, Marianne Harris, Brian Conway, Mark A. Wainberg, D. Smith, Patrick Robinson, David Hall, Maureen Myers, and Joep M. A. Lange, "A Randomized Double-Blind, Comparative Trial of the Effects of Zidovudine, Didanosine, and Nevirapine Combinations in Antiviral-Naive, AIDS-Free, HIV-Infected Patients with CD4 Cell Counts 200–600/mm^3," Abstract

no. B294, Program and Abstracts of the Eleventh International Conference on AIDS (Vancouver, B.C., July 7–12, 1996).

28. Centers for Disease Control and Prevention, *HIV Mortality: Trends (1987–2008)*, "Slide 5: Trends in Annual Age-Adjusted Rate of Death Due to HIV Disease: United States, 1987–2008," presentation notes, www.cdc.gov/hiv/topics/surveillance/resources/slides/mortality/slides/mortality.pdf (accessed January 8, 2013).

29. Eric Sawyer, "Remarks at the Opening Ceremony" (speech given at the Eleventh International Conference on AIDS, Vancouver, B.C., July 7–12, 1996).

30. Behrman, *The Invisible People*, 134.

31. In 1999, ACT UP New York drew "dozens" of members to its chapter meetings, though in 1988 the same chapter had used a larger space to accommodate meetings that drew as many as 350 people (Thomas Morgan, "Mainstream Strategy for AIDS Group," *New York Times*, July 22, 1988, B1; Chris Bull, "Still Angry after All These Years," *Advocate*, August 17, 1999).

32. Elliot Marseille, Paul B. Hofmann, and James G. Kahn, "HIV Prevention before HAART in Sub-Saharan Africa," *Lancet* 359, no. 9320 (2002): 1851.

33. Andrew Creese, Katherine Floyd, Anita Alban, and Lorna Guinness, "Cost-Effectiveness of HIV/AIDS Interventions in Africa: A Systematic Review of the Evidence," *Lancet* 359, no. 9318 (2002): 1635–1642.

34. U.S. House Committee on International Relations, *The Spread of AIDS in the Developing World: Hearing before the Committee on International Relations*, 105th Cong., 2nd sess., September 16, 1998 (Washington, D.C.: Government Printing Office, 1998), 4:74.

35. Andrew Natsios, testimony before U.S. House of Representatives Committee on International Relations, *Hearing: The United States' War on AIDS*, 107th Cong., 1st sess., Washington, D.C., June 7, 2001, http://comm docs.house.gov/committees/intlrel/hfa72978.000/hfa72978_0.HTM (accessed August 10, 2012).

36. See, for instance, the Cange Declaration, read by Nerlande Lahens in Cange, Haiti, August 24, 2001, www.pih.org/publications/entry/the-declara tion-of-cange-world-aids-day-2001 (accessed December 1, 2012).

37. Paul Farmer, Fernet Léandre, Joia Mukherjee, Rajesh Gupta, Laura Tarter, and Jim Yong Kim, "Community-Based Treatment of Advanced HIV Disease: Introducing DOT-HAART (Directly Observed Therapy with Highly Active Antiretroviral Therapy)," *Bulletin of the World Health Organization* 79, no. 12 (2001): 1145–1151.

38. World Health Organization, "Antiretroviral Therapy in Primary Health Care: Experience of the Khayelitsha Programme in South Africa [Case Study]," *Perspectives and Practice in Antiretroviral Treatment* (Geneva: World Health Organization, 2003), 5.

39. "Consensus Statement on Antiretroviral Treatment for AIDS in Poor Countries, by Individual Members of the Faculty of Harvard University," March 2001, www.cid.harvard.edu/cidinthenews/pr/consensus_aids_therapy. pdf (accessed August 8, 2012).

40. Harriet Washington, *Medical Apartheid: The Dark History of Medical Experimentation on Black Americans from Colonial Times to the Present* (New York: Doubleday, 2006). See also Philippe Bourgois and Jeff Schonberg, "Intimate Apartheid: Ethnic Dimensions of Habitus among Homeless Heroin Injectors," *Ethnography* 8, no. 1 (2007): 7–31.

41. Raymond A. Smith and Patricia D. Siplon, *Drugs into Bodies: Global AIDS Treatment Activism* (London: Praeger, 2006), 59.

42. Anne-Christine d'Adesky, *Moving Mountains: The Race to Treat Global AIDS* (London: Verso, 2004), 28–30. See also João Biehl, *Will to Live: AIDS Therapies and the Politics of Survival* (Princeton, N.J.: Princeton University Press, 2007).

43. Such compulsory licensing was approved by the World Trade Organization via the Doha Declaration in 2001. Compulsory licensing for a particular drug introduces competition into a market previously dominated by a single company that held the patent on that drug. See World Trade Organization, "Declaration on the TRIPs Agreement and Public Health," adopted November 14, 2001, by the 4th World Trade Organization Ministerial Conference in Doha, Qatar, www.wto.org/english/thewto_e/minist_e/min01_e/mindecl_trips_e.htm (accessed December 1, 2012).

44. Amy Kapczynski, Samantha Chaifetz, Zachary Katz, and Yochai Benkler, "Addressing Global Health Inequities: An Open Licensing Approach for University Innovations," *Berkeley Technology Law Journal* 20, no. 2 (2005): 1034.

45. Ibid., 1038 n. 33.

46. Office of the United States Trade Representative, "USTR Announces Results of Special 301 Annual Review," press release, April 30, 1999, http://keionline.org/ustr/1999special301 (accessed February 15, 2013).

47. Smith and Siplon, *Drugs into Bodies,* 66.

48. Behrman, *The Invisible People,* 158.

49. Ibid.

50. World Trade Organization, "Declaration on the TRIPs Agreement and Public Health."

51. Jonathan Rauch, "This Is Not Charity: How Bill Clinton, Ira Magaziner, and a Team of Management Consultants Are Creating New Markets, Reinventing Philanthropy—and Trying to Save the World," *The Atlantic,* October 2007, www.theatlantic.com/magazine/archive/2007/10/-ldquo-this-is-not-charity-rdquo/6197/ (accessed August 10, 2012).

52. Médecins Sans Frontières, "A Matter of Life and Death: The Role of Patents in Access to Essential Medicines," MSF briefing for the 4th World Trade Organization Ministerial Conference in Doha, Qatar, November 9–14, 2001.

53. *Macroeconomics and Health: Investing in Health for Economic Development,* Report of the Commission on Macroeconomics and Health, presented by Jeffrey D. Sachs, chair, to Gro Harlem Brundtland, director-general of the World Health Organization, December 20, 2001 (Geneva: World Health Organization, 2001), http://whqlibdoc.who.int/publications/2001/924154550x.pdf (accessed December 1, 2012).

54. Jeffrey Sachs and Amir Attaran, "Defining and Refining International Donor Support for Combating the AIDS Pandemic," *Lancet* 357, no. 9249 (2001): 57.

55. Sarah Ramsa, "Global Fund Makes Historic First Round of Payments," *Lancet* 359, no. 9317 (2002): 1581–1582.

56. Information about the Student Global AIDS Campaign was drawn from an interview with co-founder Adam Taylor, conducted by Luke Messac in Washington, D.C., July 23, 2007.

57. Jesse Helms, *Here's Where I Stand: A Memoir* (New York: Random House, 2005), 145.

58. U.S. Senate Committee on Foreign Relations, "Helms Praises Frist AIDS Bill," July 26, 2000, http://lobby.la.psu.edu/020_Compulsory_Licens ing/Congressional_Statements/Senate/S_Helms_072600.htm (accessed February 9, 2012).

59. A transcript of the Bono interview, which was part of the *Frontline* series *The Age of AIDS,* is available at www.pbs.org/wgbh/pages/frontline/ aids/interviews/bono.html (accessed August 5, 2012).

60. Jesse Helms, "Opinion: We Cannot Turn Away," *Washington Post,* March 24, 2002, B07.

61. Behrman, *The Invisible People,* 246.

62. "Newsmaker: George W. Bush," interview by Jim Lehrer, *MacNeil/ Lehrer NewsHour,* PBS, February 16, 2000, transcript and audio, www.pbs. org/newshour/bb/politics/jan-june00/bush_02–16.html (accessed September 2, 2012).

63. George W. Bush, "State of the Union Address," January 28, 2003, available at www.washingtonpost.com/wp-srv/onpolitics/transcripts/bushtext _012803.html (accessed December 1, 2012).

64. To view the authorizing legislation and its history, see H.R. 1298, *United States Leadership against HIV/AIDS, Tuberculosis, and Malaria Act of 2003,* 108th Cong., 1st sess., www.govtrack.us/congress/bills/108/hr1298 (accessed September 2, 2012).

65. "Gleneagles 2005: Chairman's Summary," July 8, 2005, http://web archive.nationalarchives.gov.uk/+/http://www.number10.gov.uk/Page7883 (December 1, 2012).

66. Jennifer Kates, Adam Wexler, Eric Lief, Carlos Avila, and Benjamin Gobet, "Financing the Response to AIDS in Low- and Middle-Income Countries: International Assistance from Donor Governments in 2010," Kaiser Family Foundation/UNAIDS Report, July/August 2011, www.kff.org/hivaids/ upload/7347–07.pdf (accessed February 9, 2012).

67. See World Health Organization, *World Malaria Report 2008* (Geneva: World Health Organization, 2008), http://whqlibdoc.who.int/publications/ 2008/9789241563697_eng.pdf (accessed December 1, 2012); and Roll Back Malaria Partnership (RBM), *The Global Malaria Action Plan: For a Malaria-Free World,* 2008, www.rbm.who.int/gmap/toc.pdf (accessed December 1, 2012).

68. See H.R. 5501, *Tom Lantos and Henry J. Hyde United States Global Leadership against HIV/AIDS, Tuberculosis, and Malaria Reauthoriza-*

tion Act of 2008, 110th Cong., www.govtrack.us/congress/bills/110/hr5501 (accessed September 2, 2012).

69. In November 2011, as a result of these funding shortfalls, the Global Fund canceled its eleventh round of grant applications. Since the cancellation, the Global Fund has altered its application procedure to be an iterative process rather than a round-based process. See Kaiser Family Foundation, Kaiser Daily Global Health Policy Report, "Global Fund Cancels Round 11 Grants, Approves New Strategy and Organization Plan," November 29, 2011, http:// globalhealth.kff.org/Daily-Reports/2011/November/29/GH-112911-Global -Fund-Round-11.aspx (accessed January 8, 2013).

70. Myron Cohen, Ying Q. Chen, et al., "Prevention of HIV-1 Infection with Early Antiretroviral Therapy," *New England Journal of Medicine* 365, no. 6 (2011): 493.

71. Garrett, Laurie. "Update from the Global Health Program of the Council on Foreign Relations," July 2, 2008. Council on Foreign Relations. http:// www.cfr.org/content/thinktank/GlobalHealth/GHU_FoodCrisis_Jul208.pdf.

72. David A. Walton, Paul E. Farmer, Wesler Lambert, Fernet Léandre, Serena P. Koenig, and Joia S. Mukherjee, "Integrated HIV Prevention and Care Strengthens Primary Health Care: Lessons from Rural Haiti," *Journal of Public Health Policy* 25, no. 2 (2004): 137–158.

University Students and Access to Medicines: Yale and d4t, page 124

1. The early phases of drug development, especially basic science research, are most often funded by the federal government and conducted at academic research institutions, whose ostensible missions are the production and development of knowledge for the advancement of the public good. Many U.S. academic research institutions either hold patents or otherwise participate in the development of therapeutic interventions important to global health, including the University of Minnesota (abacavir, an ARV), Emory University (3TC, an ARV), Duke University (t20, an ARV), the University of Washington (hepatitis B vaccine), and Michigan State University (cisplatin and carboplatin, two drugs central to many cancer chemotherapy regimens). The Yale experience helped to spawn student-led activism (mostly conducted under the auspices of Universities Allied for Essential Medicines) around university licensing provisions at other campuses. See Amit Khera, "The Role of Universities," presentation of Universities Allied for Essential Medicines, www.essentialmedicine .org/uploads/AmitKheraRoleOfUniversities.ppt (accessed February 15, 2013); and Dave A. Chokshi, "Improving Access to Medicines in Poor Countries: The Role of Universities," *PLoS Medicine* 3, no. 6 (2006): e136, www.plos medicine.org/article/info:doi/10.1371/journal.pmed.0030136 (accessed February 9, 2012).

2. Rahul Rajkumar, "The Role of Universities in Addressing the Access and Research Gaps," UAEM National Conference, September 2007, http:// essentialmedicine.org/sites/default/files/archive/uaemconference2007-day-1 -role-of-universities.pdf (accessed September 24, 2012).

3. A.J. Stevens and A.E. Effort, "Using Academic License Agreements to

Promote Global Social Responsibility," *Les Nouvelles: Journal of the Licensing Executives Society International* 43 (June 2008): 87.

4. Daryl Lindsey, "Amy and Goliath," *Salon.com,* May 1, 2001, www.salon.com/2001/05/01/aids_8/ (accessed December 1, 2012).

5. Donald McNeil Jr., "Yale Pressed to Help Cut Drug Costs in Africa," *New York Times,* March 12, 2001, www.nytimes.com/2001/03/12/world/yale-pressed-to-help-cut-drug-costs-in-africa.html (accessed February 15, 2013); William Prusoff, "The Scientist's Story," *New York Times,* March 19, 2001, www.nytimes.com/2001/03/19/opinion/19PRUS.html (accessed February 15, 2013).

6. "Bristol-Myers Squibb Announces Accelerated Program to Fight HIV/AIDS in Africa," press release, www.prnewswire.co.uk/cgi/news/release?id=64424 (accessed February 15, 2013).

7. Chokshi, "Improving Access to Medicines in Poor Countries."

The Politics of Global AIDS Funding in the American Heartland, page 129

1. Emily Pierce, "Nussle Feeling Heat from Locals," *Roll Call,* April 22, 2004, www.rollcall.com/issues/49_112/-5274-1.html (accessed February 15, 2013).

2. Ibid.

3. Emily Pierce, "Nussle Heeds Calls, Boosts AIDS Funds," *Roll Call,* June 1, 2004, www.rollcall.com/issues/49_130/-5700-1.html (accessed February 15, 2013).

4. Ibid. A conference committee is an ad hoc committee of leaders from both the House of Representatives and the Senate convened to resolve differences between disparate versions of the same legislation before final passage.

CHAPTER 6

Portions of this chapter—the review of tuberculosis care in central Haiti—are adapted from previously published work; see Paul Farmer, *Infections and Inequalities: The Modern Plagues* (Berkeley: University of California Press, 1999), 213–223.

1. For more information about these organizations, see their respective websites: www.doctorswithoutborders.org, www.villagehealthworks.org, www.tiyatienhealth.org, and www.nyayahealth.org (accessed September 10, 2012).

2. Laurent Dubois, *Avengers of the New World: The Story of the Haitian Revolution* (Cambridge, Mass.: Harvard University Press, 2004), 21, 19.

3. Laurent Dubois, *Haiti: The Aftershocks of History* (New York: Metropolitan Books, 2011), 47.

4. Michel-Rolph Trouillot, *Haiti, State against Nation: The Origins and Legacy of Duvalierism* (New York: Monthly Review Press, 1990), 74.

5. Dubois, *Haiti: The Aftershocks of History,* 118.

6. Rod Prince, *Haiti: Family Business* (London: Latin America Bureau, 1985), 17–20; Paul Farmer, *The Uses of Haiti* (Monroe, Maine: Common Courage Press, 1994), 71–74.

7. Prince, *Haiti: Family Business*, 17.

8. Trouillot, *Haiti, State against Nation*, 66–69, 83–88.

9. Ibid., 140–141, 144–148. On the "big push" model of development economics, see, for example, Kevin M. Murphy, Andrei Shleifer, and Robert W. Vishny, "Industrialization and the Big Push," *Journal of Political Economy* 97, no. 5 (October 1989): 1003–1026.

10. James Ferguson, *Papa Doc, Baby Doc: Haiti and the Duvaliers* (Oxford: Basil Blackwell, 1987), 40–52.

11. Trouillot, *Haiti, State against Nation*, 183.

12. Ibid., 173–177.

13. Ibid., 181–183; Peter Hallward, *Damning the Flood: Haiti and the Politics of Containment* (London: Verso, 2010), xi.

14. Farmer, *The Uses of Haiti*, 102–107.

15. As chapter 9 describes in greater detail, in March 2010, former U.S. president Bill Clinton apologized before the Senate Committee on Foreign Relations for promoting U.S. food exports that in effect ruined Haiti's rice crop. For video of Clinton's testimony, see U.S. Senate Committee on Foreign Relations, *Hearing: Building on Success: New Directions in Global Health*, March 10, 2010, www.foreign.senate.gov/hearings/building-on-success-new -directions-in-global-health (accessed September 3, 2012).

16. Paul Farmer, "The Power of the Poor in Haiti," *America* 164, no. 9 (1992): 260–267; Amy Wilentz, *The Rainy Season: Haiti since Duvalier* (New York: Simon and Schuster, 1990).

17. Farmer, *The Uses of Haiti*, 149–157; Irwin P. Stotzky, *Silencing the Guns in Haiti: The Promise of Deliberative Democracy* (Chicago: University of Chicago Press, 1997), 30–48.

18. Farmer, *The Uses of Haiti*, 360.

19. Ibid., 354–375; Paul Farmer, Mary C. Smith Fawzi, and Patrice Nevil, "Unjust Embargo of Aid for Haiti," *Lancet* 361, no. 9355 (2003): 420.

20. Paul Farmer, "Who Removed Aristide?" *London Review of Books* 26, no. 8 (2004): 28–31.

21. The first three paragraphs of this section are adapted from Farmer, *Infections and Inequalities*, 213–215.

22. Bernard Foubert, "L'habitation Lemmens à Saint-Domingue au début de la révolution," *Revue de la Société Haïtienne d'Histoire et de Géographie* 45, no. 154 (1987): 3.

23. Ary Bordes, *Évolution des sciences de la santé et de l'hygiène publique en Haïti* (Port-au-Prince: Centre d'Hygiène Familiale, 1980), 1:16–17; translation by Paul Farmer.

24. World Bank, *World DataBank World Development Indicators (WDI) and Global Development Finance (GDF)*, 2009, http://databank.worldbank .org/ddp/home.do?Step=3&id=4 (accessed September 26, 2012).

25. United Nations, Office of the Secretary-General's Special Adviser on Community-Based Medicine and Lessons from Haiti, "Key Statistics: Facts and Figures about the 2010 Earthquake in Haiti," www.lessonsfromhaiti.org/ lessons-from-haiti/key-statistics/ (accessed March 5, 2013).

26. UNICEF, "At a Glance: Haiti," www.unicef.org/infobycountry/haiti_statistics.html (accessed September 10, 2012).

27. Farmer, *Infections and Inequalities,* 215.

28. Library of Congress, Federal Research Division, "Country Profile: Haiti," May 2006, lcweb2.loc.gov/frd/cs/profiles/Haiti.pdf (accessed September 2, 2012).

29. Association of American Medical Colleges, Center for Workforce Studies, *2011 State Physician Workforce Data Release, March 2011* (Washington, D.C.: AAMC, 2011), https://www.aamc.org/download/181238/data/state_databook_update.pdf (accessed September 26, 2012).

30. Paul Farmer, *Partner to the Poor: A Paul Farmer Reader,* ed. Haun Saussy (Berkeley: University of California Press, 2010), 100.

31. Joint United Nations Programme on HIV/AIDS (UNAIDS), *2004 Report on the Global AIDS Epidemic: 4th Global Report* (Geneva: UNAIDS, 2004), annex, www.globalhivmeinfo.org/DigitalLibrary/Digital%20Library/UNAIDSGlobalReport2004_en.pdf (accessed September 3, 2012).

32. The full mission statement reads:

> Our mission is a preferential option for the poor in health care. By establishing long-term relationships with sister organizations based in settings of poverty, Partners In Health strives to achieve two overarching goals: to bring benefits of modern medical science to those most in need of them and to serve as an antidote to despair. We draw on the resources of the world's leading medical and academic institutions and on the lived experience of the world's poorest and sickest communities. At its root, our mission is both medical and moral. It is based on solidarity, rather than charity alone. When our patients are ill and have no access to care, our team of health professionals, scholars, and activists will do whatever it takes to make them well—just as we would do if a member of our own families, or we ourselves, were ill.

33. See Tracy Kidder, *Mountains Beyond Mountains* (New York: Random House, 2003), 300.

34. Paul Farmer, *AIDS and Accusation: Haiti and the Geography of Blame* (Berkeley: University of California Press, 1992), 22–27.

35. This recounting of Acéphie's story is adapted from Farmer, *Partner to the Poor,* 330–332.

36. See, for example, Paul Farmer, "An Anthropology of Structural Violence," *Current Anthropology* 45, no. 3 (2004): 305–326.

37. Johanna Daily, Paul Farmer, Joe Rhatigan, Joel Katz, and Jennifer Furin, "Women and HIV Infection," in *Women, Poverty, and AIDS: Sex, Drugs, and Structural Violence,* ed. Paul Farmer, Margaret Connors, and Janie Simmons (Monroe, Maine: Common Courage Press, 1996), 125–144.

38. Parts of this section are adapted from Farmer, *Infections and Inequalities,* 213–223.

39. Helen Jean Coleman Wiese, "The Interaction of Western and Indigenous Medicine in Haiti in Regard to Tuberculosis," PhD diss., Department of Anthropology, University of North Carolina, Chapel Hill, 1971, 38.

40. Service d'Hygiène, *Notes bio-bibliographique: Médecins et naturalistes de l'ancienne colonie française de Saint-Domingue* (Port-au-Prince: Imprimerie de l'État, 1933), 12.

41. Médéric Louis Élie Moreau de Saint-Méry, *Description topographique, physique, civile, politique et historique de la partie française de l'isle Saint-Domingue (1797–1798)*, ed. Blanche Maurel and Etienne Taillemite (Paris: Société de l'Histoire des Colonies Françaises and Librairie Larose, 1984), 1068.

42. Frantz Tardo-Dino, *Le collier de servitude: La condition sanitaire des esclaves aux Antilles françaises du XVIIe au XIXe siècle* (Paris: Éditions Caribéennes, 1985), 198.

43. Wiese, "Interaction of Western and Indigenous Medicine," 40.

44. James Graham Leyburn, *The Haitian People*, rev. ed., with introduction by Sidney Mintz (New Haven, Conn.: Yale University Press, 1966), 275.

45. United Nations, *Mission to Haiti: Report of the United Nations Mission of Technical Assistance to the Republic of Haiti* (Lake Success, N.Y.: United Nations, 1949), 70–72.

46. Pan American Health Organization, *Reported Cases of Notifiable Diseases in the Americas*, Scientific Publication no. 149 (Washington, D.C.: PAHO, 1967), 290.

47. For a review of these data, see Rachel Feilden, James Allman, Joel Montague, and Jon Rohde, *Health, Population, and Nutrition in Haiti: A Report Prepared for the World Bank* (Boston: Management Sciences for Health, 1981).

48. Julio Desormeaux, Michael P. Johnson, Jacqueline S. Coberly, Phyllis Losikoff, Erika Johnson, Robin Huebner, Lawrence Geiter, Homer Davis, Joan Atkinson, Richard E. Chaisson, Reginald Boulos, and Neal A. Halsey, "Widespread HIV Counseling and Testing Linked to a Community-Based Tuberculosis Control Program in a High-Risk Population," *Bulletin of the Pan American Health Organization* 30, no. 1 (1996): 1–8; Jean William Pape and Warren D. Johnson Jr., "Epidemiology of AIDS in the Caribbean," *Baillière's Clinical Tropical Medicine and Communicable Diseases* 3, no. 1 (1988): 31–42; Richard Long, Marcella Scalcini, George Carré, Elizabeth Philippe, Earl Hershfield, Laila Sekla, and Walter Stackiw, "Impact of Human Immunodeficiency Virus Type 1 on Tuberculosis in Rural Haiti," *American Review of Respiratory Disease* 143, no. 1 (1991): 69–73.

49. Marcella Scalcini, George Carré, Michel Jean-Baptiste, Earl Hershfield, Shirley Parker, Joyce Wolfe, Katherina Nelz, and Richard Long, "Antituberculous Drug Resistance in Central Haiti," *American Review of Respiratory Disease* 142, no. 3 (1990): 508–511. See also Paul Farmer, Jaime Bayona, Mercedes Becerra, J. Daily, Jennifer J. Furin, D. Garcia, Jim Yong Kim, Carole Mitnick, Edward Nardell, Maxi Raymonville, Sonya Sunhi Shin, and P. Small, "Poverty, Inequality, and Drug Resistance: Meeting Community Needs in the Global Era," in *Proceedings of the International Union against Tuberculosis and Lung Disease, North American Region Conference*, Chicago, February 27–March 2, 1997, 88–101.

50. Scalini et al., "Antituberculosis Drug Resistance in Central Haiti."

51. Paul Shears, *Tuberculosis Control Programmes in Developing Countries* (Oxford: Oxfam Publishing, 1988).

52. Helen Jean Coleman Wiese, "Tuberculosis in Rural Haiti," *Social Science and Medicine* 8, no. 6 (1974): 359–362.

388 | Notes to Chapter 6

53. Rifampin has since replaced streptomycin in the initial treatment of adults with tuberculosis. The clinic also stocks second-line drugs for culture-proven cases of MDRTB.

54. One patient who initially lived in Sector 1 later moved out of the catchment area and was no longer served by a community health worker. This patient, rumored to have died some months after leaving the area, is not considered in any of the data analysis of either group.

55. For a concise review of this methodology, see Arthur Kleinman, Leon Eisenberg, and Byron Good, "Culture, Illness, and Care: Clinical Lessons from Anthropologic and Cross-Cultural Research," *Annals of Internal Medicine* 88, no. 2 (1978): 251–258. For an assessment of the methodology's limitations, see Arthur Kleinman, *Writing at the Margin: Discourse between Anthropology and Medicine* (Berkeley: University of California Press, 1985), 5–15. See also Arthur Kleinman, "From Illness as Culture to Caregiving as Moral Experience," *New England Journal of Medicine*, 368 (2013): 1376–1377.

56. The preponderance of women waned over subsequent years, suggesting that the female patients in our study represented a backlog of untreated women who had faced significant barriers to care.

57. The presence of acid-fast bacilli in a sputum sample usually signals the presence of active pulmonary tuberculosis. Although it is an imperfect test for tuberculosis—as all patients with extrapulmonary disease and many with pulmonary disease will have falsely negative smears—sputum microscopy is the standard test in most settings in the developing world, including Haiti. It is an outmoded diagnostic and needs to be replaced or at least supplemented by others, especially in settings with high rates of HIV co-infection and drug resistance, as discussed in chapter 9.

58. Paul Farmer, "Sending Sickness: Sorcery, Politics, and Changing Concepts of AIDS in Rural Haiti," *Medical Anthropology Quarterly* 4, no. 1 (1990): 6–27.

59. See Paul Farmer, Simon Robin, St. Luc Ramilus, and Jim Yong Kim, "Tuberculosis, Poverty, and 'Compliance': Lessons from Rural Haiti," *Seminars in Respiratory Infections* 6, no. 4 (1991): 254–260.

60. Paul Farmer, Fernet Léandre, Joia S. Mukherjee, Marie Sidonise Claude, Patrice Nevil, Mary C. Smith Fawzi, Serena P. Koenig, Arachu Castro, Mercedes C. Becerra, Jeffrey Sachs, Amir Attaran, and Jim Yong Kim, "Community-Based Approaches to HIV Treatment in Resource-Poor Settings," *Lancet* 358, no. 9279 (2001): 404–409.

61. Joia S. Mukherjee, Louise Ivers, Fernet Léandre, Paul Farmer, and Heidi Behforouz, "Antiretroviral Therapy in Resource-Poor Settings: Decreasing Barriers to Access and Promoting Adherence," *Journal of Acquired Immune Deficiency Syndromes* 43, suppl. 1 (December 1, 2006): S123–S126.

62. Andrew Natsios, testimony before U.S. House of Representatives Committee on International Relations, *Hearing: The United States' War on AIDS*, 107th Cong., 1st sess., Washington, D.C., June 7, 2001, http://commdocs .house.gov/committees/intlrel/hfa72978.000/hfa72978_0.HTM (accessed February 15, 2013).

63. Joia S. Mukherjee, Fernet Léandre, Wesler Lambert, Chloe Gans-

Rugebregt, Patrice Nevil, Alice Yang, Michael Seaton, Maxi Raymonville, Paul Farmer, and Louise Ivers, "Excellent Outcomes, High Retention in Treatment, and Low Rate of Switch to Second Line ART in Community Based HIV Treatment Program in Haiti" (presented at Seventeenth International AIDS Conference, Mexico City, August 3–8, 2008).

64. Joia Mukherjee, Margaly Colas, Paul Farmer, Fernet Léandre, Wesler Lambert, Maxi Raymonville, Serena Koenig, David Walton, Patrice Nevil, Nirlande Louissant, and Cynthia Orélus, "Access to Antiretroviral Treatment and Care: The Experience of the HIV Equity Initiative, Cange, Haiti [Case Study]," *Perspectives and Practice in Antiretroviral Treatment* (Geneva: World Health Organization, 2003), www.who.int/hiv/pub/prev_care/en/Haiti_E.pdf (accessed December 28, 2012).

65. David Coetzee, Katherine Hildebrand, et al., "Outcomes after Two Years of Providing Antiretroviral Treatment in Khayelitsha, South Africa," *AIDS* 18, no. 6 (2004): 887–895.

66. "Consensus Statement on Antiretroviral Treatment for AIDS in Poor Countries, by Individual Members of the Faculty of Harvard University," March 2001, www.cid.harvard.edu/cidinthenews/pr/consensus_aids_therapy. pdf (accessed August 8, 2012).

67. See, for example, Jeffrey Sachs, "Weapons of Mass Salvation," *Economist,* October 24, 2002, 73–74.

68. Anthony S. Fauci, "The Expanding Global Health Agenda: A Welcome Development," *Nature Medicine* 13, no. 10 (October 2007): 1169–1171.

69. Jim Yong Kim and Charlie Gilks, "Scaling Up Treatment—Why We Can't Wait," *New England Journal of Medicine* 353, no. 22 (2005): 2392–2394.

70. Martha Ainsworth and Waranya Teokul, "Breaking the Silence: Setting Realistic Priorities for AIDS Control in Less-Developed Countries," *Lancet* 356, no. 9223 (2000): 55–59.

71. Patrice Severe et al., "Antiretroviral Therapy in a Thousand Patients with AIDS in Haiti," *New England Journal of Medicine* 353 (2005): 2325–2334.

72. David A. Walton, Paul E. Farmer, Wesler Lambert, Fernet Léandre, Serena P. Koenig, and Joia S. Mukherjee, "Integrated HIV Prevention and Care Strengthens Primary Health Care: Lessons from Rural Haiti," *Journal of Public Health Policy* 25, no. 2 (2004): 145.

73. For a review of these data and their provenance and for an assessment of claims of causality regarding such conclusions, see Paul Farmer, Cameron T. Nutt, et al., "Reduced Premature Mortality in Rwanda: Lessons from Success," *British Medical Journal* 346 (2013): f65. Neal Emery has written a concise and readable summary of our report in the *Atlantic Monthly* ("Rwanda's Historic Health Recovery: What the U.S. Might Learn," 20 February 2013).

74. See, for example, David Dagan, "The Cleanest Place in Africa," *Foreign Policy,* October 19, 2011, www.foreignpolicy.com/articles/2011/10/19/rwanda_the_cleanest_place_in_africa (accessed September 10, 2012); and "Africa Rising: The Hopeful Continent," *Economist,* December 3, 2011, www.economist.com/node/21541015 (accessed September 10, 2012).

75. Rwanda shares many historical similarities with its neighbor Burundi,

a small mountainous country to its south with a history of political violence. During its precolonial era, Burundi, too, was a single kingdom with a single language.

76. Jan Vansina, *Antecedents to Modern Rwanda: The Nyiginya Kingdom* (Madison: University of Wisconsin Press, 2004), 126–139.

77. Mahmood Mamdani, *When Victims Become Killers: Colonialism, Nativism, and the Genocide in Rwanda* (Princeton, N.J.: Princeton University Press, 2001), 50–59.

78. Vansina, *Antecedents to Modern Rwanda*, 134.

79. Frederick Cooper, *Africa since 1940: The Past of the Present* (Cambridge: Cambridge University Press, 2002), 8; Peter Uvin, *Aiding Violence: The Development Enterprise in Rwanda* (West Hartford, Conn.: Kumarian Press, 1998), 14–15.

80. Mamdani, *When Victims Become Killers*, 53–54, 70.

81. Philip Gourevitch, *We Wish to Inform You That Tomorrow We Will Be Killed with Our Families: Stories from Rwanda* (New York: Farrar, Straus and Giroux, 1998), 59. For one example of the phrase "age-old animosity" used in reference to Hutus and Tutsis in Rwanda, see James C. McKinley Jr., "In Congo, Fighting Outlasts Defeat of Mobutu," *New York Times,* October 13, 1997, http://partners.nytimes.com/library/world/101397congo-kabila.html (accessed September 10, 2012).

82. Mamdani, *When Victims Become Killers*, chap. 2.

83. Vansina, *Antecedents to Modern Rwanda*, 215.

84. C.G. Seligman and Brenda Z. Seligman, *Pagan Tribes of the Nilotic Sudan* (London: Routledge, 1932), 4.

85. Gourevitch, *We Wish to Inform You*, 56.

86. Jacques J. Maquet and Marcel d'Hertefelt, *Élections en société féodale: une étude sur l'introduction du vote populaire au Ruanda-Urundi* (Brussels: Académie Royale des Sciences Coloniales, 1958), 86.

87. Gourevitch, *We Wish to Inform You*, 57.

88. Catharine Newbury, *The Cohesion of Oppression: Clientship and Ethnicity in Rwanda, 1860–1960* (New York: Columbia University Press, 1989), 209, 191.

89. Gourevitch, *We Wish to Inform You*, 60.

90. Newbury, *The Cohesion of Oppression*, 197.

91. Gourevitch, *We Wish to Inform You*, 63.

92. Uvin, *Aiding Violence*, 54, 124.

93. A. Nkeshimana, "Vulgarisation agricole: Défiance d'un système," *Dialogue* 123 (1987): 83–86, quoted in ibid., 151.

94. Uvin, *Aiding Violence*, 45; Farmer, *Partner to the Poor*, 415.

95. Fiona Terry, *Condemned to Repeat? The Paradox of Humanitarian Action* (Ithaca, N.Y.: Cornell University Press, 2002), 155.

96. Scott Straus, *The Order of Genocide: Race, Power, and War in Rwanda* (Ithaca, N.Y.: Cornell University Press, 2006), 118.

97. See Roméo Dallaire, *Shake Hands with the Devil: The Failure of Humanity in Rwanda* (New York: Carroll and Graf, 2003).

98. Linda Polman, *The Crisis Caravan: What's Wrong with Humanitarian Aid?* (New York: Metropolitan Books, 2010), 27.

99. Terry, *Condemned to Repeat?* 163.

100. A.K. Siddique, K. Akram, K. Zaman, S. Laston, A. Salam, R.N. Majumdar, M.S. Islam, and N. Fronczak, "Why Treatment Centres Failed to Prevent Cholera Deaths among Rwandan Refugees in Goma, Zaire," *Lancet* 345, no. 8946 (1995): 359–361.

101. Gourevitch, *We Wish to Inform You*, 161.

102. Stephen Kinzer, *A Thousand Hills: Rwanda's Rebirth and the Man Who Dreamed It* (Hoboken, N.J.: Wiley, 2008), 226.

103. U.S. State Department, Bureau of Democracy, Human Rights, and Labor, "2010 Human Rights Report: Rwanda," *2010 Country Reports on Human Rights Practices*, April 8, 2011, 12, www.state.gov/j/drl/rls/hrrpt/2010/af/154364.htm (accessed August 13, 2012).

104. Republic of Rwanda, Ministry of Finance and Economic Planning, *Rwanda Vision 2020*, July 2000, www.gesci.org/assets/files/Rwanda_Vision_2020.pdf (accessed February 15, 2013).

105. Josh Ruxin, "Rwanda 15 Years On," *New York Times*, April 11, 2009.

106. Daniel Isenberg, "The Big Idea: How to Start an Entrepreneurial Revolution," *Harvard Business Review*, June 2010.

107. This referred to the use of HIV as a weapon of war; during the genocide, men presumed to be HIV-positive were ordered to rape targeted women. Elisabeth Rehn and Ellen Johnson Sirleaf, *Women, War, and Peace: The Independent Experts' Assessment on the Impact of Armed Conflict on Women and Women's Role in Peace-Building* (New York: United Nations Development Fund for Women, 2002), 52.

108. Unpublished data from Partners In Health, presented by Paul Farmer in a lecture, Anthropology 1825, Harvard University, Fall 2008. Trends suggested by these preliminary data were confirmed on a larger scale in short order. See Michael Rich et al., "Excellent Clinical Outcomes and High Retention in Care Among Adults in a Community-Based HIV Treatment Program in Rural Rwanda," *Journal of Acquired Immune Deficiency Syndromes* 59, no. 3 (2012): e35–e42; see also Molly F. Franke et al., "Malaria Parasitemia and CD4 T Cell Count, Viral Load, and Adverse HIV Outcomes among HIV-Infected Pregnant Women in Tanzania," *American Journal of Tropical Medicine and Hygiene* 82, no. 4 (2010): 556–562.

109. The Antiretroviral Therapy (ART) Cohort Collaboration, "HIV Treatment Response and Prognosis in Europe and North America in the First Decade of Highly Active Antiretroviral Therapy: A Collaborative Analysis," *Lancet* 368, no. 9534 (2006): 451–458, esp. 453, table 2.

110. Government of Rwanda, Ministry of Health; Partners In Health; and Clinton Foundation, *Rwanda Rural Health Care Plan: A Comprehensive Approach to Rural Health*, November 2007, 30–36.

111. Government of Rwanda, Ministry of Health, *Health Sector Strategic Plan: July 2009–June 2012*, 34, http://transition.usaid.gov/rw/our_work/for_partners/images/rwandahealthsectorstrategicplanii.pdf (accessed September 2, 2012).

112. Government of Rwanda, Ministry of Health; Partners In Health; and Clinton Foundation, *Rwanda Rural Health Care Plan,* 14.

113. Claude Sekabaraga, Agnes Soucat, F. Diop, and G. Martin, "Innovative Financing for Health in Rwanda: A Report of Successful Reforms," *Improving Human Development Outcomes with Innovative Policies* (Washington, D.C.: World Bank, 2011), http://siteresources.worldbank.org/AFRICA EXT/Resources/258643–1271798012256/Rwanda-health.pdf (accessed March 31, 2012).

114. PIH supplemented existing grants from the Global Fund to Fight AIDS, Tuberculosis and Malaria as well as other public and private funds for *mutuelle* premiums for vulnerable populations.

115. Chunling Lu, Brian Chin, Jiwon Lee Lewandowski, Paulin Basinga, Lisa R. Hirschhorn, Kenneth Hill, Megan Murray, and Agnes Binagwaho, "Towards Universal Health Coverage: An Evaluation of Rwanda *Mutuelles* in Its First Eight Years," *PLoS ONE* 7, no. 6 (2012): e39282, www.plosone.org/ article/info%3Adoi%2F10.1371%2Fjournal.pone.0039282 (accessed September 20, 2012).

116. See, for example, Uvin, *Aiding Violence.*

117. Aaron D. A. Shakow, Gene Bukhman, Olumuyiwa Adebona, Jeremy Greene, Jean de Dieu Ngirabega, Agnès Binagwaho, "Transforming South–South Technical Support to Fight Noncommunicable Diseases," *Global Heart* 7, no. 1 (2012): 35–45.

118. In Burundi, the sister organization is Village Health Works; see Natasha Rybak, "'Village Health Works' in Burundi," *Medicine and Health, Rhode Island* 90, no. 11 (2007): 356–357; see also Tracy Kidder, *Strength in What Remains: A Journey of Remembrance and Forgiveness* (New York: Random House, 2009). In Liberia, the sister organization is Tiyatien Health; see R. Panjabi, O. Aderibigbe, W. Quitoe, et al., "Towards Universal Outcomes: A Community-Based Approach to Improve HIV Care in Post-Conflict Liberia," abstract no. CDB0306, Seventeenth International AIDS Conference, Mexico City, August 3–8, 2008, www.iasociety.org/Abstracts/A200717482. aspx (accessed September 10, 2012).

119. "Haiti," *New York Times,* December 24, 2012, http://topics.nytimes .com/top/news/international/countriesandterritories/haiti/index.html (accessed February 15, 2013).

120. United Nations, Office of the Secretary-General's Special Adviser on Community-Based Medicine and Lessons from Haiti, "Key Statistics: Facts and Figures about the 2010 Earthquake in Haiti," www.lessonsfromhaiti.org/ lessons-from-haiti/key-statistics/ (accessed March 5, 2013).

121. Eduardo A. Cavallo, Andrew Powell, and Oscar Becerra, *Estimating the Direct Economic Damage of the Earthquake in Haiti,* Inter-American Development Bank Working Paper, Series IDB-WP-163, February 2010.

122. Rudy Roberts, *Responding in a Crisis: The Role of National and International Health Workers—Lessons from Haiti* (London: Merlin, August 2010).

123. United Nations, Office of the Secretary-General's Special Adviser on Community-Based Medicine and Lessons from Haiti, "Key Statistics: Facts

and Figures about the 2010 Earthquake in Haiti," www.lessonsfromhaiti.org/lessons-from-haiti/key-statistics/ (accessed March 5, 2013).

124. United Nations, Office of the Secretary-General's Special Adviser on Community-Based Medicine and Lessons from Haiti, "Assistance Tracker," www.lessonsfromhaiti.org/assistance-tracker/ (accessed April 30, 2013).

125. Paul Farmer, *Haiti after the Earthquake* (New York: PublicAffairs, 2011), 122.

126. United Nations, Office of the Secretary-General's Special Adviser on Community-Based Medicine and Lessons from Haiti, "Key Statistics: Aid to Haiti after the January 12, 2010, Earthquake," www.lessonsfromhaiti.org/lessons-from-haiti/key-statistics/ (accessed April 30, 2013).

127. Jean-Max Bellerive and Bill Clinton, "Finishing Haiti's Unfinished Work," *New York Times,* July 11, 2010, www.nytimes.com/2010/07/12/opinion/12clinton-1.html (accessed August 13, 2012).

128. International Organization for Migration, "Displacement Tracking Matrix," http://iomhaitidataportal.info/dtm/ (accessed November 19, 2012).

129. Centers for Disease Control and Prevention, "Update: Outbreak of Cholera—Haiti, 2010," *Morbidity and Mortality Weekly Report (MMWR)* 59, no. 48 (December 10, 2010): 1586–1590.

130. Dorothy E. Logie, Michael Rowson, and Felix Ndagije, "Innovations in Rwanda's Health System: Looking to the Future," *Lancet* 372, no. 9634 (2008): 256–261.

131. Claire Devlin and Robert Elgie, "The Effect of Increased Women's Representation in Parliament: The Case of Rwanda," *Parliamentary Affairs* 61, no. 2 (2008): 237–254.

Health Care Delivery Model, pages 160–161

1. Amartya Sen, "Missing Women: Social Inequality Outweighs Women's Survival Advantage in Asia and North Africa," *British Medical Journal* 304, no. 6287 (1992): 587–588.

CHAPTER 7

1. Livia Montana, Melissa Neuman, and Vinod Mishra, *Spatial Modeling of HIV Prevalence in Kenya,* Demographic and Health Research, U.S. Agency for International Development, DHS Working Paper 27 (2007), 15, www.measuredhs.com/pubs/pdf/WP27/WP27.pdf (accessed October 12, 2012).

2. Sudhir Anand and Amartya K. Sen, "Concepts of Human Development and Poverty: A Multidimensional Perspective," in *Human Development Papers 1997: Poverty and Human Development* (New York: United Nations Development Programme, 1997), 1–20; Jeffrey D. Sachs, "Health in the Developing World: Achieving the Millennium Development Goals," *Bulletin of the World Health Organization* 82, no. 12 (2004): 947–949; Paul Farmer, *Infections and Inequalities: The Modern Plagues* (Berkeley: University of California Press, 1999).

3. Paul E. Farmer, Simon Robin, St. Luc Ramilus, and Jim Yong Kim,

"Tuberculosis, Poverty, and 'Compliance': Lessons from Rural Haiti," *Seminars in Respiratory Infections* 6, no. 4 (1991): 254–260.

4. See, for example, Amit Chattopadhyay and Rosemary G. McKaig, "Social Development of Commercial Sex Workers in India: An Essential Step in HIV/AIDS Prevention," *AIDS Patient Care and STDs* 18, no. 3 (2004): 159–168.

5. See chapter 8 of this volume for a more detailed discussion of the barriers to seeking care for mental health needs. On stigma associated with neglected tropical diseases, see chapter 11 as well as Peter J. Hotez, David H. Molyneux, Alan Fenwick, Jacob Kumaresan, Sonia Ehrlich Sachs, Jeffrey D. Sachs, and Lorenzo Savioli, "Control of Neglected Tropical Diseases," *New England Journal of Medicine* 357, no. 10 (2007): 1018–1027.

6. Paul Farmer, "Sending Sickness: Sorcery, Politics, and Changing Concepts of AIDS in Rural Haiti," *Medical Anthropology Quarterly* 4, no. 1 (1990): 6–27; Paul Farmer, "Bad Blood, Spoiled Milk: Bodily Fluids as Moral Barometers in Rural Haiti," *American Ethnologist* 15, no. 1 (1988): 62–83.

7. For an overview of the divergent perspectives on remunerating community health workers, see Uta Lehmann and David Sanders, *Community Health Workers: What Do We Know about Them?* (Geneva: World Health Organization, 2007), www.who.int/hrh/documents/community_health_workers .pdf (accessed October 12, 2012); Paul E. Farmer, Fernet Léandre, Joia S. Mukherjee, Marie Sidonise Claude, Patrice Nevil, Mary C. Smith-Fawzi, Serena P. Koenig, Arachu Castro, Mercedes C. Becerra, Jeffrey Sachs, Amir Attaran, and Jim Yong Kim, "Community-Based Approaches to HIV Treatment in Resource-Poor Settings," *Lancet* 358, no. 9279 (2001): 404–409; Joseph W. Carlson, Evan Lyon, David Walton, Wai-Chin Foo, Amy C. Sievers, Lawrence N. Shulman, Paul Farmer, Vania Nosé, and Danny A. Milner Jr., "Partners in Pathology: A Collaborative Model to Bring Pathology to Resource Poor Settings," *American Journal of Surgical Pathology* 34, no. 1 (2010): 118–123.

8. Michael E. Porter, "What Is Value in Health Care?" *New England Journal of Medicine* 363, no. 26 (2010): 2477–2481; Michael E. Porter and Elizabeth Olmsted Teisberg, *Redefining Health Care: Creating Value-Based Competition on Results* (Boston: Harvard Business Review Press, 2006).

9. Porter and Teisberg, *Redefining Health Care*, 203–206.

10. Michael E. Porter, "A Strategy for Health Care Reform: Toward a Value-Based System," *New England Journal of Medicine* 361, no. 2 (2009): 109–112.

11. Elizabeth L. Corbett, Catherine J. Watt, Neff Walker, Dermot Maher, Brian G. Williams, Mario C. Raviglione, and Christopher Dye, "The Growing Burden of Tuberculosis: Global Trends and Interactions with the HIV Epidemic," *Archives of Internal Medicine* 163, no. 9 (2003): 1009–1021.

12. See, for example, Paul Farmer, *Pathologies of Power: Health, Human Rights, and the New War on the Poor* (Berkeley: University of California Press, 2003).

13. See, for example, Phyllida Travis, Sara Bennett, Andy Haines, Tikki Pang, Zulfiqar Bhutta, Adnan A. Hyder, Nancy R. Pielemeier, Anne Mills, and Timothy Evans, "Overcoming Health-Systems Constraints to Achieve the Millennium Development Goals," *Lancet* 364, no. 9437 (2004): 900–906; and Jef-

frey D. Sachs, "Beware False Tradeoffs," *Foreign Affairs Roundtable,* January 23, 2007, www.foreignaffairs.com/discussions/roundtables/how-to-promote-global-health (accessed October 12, 2012). See also Paul Farmer, *Haiti after the Earthquake* (New York: PublicAffairs, 2011).

14. World Bank, *World Development Report 1993: Investing in Health* (Oxford: Oxford University Press, 1993), 116; *Macroeconomics and Health: Investing in Health for Economic Development,* Report of the Commission on Macroeconomics and Health, presented by Jeffrey D. Sachs, chair, to Gro Harlem Brundtland, director-general of the World Health Organization, December 20, 2001 (Geneva: World Health Organization, 2001), http://whqlibdoc.who.int/publications/2001/924154550x.pdf (accessed October 12, 2012); Matt Bonds, "A Note from the Millennium Villages Project, Rwanda: Breaking the Disease-Driven Poverty Trap," *Consilience: The Journal of Sustainable Development,* no. 1 (2008): 98–111.

15. See, for example, Alex de Waal, *AIDS and Power: Why There Is No Political Crisis—Yet* (London: Zed Books, 2006).

16. Edward Miguel and Michael Kremer, "Worms: Identifying Impacts on Education and Health in the Presence of Treatment Externalities," *Econometrica* 72 (2004): 159–217; Catherine Nokes, Sally M. Grantham-McGregor, Anthony W. Sawyer, Edward S. Cooper, and Donald A.P. Bundy, "Parasitic Helminth Infection and Cognitive Function in School Children," *Proceedings: Biological Sciences* 247, no. 1319 (1992): 77–81.

17. World Health Organization, *Everybody's Business: Strengthening Health Systems to Improve Health Outcomes* (Geneva: World Health Organization, 2007), www.who.int/healthsystems/strategy/everybodys_business.pdf (accessed October 10, 2012).

18. Ibid. Modern information systems are one pillar of effective and efficient health care delivery. Harnessing innovations in information technologies, from electronic medical records to mobile health technologies, can enhance health system performance at low cost. Strong surveillance and information systems can detect emerging threats and enable health care workers to respond rapidly. For a review, see Hamish Fraser, Paul Biondich, Deshen Moodley, Sharon Choi, Burke W. Mamlin, and Peter Szolovits, "Implementing Electronic Medical Record Systems in Developing Countries," *Informatics in Primary Care* 13, no. 2 (2005): 83–95.

19. Julio Frenk, "The Global Health System: Strengthening National Health Systems as the Next Step for Global Progress," *PLoS Medicine* 7, no. 1 (2010): e1000089.

20. Arthur Kleinman, "The Art of Medicine. Catastrophe and Caregiving: The Failure of Medicine as an Art," *Lancet* 371, no. 9606 (2008): 22–23.

21. World Health Organization, "Polio Eradication: Now More Than Ever, Stop Polio Forever," January 15, 2004, www.who.int/features/2004/polio/en/ (accessed October 15, 2012).

22. World Health Organization, "Poliomyelitis: Fact Sheet No. 114," October 2012, www.who.int/mediacentre/factsheets/fs114/en/ (accessed January 22, 2013).

23. Isao Arita, Miyuki Nakane, and Frank Fenner, "Public Health: Is Polio

Eradication Realistic?" *Science* 312, no. 5775 (May 12, 2006): 852–854; Associated Press, "Is It Time to Give Up on Eradicating Polio?" March 1, 2007, www.msnbc.msn.com/id/17405219/ns/health-infectious_diseases (accessed October 10, 2012).

24. Julio Frenk, "Bridging the Divide: Global Lessons from Evidence-Based Health Policy in Mexico," *Lancet* 368, no. 9539 (2006): 954–961.

25. Farmer, Léandre, et al., "Community-Based Approaches to HIV Treatment in Resource-Poor Settings"; David A. Walton, Paul E. Farmer, Wesler Lambert, Fernet Léandre, Serena P. Koenig, and Joia S. Mukherjee, "Integrated HIV Prevention and Care Strengthens Primary Health Care: Lessons from Rural Haiti," *Journal of Public Health Policy* 25, no. 2 (2004): 137–158.

26. Frenk, "Bridging the Divide."

27. See Jim Yong Kim, Joyce V. Millen, Alec Irwin, and John Gershman, eds., *Dying for Growth: Global Inequality and the Health of the Poor* (Monroe, Maine: Common Courage Press, 2000).

28. Médecins Sans Frontières, *No Cash, No Care: How "User Fees" Endanger Health,* MSF Briefing Paper on Financial Barriers to Healthcare, March 2008, 6, 23, www.msf.org/msf/fms/article-images/2008-00/Nocash NocareMSFapril2008.pdf (accessed October 10, 2012); Rob Yates, "The Removal of Health User Fees in Africa—Key Lessons from Sierra Leone," One World Link, January 12, 2011, http://ebookbrowse.com/one-world-link-jan -2011-1-talk-by-rob-yates-dfid-pps-d110597915 (accessed October 12, 2012).

29. See, for example, Jason Beaubien, "State-of-the-Art Hospital Offers Hope for Haiti," *National Public Radio,* January 27, 2012, www.npr.org/ 2012/01/27/145909633/state-of-the-art-hospital-offers-hope-for-haiti (accessed October 10, 2012). This article notes that the new hospital built by Partners In Health and the Haitian Ministry of Health in Mirebalais, the largest city in Haiti's Central Plateau, also has a CAT scanner—the first in rural Haiti and in the public-sector health system.

30. Jeffrey D. Sachs, *The End of Poverty: Economic Possibilities for Our Time* (New York: Penguin, 2005); Thomas W. Pogge, "Human Rights and Global Health: A Research Program," *Metaphilosophy* 36, nos. 1–2 (January 2005): 182–209.

31. "The Paris Declaration on Aid Effectiveness and the Accra Agenda for Action, 2005/2008," Organisation for Economic Co-operation and Development (OECD), www.oecd.org/development/aideffectiveness/34428351.pdf (accessed October 10, 2012).

32. For more on the concept of health as a human right, see chapter 9.

33. PEPFAR, for example, does not in principle support programs that engage with commercial sex workers, who are highly vulnerable to HIV infection. This policy reflects domestic political pressures in the United States that construe, or misconstrue, sex work not as a product of structural violence—poverty and joblessness, gender disparities, urbanization—but of choice. For more on the politics of U.S. support for global AIDS programs, see John W. Dietrich, "The Politics of PEPFAR: The President's Emergency Plan for AIDS Relief," *Ethics and International Affairs* 21, no. 3 (Fall 2007): 277–292; and Peter Piot, Michel Kazatchkine, Mark Dybul, and Julian Lob-Levyt, "AIDS:

Lessons Learnt and Myths Dispelled," *Lancet* 374, no. 9685 (2009): 260–263. Providing sex workers with access to prevention and treatment services is an essential part of slowing AIDS epidemics—as Thailand's national AIDS program exemplifies. See, for example, Sarun Charumilind, Sachin H. Jain, and Joseph Rhatigan, "HIV in Thailand: The 100% Condom Program," HBS no. GHD-001 (Boston: Harvard Business School Publishing, 2011), Global Health Delivery Online, www.ghdonline.org/cases/ (accessed October 10, 2012).

34. Erika Bolstad and Jacqueline Charles, "Haiti Prime Minister Conille: Donor Aid Needs Revision," *Miami Herald,* February 9, 2012, www.miami herald.com/2012/02/08/2630579/haiti-prime-minister-conille-donor.html (accessed October 12, 2012).

35. Puthenveetil G.K. Panikar, "Resources Not the Constraint on Health Improvement: A Case Study of Kerala," *Economic and Political Weekly* 14, no. 44 (1979): 1803.

36. Kavumpurathu R. Thankappan, "Some Health Implications of Globalization in Kerala, India," *Bulletin of the World Health Organization* 79, no. 9 (2001): 892–893.

37. Ibid.

38. In 2010, health spending in the United States was $8,362 per capita; for this figure and the 2000 data on health spending, see "Health Expenditure per Capita (current US$)," World Bank Databank, 2013, http://data.worldbank .org/indicator/SH.XPD.PCAP (accessed January 30, 2013). The 2000 data on infant mortality and life expectancy in the United States are drawn from Thankappan, "Some Health Implications of Globalization," 892. For a useful breakdown of U.S. health care costs, see Meena Seshamani, "Escalating Health Care Costs," Health Reform, Department of Health and Human Services, March 2009.

39. Panikar, "Resources Not the Constraint," 1803.

40. Thankappan, "Some Health Implications of Globalization," 892.

41. Ibid.

42. Murphy Halliburton, "Suicide: A Paradox of Development in Kerala," *Economic and Political Weekly* 33, nos. 36–37 (1998): 2341–2346; Amartya Sen, "Health: Perception versus Observation," *British Medical Journal* 324, no. 7342 (2002): 860–861.

43. Sen, "Health: Perception versus Observation."

44. See Paul Farmer, "Social Medicine and the Challenge of Biosocial Research," in *Innovative Structures in Basic Research: Ringberg Symposium, 4–7 October 2000* (Munich: Generalverwaltung der Max-Planck-Gesellschaft, Referat Press- und Öffentlichkeitsarbeit, 2002), 55–73, http://xserve02 .mpiwg-berlin.mpg.de/ringberg/talks/farmer/farmer.html (accessed October 12, 2012).

45. In 2001, World Bank president James Wolfensohn officially praised the Cuban health system for doing a "great job" (quoted in Pol De Vos, "'No One Left Abandoned': Cuba's National Health System since the 1959 Revolution," *International Journal of Health Services* 35, no. 1 [2005]: 189).

With a GDP of only $1,100 per capita in 2000, Cuba had a life expectancy of seventy-six years, a maternal mortality rate of 29 per 100,000 live births, and an infant mortality rate of 7 per 1,000 live births. Mexico's GDP is five times larger than Cuba's, and yet its indicators are seventy-three years for life expectancy, 109 deaths per 100,000 live births for maternal mortality, and 24 deaths per 1,000 live births for infant mortality.

Cuba's health indicators are in fact strikingly similar to those of another of its neighbors: the United States, which had a life expectancy of seventy-seven years, a maternal mortality rate of 8 per 100,000 live births, and an infant mortality rate of 9 per 1,000 live births that same year. GDP per capita in the United States is more than thirty-five times that of Cuba. See De Vos, "'No One Left Abandoned.'" Data for U.S. life expectancy, child mortality, and GDP in 2000 come from World Bank, *World Development Report 2003: Sustainable Development in a Dynamic World: Transforming Institutions, Growth, and Quality of Life* (Oxford: Oxford University Press, 2003). The figure for U.S. maternal mortality is for 1998 and comes from World Bank, *World Development Report 2000/2001: Attacking Poverty* (Oxford: Oxford University Press, 2001).

46. Jerry M. Spiegel and Annalee Yassi, "Lessons from the Margins of Globalization: Appreciating the Cuban Health Paradox," *Journal of Public Health Policy* 25, no. 1 (2004): 97.

47. De Vos, "'No One Left Abandoned,'" 193.

48. Spiegel and Yassi, "Lessons from the Margins of Globalization," 96, 88.

49. Farmer, *Haiti after the Earthquake,* 175 and passim.

50. *Rwanda National HIV and AIDS Monitoring and Evaluation Plan, 2006–2009,* National AIDS Control Commission (Rwanda), 2006, http://test .aidsportal.org/atomicDocuments/AIDSPortalDocuments/rwanda%20m%20 and%20e.pdf (accessed October 12, 2012).

51. Ranu S. Dhillon, Matthew H. Bonds, Max Fraden, Donald Ndahiro, and Josh Ruxin, "The Impact of Reducing Financial Barriers on Utilisation of a Primary Health Care Facility in Rwanda," *Global Public Health* 7, no. 1 (2012): 72.

52. Fabienne Shumbusho, Johan van Griensven, David Lowrance, Innocent Turate, Mark A. Weaver, Jessica Price, and Agnes Binagwaho, "Task Shifting for Scale-Up of HIV Care: Evaluation of Nurse-Centered Antiretroviral Treatment at Rural Health Centers in Rwanda," *PLoS Medicine* 6, no. 10 (2009): e1000163.

53. Jessica E. Price, Jennifer Asuka Leslie, Michael Welsh, and Agnes Binagwaho, "Integrating HIV Clinical Services into Primary Health Care in Rwanda: A Measure of Quantitative Effects," *AIDS Care* 21, no. 5 (2009): 608–614.

54. See, for example, Farmer, *Haiti after the Earthquake,* 369.

55. See Paul Collier, *The Bottom Billion: Why the Poorest Countries Are Failing and What Can Be Done about It* (New York: Oxford University Press, 2007), chap. 7; see also Farmer, *Haiti after the Earthquake.*

56. Laurie Garrett, "The Challenge of Global Health," *Foreign Affairs* 86, no. 1 (February 2007): 14–38, www.foreignaffairs.com/articles/62268/laurie -garrett/the-challenge-of-global-health (accessed October 12, 2012).

57. Clinton Foundation, "Our Work in Africa," http://africa.clintonfounda tion.org/our_work.php (accessed March 27, 2011).

58. World Health Organization, *World Health Report 2006: Working Together for Health* (Geneva: World Health Organization, 2006), xv, xix.

59. The United States, for example, may face a deficit of eight hundred thousand nurses and two hundred thousand doctors by 2020 if health care training continues at the current rate. See Garrett, "The Challenge of Global Health"; U.S. Department of Health and Human Services, *Projected Supply, Demand, and Shortages of Registered Nurses, 2000–2020* (Washington, D.C.: Health Resources and Services Administration, 2002), 13; and Richard A. Cooper, "Weighing the Evidence for Expanding Physician Supply," *Annals of Internal Medicine* 141, no. 9 (2004): 705–714.

60. World Health Organization, *World Health Report 2006,* xvii.

61. A.S. Muula, "Case for Clinical Officers and Medical Assistants in Malawi," *Croatian Medical Journal* 50, no. 1 (2009): 77–78.

62. Garrett, "The Challenge of Global Health."

63. World Health Organization, *World Health Report 2006,* 44.

64. Fitzhugh Mullan, Seble Frehywot, et al., "Medical Schools in Sub-Saharan Africa," *Lancet* 377, no. 9771 (2011): 1113–1121; Fitzhugh Mullan, "The Metrics of the Physician Brain Drain," *New England Journal of Medicine* 353, no. 17 (2005): 1810–1818.

65. World Health Organization, *World Health Report 2006,* 46.

66. Ibid., 42.

67. Ibid., 146.

68. Luis Huicho, Robert W. Scherpbier, A. Mwansa Nkowane, Cesar G. Victora, and the Multi-Country Evaluation of IMCI Study Group, "How Much Does Quality of Child Care Vary between Health Workers with Different Durations of Training? An Observational Multicountry Study," *Lancet* 372, no. 9642 (2008): 910–916.

69. Heidi L. Behforouz, Paul E. Farmer, and Joia S. Mukherjee, "From Directly Observed Therapy to *Accompagnateurs:* Enhancing AIDS Treatment Outcomes in Haiti and in Boston," *Clinical Infectious Diseases* 38, no. 5, suppl. (2004): S429–S436.

70. Walton, Farmer, et al., "Integrated HIV Prevention and Care Strengthens Primary Health Care."

71. *One Million Community Health Workers: Technical Task Force Report,* Earth Institute, Columbia University, 2011, www.millenniumvillages .org/files/2011/06/1mCHW_TechnicalTaskForceReport.pdf (accessed October 12, 2012).

72. Garrett, "The Challenge of Global Health."

73. Giuseppe Raviola, M'Imunya Machoki, Esther Mwaikambo, and Mary Jo DelVecchio Good, "HIV, Disease Plague, Demoralization, and 'Burnout': Resident Experience of the Medical Profession in Nairobi, Kenya," *Culture, Medicine, and Psychiatry* 26, no. 1 (2002): 55–86.

74. Suwit Wibulpolprasert, "The Inequitable Distribution of Doctors: Can It Be Solved?" *Human Resources for Health and Development* 3, no. 1 (January 1999): 2–39, www.moph.go.th/ops/hrdj/hrdj6/pdf31/INEQUIT.PDF (accessed January 30, 2013).

75. Ibid.

76. Garrett, "The Challenge of Global Health."

77. Barbara Stilwell, Khassoum Diallo, Pascal Zurn, Marko Vujicic, Orvill Adams, and Mario Dal Poz, "Migration of Health-Care Workers from Developing Countries: Strategic Approaches to Its Management," *Bulletin of the World Health Organization* 82, no. 8 (August 2004): 595–600.

78. See, for example, Roger Bate and Kathryn Boateng, "Honesty Is a Virtue," *Foreign Affairs Roundtable,* January 24, 2007, www.foreignaffairs.com/discussions/roundtables/how-to-promote-global-health (accessed October 15, 2012). Laurie Garrett in return calls Bate's and Boateng's critique an "unfair swipe . . . against poor countries" and notes that "nearly every one of the targeted countries has significantly increased the percentage of its GDP spent on health over the last three years. So their criticism is out of date" (Garrett, "The Song Remains the Same," *Foreign Affairs Roundtable,* January 24, 2007, www.foreignaffairs.com/discussions/roundtables/how-to-promote -global-health [accessed October 15, 2012]).

79. Paul Farmer notes that the entire budgets for the ministries of health in Malawi and Haiti are both less than the budget of the Brigham and Women's Hospital in Boston (Farmer, "Challenging Orthodoxies: The Road Ahead for Health and Human Rights," *Health and Human Rights: An International Journal* 10, no. 1 [2008]: 7).

Case Brief 1. Polio in Uttar Pradesh: Local Context Matters, page 187

1. Adapted from Andrew Ellner, Sachin H. Jain, Joseph Rhatigan, and Daniel Blumenthal, "Polio Elimination in Uttar Pradesh," HBS no. GHD-005 (Boston: Harvard Business School Publishing, 2011), Global Health Delivery Online, www.ghdonline.org/cases/ (accessed October 10, 2012).

2. Ibid.; see also Government of Uttar Pradesh, "Human Development," chap. 5 in *Annual Plan for 2006–2007 for the State of Uttar Pradesh,* ed. Planning Department (Government of Uttar Pradesh, 2005).

3. Ellner, Jain, et al., "Polio Elimination in Uttar Pradesh." See also Rob Stephenson and Amy Ong Tsui, "Contextual Influences on Reproductive Health Service Use in Uttar Pradesh, India," *Studies in Family Planning* 33, no. 4 (2002): 312.

4. Nicholas C. Grassly, Christophe Fraser, Jay Wenger, Jagadish M. Deshpande, Roland W. Sutter, David L. Heymann, and R. Bruce Aylward, "New Strategies for the Elimination of Polio from India," *Science* 314, no. 5802 (November 17, 2006): 1150–1153.

5. "Infected Districts, 2000–2005," National Polio Surveillance Project, 2012, www.npspindia.org/infecteddistricts.asp (accessed October 10, 2012). See also Ellner, Jain, et al., "Polio Elimination in Uttar Pradesh."

Case Brief 2. AMPATH HIV Care: A Care Delivery Value Chain, page 191

1. Adapted from Peter Park, Arti Bhatt, and Joseph Rhatigan, "The Academic Model for the Prevention and Treatment of HIV/AIDS," HBS no. GHD-

013 (Boston: Harvard Business School Publishing, 2011), Global Health Delivery Online, www.ghdonline.org/cases/ (accessed October 10, 2012).

Case Brief 3. BRAC's Rural Tuberculosis Program:
Shared Delivery Infrastructure, page 193

1. Adapted from Maria May, Joseph Rhatigan, and Richard Cash, "BRAC's Tuberculosis Program: Pioneering DOTS Treatment for TB in Rural Bangladesh," HBS no. GHD-010 (Boston: Harvard Business School Publishing, 2011), Global Health Delivery Online, www.ghdonline.org/cases/ (accessed October 10, 2012).

Case Brief 4. A to Z Textile Mills Ltd.: Improving Health and the Economy, page 195

1. Pedro L. Alonso, Steve W. Lindsay, Joanna R.M. Armstrong Schellenberg, Andres de Francisco, F.C. Shenton, Brian M. Greenwood, M. Conteh, K. Cham, Allan G. Hill, Patricia H. David, Greg Fegan, and A.J. Hall, "The Effect of Insecticide-Treated Bed Nets on Mortality of Gambian Children," *Lancet* 337, no. 8756 (1991): 1499–1502.

2. Adapted from William Rodriguez and Kileken ole-MoiYoi, "Building Local Capacity for Health Commodity Manufacturing: A to Z Textile Mills Ltd.," HBS no. GHD-009 (Boston: Harvard Business School Publishing, 2011), Global Health Delivery Online. www.ghdonline.org/cases/ (accessed October 12, 2012).

The U.S. Health System, page 204

1. Alan M. Garber and Jonathan Skinner, "Is American Health Care Uniquely Inefficient?" *Journal of Economic Perspectives* 22, no. 4 (2008): 27.

2. Gerard F. Anderson and Bianca K. Frogner, "Health Spending in OECD Countries: Obtaining Value per Dollar," *Health Affairs* 27, no. 6 (2008): 1718.

3. U.S. Census Bureau, "Income, Poverty, and Health Insurance Coverage in the United States: 2010," press release, September 13, 2011, www.census.gov/newsroom/releases/archives/income_wealth/cb11–157.html (accessed October 12, 2012).

4. Institute of Medicine, Committee on the Consequences of Uninsurance, *Hidden Costs, Value Lost: Uninsurance in America* (Washington, D.C.: National Academies Press, 2003), 1–11.

5. Peter Singer, "Why We Must Ration Health Care," *New York Times,* July 15, 2009, www.nytimes.com/2009/07/19/magazine/19healthcare-t.html ?pagewanted=all (accessed January 23, 2013).

6. There is a lively debate about the effects of health care spending in the United States. David Cutler argues in *Your Money or Your Life: Strong Medicine for America's Healthcare System* (New York: Oxford University Press, 2004) that the substantial improvements in the U.S. health system over the last fifty years in large part justify the high costs. By contrast, in their article "Is American Health Care Uniquely Inefficient?" Alan Garber and Jonathan

Skinner bemoan the inefficiencies and unsustainable rising costs of the U.S. health system.

7. See Gerard F. Anderson and Jean-Pierre Poullier, "Health Spending, Access, and Outcomes: Trends in Industrialized Countries," *Health Affairs* 18, no. 3 (1999): 178–192; and Marcia Clemmitt, "U.S. Spends a Lot on Health But Doesn't Know What It Buys," *Medicine and Health* 54, no. 22, suppl. (May 29, 2000): 1–4.

8. World Health Organization, *World Health Report 2000—Health Systems: Improving Performance* (Geneva: World Health Organization, 2000), 155. The United States ranked behind countries as diverse as Italy (rated 2), Japan (10), Saudi Arabia (26), Canada (30), and Costa Rica (36).

9. As Garber and Skinner caution, "Cross-country comparisons of expenditures and health outcomes are common but are also of limited value because of our inability to control adequately for underlying health differences across countries—for example, that Americans are more likely to have diabetes or to be obese compared to the English" ("Is American Health Care Uniquely Inefficient?" 28).

10. Christopher J. L. Murray and Julio Frenk, "Ranking 37th—Measuring the Performance of the U.S. Health Care System," *New England Journal of Medicine* 362, no. 2 (2010): 98–99.

CHAPTER 8

1. Giuseppe Raviola, Anne E. Becker, and Paul Farmer, "A Global Scope for Global Health—Including Mental Health," *Lancet* 378, no. 9803 (2011): 1613–1615.

2. See, for example, Martin Prince, Vikram Patel, Shekhar Saxena, Mario Maj, Joanna Maselko, Michael R. Phillips, and Atif Rahman, "No Health without Mental Health," *Lancet* 370, no. 9590 (2007): 859–877.

3. Byron J. Good, *Medicine, Rationality, and Experience: An Anthropological Perspective* (New York: Cambridge University Press, 1994), 116–128.

4. A CDC study analyzing data from 2006–2008 found that nearly 1 in 10 Americans suffer from depression; see Centers for Disease Control and Prevention, "Current Depression among Adults: United States, 2006 and 2008," *Morbidity and Mortality Weekly Report (MMWR)* 59, no. 38 (October 1, 2010): 1229–1235.

5. Allan V. Horwitz and Jerome C. Wakefield, *The Loss of Sadness: How Psychiatry Transformed Normal Sorrow into Depressive Disorder* (New York: Oxford University Press, 2007), 4; Arthur Kleinman, *Rethinking Psychiatry: From Cultural Category to Personal Experience* (New York: Free Press, 1988), 53–75.

6. Centers for Disease Control and Prevention, National Center for Health Statistics, *Health, United States, 2007: With Chartbook on Trends in the Health of Americans* (Washington, D.C.: U.S. Government Printing Office, 2007), 88, www.cdc.gov/nchs/data/hus/hus07.pdf#summary%20 (accessed October 16, 2012).

7. Horwitz and Wakefield, *The Loss of Sadness*, 6.

8. See Louis Menand, "Head Case: Can Psychiatry Be a Science?" *New Yorker*, March 1, 2010, www.newyorker.com/arts/critics/atlarge/2010/03/01/100301crat_atlarge_menand (accessed September 18, 2012). "Me-too" drugs are alternate versions of existing medications that have slightly modified chemical structures; such drugs allow a pharmaceutical company to capture market share of a successful, but still patented, drug manufactured and sold by a competitor.

9. Arthur Kleinman, "Culture, Bereavement, and Psychiatry," *Lancet* 379, no. 9816 (2012): 608–609.

10. Hans-Ulrich Wittchen and Frank Jacobi, "Size and Burden of Mental Disorders in Europe: A Critical Review and Appraisal of 27 Studies," *European Neuropsychopharmacology* 15, no. 4 (2005): 357–376.

11. See, for example, Amy Schulz, Barbara Israel, David Williams, Edith Parker, Adam Becker, and Sherman James, "Social Inequalities, Stressors, and Self Reported Health Status among African American and White Women in the Detroit Metropolitan Area," *Social Science and Medicine* 51, no. 11 (2000): 1639–1653; Kenneth Wells, Ruth Klap, Alan Koike, and Cathy Sherbourne, "Ethnic Disparities in Unmet Need for Alcoholism, Drug Abuse, and Mental Health Care," *American Journal of Psychiatry* 158, no. 12 (2001): 2027–2032; Anne E. Becker, Debra L. Franko, Alexandra Speck, and David B. Herzog, "Ethnicity and Differential Access to Care for Eating Disorder Symptoms," *International Journal of Eating Disorders* 33, no. 2 (2003): 205–212.

12. WHO World Mental Health Survey Consortium, "Prevalence, Severity, and Unmet Need for Treatment of Mental Disorders in the World Health Organization World Mental Health Surveys," *Journal of the American Medical Association* 291, no. 21 (2004): 2581–2590.

13. World Health Organization, *The Global Burden of Disease: 2004 Update* (Geneva: World Health Organization, 2008), 62, www.who.int/healthinfo/global_burden_disease/GBD_report_2004update_full.pdf (accessed November 26, 2012).

14. Christopher J.L. Murray and Alan D. Lopez, "Alternative Projections of Mortality and Disability by Cause, 1990–2020: Global Burden of Disease Study," *Lancet* 349, no. 9064 (1997): 1501–1502.

15. Vikram Patel, "Alcohol Use and Mental Health in Developing Countries," *Annals of Epidemiology* 17, no. 5, suppl. (2007): S87.

16. Schulz, Israel, et al., "Social Inequalities, Stressors, and Self Reported Health Status."

17. See *The Lancet* Series on Global Mental Health, London, September 2007, www.thelancet.com/series/global-mental-health (accessed October 15, 2012).

18. Prince, Patel, et al., "No Health without Mental Health," 868. One sorry manifestation of the effects of such co-morbidity was the presumed first cholera case in Haiti: researchers believe that a twenty-eight-year-old man with a history of severe untreated psychiatric disease was the first Haitian to get sick from cholera; he died at home in the Artibonite River Valley on October 13, 2010. See Louise C. Ivers and David A. Walton, "The 'First' Case of

Cholera in Haiti: Lessons for Global Health," *American Journal of Tropical Medicine and Hygiene* 86, no. 1 (2012): 36–38.

19. Prince, Patel, et al., "No Health without Mental Health," 868.

20. Ibid.; World Health Organization, *World Health Report 2001—Mental Health: New Understanding, New Hope* (Geneva: World Health Organization, 2001), www.who.int/whr/2001/en/whr01_en.pdf (accessed October 15, 2012).

21. WHO World Mental Health Survey Consortium, "Prevalence, Severity, and Unmet Need."

22. Vikram Patel and Arthur Kleinman, "Poverty and Common Mental Disorders in Developing Countries," *Bulletin of the World Health Organization* 81, no. 8 (2003): 609.

23. Raviola, Becker, and Farmer, "A Global Scope for Global Health."

24. Robert Desjarlais, Leon Eisenberg, Byron Good, and Arthur Kleinman, eds., *World Mental Health: Problems and Priorities in Low-Income Countries* (Oxford: Oxford University Press, 1996), 31.

25. Ibid., 183. For more on the social consequences of the gender bias against women, see Amartya Sen, "Missing Women: Social Inequality Outweighs Women's Survival Advantage in Asia and North Africa," *British Medical Journal* 304, no. 6827 (1992): 587–588.

26. World Health Organization, *World Health Report 2001—Mental Health,* 36.

27. For statistics on suicide as a leading cause of death among young adults in China and Europe, see ibid., 39. For U.S. statistics, see Centers for Disease Control and Prevention, National Center for Injury Prevention and Control, *Web-Based Injury Statistics Query and Reporting System,* www.cdc.gov/injury/wisqars/index.html (accessed September 18, 2012).

28. Vikram Patel, Benedetto Saraceno, and Arthur Kleinman, "Beyond Evidence: The Moral Case for International Mental Health," *American Journal of Psychiatry* 163, no. 8 (2006): 1313.

29. Ibid.

30. Ibid., 1314. This view has been disputed, however. For example, in his book *Crazy Like Us: The Globalization of the American Psyche* (New York: Free Press, 2010), Ethan Watters contends that promulgating a strictly biological understanding of mental illness may at times increase stigma.

31. Desjarlais, Eisenberg, et al., *World Mental Health,* 54.

32. Tami L. Mark, Rosanna M. Coffey, Rita Vandivort-Warren, Hendrick J. Harwood, Edward C. King, and the MHSA Spending Estimates Team, "Trends: U.S. Spending for Mental Health and Substance Abuse Treatment, 1991–2001," *Health Affairs* 24 (2005): 133; Thomas Insel, "Assessing the Economic Costs of Serious Mental Illness," *American Journal of Psychiatry* 165, no. 6 (2008): 663–665.

33. Desjarlais, Eisenberg, et al., *World Mental Health,* 30. The programs referenced were responses to natural disasters, but the authors suggest that the examples serve as a model for the implementation of mental health care services in resource-poor health systems.

34. Details about the Nepal Community Mental Health Project are drawn from Sarah Acland, "Mental Health Services in Primary Care: The Case of

Nepal," in *World Mental Health Casebook: Social and Mental Health Programs in Low-Income Countries,* ed. Alex Cohen, Arthur Kleinman, and Benedetto Saraceno (New York: Kluwer Academic/Plenum, 2002), 121–153.

35. Ibid., 129.

36. Ibid., 141.

37. T. Adeoye Lambo, "Patterns of Psychiatric Care in Developing African Countries: The Nigerian Village Program," in *International Trends in Mental Health,* ed. Henry P. David (New York: McGraw-Hill, 1966), 147–153; Olabisi A. Odejide, L. Kola Oyewunmi, and Jude U. Ohaeri, "Psychiatry in Africa," *American Journal of Psychiatry* 146, no. 6 (1989): 708–716.

38. Alberto Minoletti and Alessandra Zaccaria, "Plan Nacional de Salud Mental en Chile: 10 Años de Experiencia," *Revista Panamericana de Salud Publica* 18, nos. 4–5 (2005): 346–358. See also Graciela Rojas, Rosemarie Fritsch, Jaime Solis, Enrique Jadresic, Cristóbal Castillo, Marco González, Viviana Guajardo, Glyn Lewis, Tim J. Peters, and Ricardo Araya, "Treatment of Postnatal Depression in Low-Income Mothers in Primary-Care Clinics in Santiago, Chile: A Randomised Controlled Trial," *Lancet* 370, no. 9599 (2007): 1629–1637; Ricardo Araya, Graciela Rojas, Rosemarie Fritsch, Jorge Gaete, Maritza Rojas, Greg Simon, and Tim J. Peters, "Treating Depression in Primary Care in Low-Income Women in Santiago, Chile: A Randomised Controlled Trial," *Lancet* 361, no. 9362 (2003): 995–1000.

39. Raviola, Becker, and Farmer, "A Global Scope for Global Health."

40. Giuseppe Raviola, Eddy Eustache, Catherine Oswald, and Gary Belkin, "Mental Health Response in Haiti in the Aftermath of the 2010 Earthquake: A Case Study for Building Long-Term Solutions," *Harvard Review of Psychiatry* 20, no. 1 (2012): 71.

41. World Health Organization, *mhGAP Intervention Guide for Mental, Neurological, and Substance Use Disorders in Non-Specialized Health Settings: Mental Health GAP Action Programme (mhGAP)* (Geneva: World Health Organization, 2010), www.who.int/mental_health/publications/mh GAP_intervention_guide/en/index.html (accessed September 18, 2012).

42. Vikram Patel, Gregory Simon, Neerja Chowdhary, Sylvia Kaaya, and Ricardo Araya, "Packages of Care for Depression in Low- and Middle-Income Countries," *PLoS Medicine* 6, no. 10 (2009): e1000159; Vikram Patel and Martin Prince, "Global Mental Health: A New Global Health Field Comes of Age," *Journal of the American Medical Association* 303, no. 19 (2010): 1976–1977; Dan Chisholm, Crick Lund, and Shekhar Saxena, "Cost of Scaling Up Mental Healthcare in Low- and Middle-Income Countries," *British Journal of Psychiatry* 191 (2007): 528–535.

43. Gary S. Belkin, Jurgen Unützer, Ronald C. Kessler, Helen Verdeli, Giuseppe Raviola, Katherine Sachs, Catherine Oswald, and Eddy Eustache, "Scaling Up for the 'Bottom Billion': '5 × 5' Implementation of Community Mental Health Care in Low-Income Regions," *Psychiatric Services* 62, no. 12 (2011): 1494–1502.

44. Arthur Kleinman, *Writing at the Margin: Discourse between Anthropology and Medicine* (Berkeley: University of California Press, 1995), 38. See also Arthur Kleinman, "Medicalization and the Clinical Praxis of Medical

Systems," in *The Use and Abuse of Medicine,* ed. Marten W. De Vries, Robert L. Berg, and Mack Lipkin Jr. (New York: Praeger Scientific, 1982), 42–49.

45. Kleinman, *Writing at the Margin,* 182.

46. See, for example, Patel and Kleinman, "Poverty and Common Mental Disorders in Developing Countries."

47. Vikram Patel and Athula Sumathipala, "International Representation in Psychiatric Literature," *British Journal of Psychiatry* 178 (2001): 407.

48. Watters, *Crazy Like Us.* See also Arthur Kleinman, *The Illness Narratives: Suffering, Healing, and the Human Condition* (New York: Basic Books, 1988).

49. Watters, *Crazy Like Us,* 2–64.

50. See, for example, Arthur Kleinman, Veena Das, and Margaret Lock, eds. *Social Suffering* (Berkeley: University of California Press, 1997).

51. Kleinman, *The Illness Narratives,* 128.

52. Kleinman, *Rethinking Psychiatry,* 11.

53. Ibid., 49.

54. Dean T. Jamison, Joel G. Breman, Anthony R. Measham, George Alleyne, Mariam Claeson, David B. Evans, Prabhat Jha, Anne Mills, and Philip Musgrove, eds., *Priorities in Health: Disease Control Priorities Project* (Washington, D.C.: World Bank, 2006), 43.

55. The 1993 *World Development Report* found that mental illness accounted for more than 8.1 percent of the global burden of disease, as measured in DALYs; see World Bank, *World Development Report 1993: Investing in Health* (Oxford: Oxford University Press, 1993).

56. Christopher J.L. Murray, "Quantifying the Burden of Disease: The Technical Basis for Disability-Adjusted Life Years," *Bulletin of the World Health Organization* 72, no. 3 (1994): 429.

57. Ibid., 439.

58. Ibid., 434–436.

59. As the authors explain, "If individuals are forced to choose between saving a year of life for a 2 year-old and saving it for a 22 year-old, most prefer to save the 22 year-old"; see Christopher J.L. Murray and Alan D. Lopez, eds., *The Global Burden of Disease: A Comprehensive Assessment of Mortality and Disability from Diseases, Injuries, and Risk Factors in 1990 and Projected to 2020,* vol. 1, Global Burden of Disease and Injury Series (Cambridge, Mass.: Harvard University Press, 1996), 13.

60. Sudhir Anand and Kara Hanson, "Disability-Adjusted Life Years: A Critical Review," *Journal of Health Economics* 16, no. 6 (1997): 691.

61. Murray, "Quantifying the Burden of Disease," 431–433.

62. Ibid., 429.

63. Richard S. Cooper, Babatunde Osotimehin, Jay S. Kaufman, and Terrence Forrester, "Disease Burden in Sub-Saharan Africa: What Should We Conclude in the Absence of Data?" *Lancet* 351, no. 9097 (1998): 209.

64. World Health Organization, *World Health Report 2000—Health Systems: Improving Performance* (Geneva: World Health Organization, 2000).

65. Elizabeth Lowry, "Strong Medicine," *University of Washington*

Alumni Magazine, December 2007, 4, www.washington.edu/alumni/columns/dec07/content/view/79/1 (accessed October 15, 2012).

66. Julio Frenk, "Bridging the Divide: Global Lessons from Evidence-Based Health Policy in Mexico," *Lancet* 368, no. 9539 (2006): 954–961.

67. Gary King, Emmanuela Gakidou, Kosuke Imai, Jason Lakin, Ryan T. Moore, Clayton Nall, Nirmala Ravishankar, Manett Vargas, Martha María Téllez-Rojo, Juan Eugenio Hernández Ávila, Mauricio Hernández Ávila, and Héctor Hernández Llamas, "Public Policy for the Poor? A Randomised Assessment of the Mexican Universal Health Insurance Programme," *Lancet* 373, no. 9673 (2009): 1447–1454.

68. Arthur Kleinman, "A Critique of Objectivity in International Health," in Kleinman, *Writing at the Margin,* 81.

69. Amartya Sen, "Objectivity and Position: Assessment of Health and Well-Being," in *Health and Social Change in International Perspective,* ed. Lincoln C. Chen, Arthur Kleinman, and Norma C. Ware (Cambridge, Mass.: Harvard School of Public Health, 1994), 123.

70. Arthur Kleinman, Veena Das, and Margaret Lock, "Introduction," in Kleinman, Das, and Lock, *Social Suffering,* ix.

71. See, for example, Andreu Mas-Colell, Michael D. Whinston, and Jerry R. Green, *Microeconomic Theory* (New York: Oxford University Press, 1995), chap. 3.

72. Murray, "Quantifying the Burden of Disease," 431.

73. Ibid., 434.

74. Ibid., 432.

75. Anand and Hanson, "Disability-Adjusted Life Years," 687.

76. Ibid., 688.

77. Murray, "Quantifying the Burden of Disease," 434.

78. Anand and Hanson, "Disability-Adjusted Life Years," 690.

79. Murray, "Quantifying the Burden of Disease," 435.

80. Prince, Patel, et al., "No Health without Mental Health."

81. World Bank, *World Development Report 1993,* iii, 5.

82. Marian Goble, Michael D. Iseman, Lorie A. Madsen, Dennis Waite, Lynn Ackerson, and C. Robert Horsburgh Jr., "Treatment of 171 Patients with Pulmonary Tuberculosis Resistant to Isoniazid and Rifampin," *New England Journal of Medicine* 328, no. 8 (1993): 527–532.

83. World Health Organization, *Multidrug and Extensively Drug-Resistant TB (M/XDR-TB): 2010 Global Report on Surveillance and Response,* Report no. WHO/HTM/TB/2010.3 (Geneva: World Health Organization, 2010), http://whqlibdoc.who.int/publications/2010/9789241599191_eng.pdf (accessed September 20, 2012).

84. Salmaan Keshavjee and Paul E. Farmer, "Picking Up the Pace: Scale-Up of MDR Tuberculosis Treatment Programs," *New England Journal of Medicine* 363, no. 19 (2010): 1781–1784.

85. See, for example, Jim Yong Kim, Joia S. Mukherjee, Michael L. Rich, Kedar Mate, Jaime Bayona, and Mercedes C. Becerra, "From Multidrug-Resistant Tuberculosis to DOTS Expansion and Beyond: Making the Most of a Paradigm Shift," *Tuberculosis* 83, nos. 1–3 (2003): 59–65; Keshavjee and

Farmer, "Picking Up the Pace"; Salmaan Keshavjee, Kwonjune Seung, et al., "Stemming the Tide of Multidrug-Resistant Tuberculosis: Major Barriers to Addressing the Growing Epidemic," in Institute of Medicine, *Addressing the Threat of Drug-Resistant Tuberculosis: A Realistic Assessment of the Challenge. Workshop Summary* (Washington, D.C.: National Academies Press, 2009), 139–236, www.iom.edu/~/media/Files/Activity%20Files/Research/DrugForum/IOM_MDRTB_whitepaper_2009_01_14_FINAL_Edited.pdf (accessed October 15, 2012); Eva Nathanson, Paul Nunn, Mukund Uplekar, Katherine Floyd, Ernesto Jaramillo, Knut Lönnroth, Diana Weil, and Mario Raviglione, "MDR Tuberculosis—Critical Steps for Prevention and Control," *New England Journal of Medicine* 363, no. 11 (2010): 1050–1058.

86. Thomas R. Frieden, Paula I. Fujiwara, Rita M. Washko, and Margaret A. Hamburg, "Tuberculosis in New York City—Turning the Tide," *New England Journal of Medicine* 333, no. 4 (1995): 229–233; Centers for Disease Control and Prevention, "National Action Plan to Combat Multidrug-Resistant Tuberculosis: Meeting the Challenge of Multidrug-Resistant Tuberculosis. Summary of a Conference; Management of Persons Exposed to Multidrug-Resistant Tuberculosis," *Morbidity and Mortality Weekly Report (MMWR)* 41, no. RR-11 (June 19, 1992): 1–71.

87. Arata Kochi, "Tuberculosis Control—Is DOTS the Health Breakthrough of the 1990s?" *World Health Forum* 18, nos. 3–4 (1997): 225–232; World Health Organization, *Treatment of Tuberculosis: Guidelines for National Programmes* (Geneva: World Health Organization, 1997).

88. World Bank, *World Development Report 1993*, 63.

89. World Health Organization, "WHO Global Tuberculosis Program," *TB Treatment Observer*, no. 2 (March 24, 1997).

90. Mercedes C. Becerra, Jonathan Freeman, Jaime Bayona, Sonya S. Shin, Jim Yong Kim, Jennifer J. Furin, Barbara Werner, Alexander Sloutsky, Ralph Timperi, Paul E. Farmer, et al., "Using Treatment Failure under Effective Directly Observed Short-Course Chemotherapy Programs to Identify Patients with Multidrug-Resistant Tuberculosis," *International Journal of Tuberculosis and Lung Disease* 4, no. 2 (2000): 108–114.

91. Paul Farmer, "Social Medicine and the Challenge of Biosocial Research," in *Innovative Structures in Basic Research: Ringberg Symposium 4–7 October 2000* (Munich: Generalverwaltung der Max-Planck-Gesellschaft, Referat Press- und Öffentlichkeitsarbeit, 2002), 55–73, http://xserve02.mpiwg-berlin.mpg.de/ringberg/talks/farmer/farmer.html (accessed October 12, 2012).

92. Kwonjune J. Seung, Irina E. Gelmanova, Gennadiy G. Peremitin, Vera T. Golubchikova, Vera E. Pavlova, Olga B. Sirotkina, Galina V. Yanova, and Aivar K. Strelis, "The Effect of Initial Drug Resistance on Treatment Response and Acquired Drug Resistance during Standardized Short-Course Chemotherapy for Tuberculosis," *Clinical Infectious Diseases* 39, no. 9 (2004): 1321–1328; Paul E. Farmer and Jim Yong Kim, "Resurgent TB in Russia: Do We Know Enough to Act?" *European Journal of Public Health* 10, no. 2 (2000): 150–153; Paul E. Farmer, Alexander S. Kononets, Sergei E. Borisov, Alex Goldfarb, Timothy Healing, and Martin McKee, "Recrudescent Tuberculosis in the

Russian Federation," in *The Global Impact of Drug-Resistant Tuberculosis,*
by Harvard Medical School and Open Society Institute (Boston: Program in
Infectious Disease and Social Change, Department of Social Medicine, Harvard Medical School, 1999), 39–83; Rudi Coninx, Gaby E. Pfyffer, Christine Mathieu, D. Savina, Martine Debacker, Fizuli Jafarov, I. Jabrailov, Ali
Ismailov, Fuad Mirzoev, Rodolphe de Haller, and Françoise Portaels, "Drug
Resistant Tuberculosis in Prisons in Azerbaijan: Case Study," *British Medical Journal* 316 (1998): 1423–1425; Michael E. Kimerling, Hans Kluge, Nata-
lia Vezhnina, Tiziana Iacovazzi, Tine Demeulenaere, Françoise Portaels, and
Francine Matthys, "Inadequacy of the Current WHO Re-Treatment Regimen
in a Central Siberian Prison: Treatment Failure and MDR-TB," *International
Journal of Tuberculosis and Lung Disease* 3, no. 5 (1999): 451–453; Centers
for Disease Control and Prevention, "Primary Multidrug-Resistant Tuberculosis—Ivanovo Oblast, Russia, 1999," *Morbidity and Mortality Weekly Report
(MMWR)* 48, no. 30 (August 6, 1999): 661–663; Michael E. Kimerling, "The
Russian Equation: An Evolving Paradigm in Tuberculosis Control," *International Journal of Tuberculosis and Lung Disease* 4, suppl. 2 (2000): S160-S167.

93. Jaime Aréstegui Benavente, Gilberto Martinez Freitas, and Ana Maria
Yamunaque Morales, "Seminario taller nacional: Evaluación del programa de
control de tuberculosis ano 1991," in *Seminario Sub Regional Andino de Evaluación y Control de Tuberculosis,* ed. Ministerio de Salud (Lima: República
del Perú, Programa Nacional de Control de la Tuberculosis, 1992), 47.

94. World Health Organization, *Groups at Risk: WHO Report on the
Tuberculosis Epidemic 1996* (Geneva: World Health Organization, 1996), 2
(emphasis added).

95. World Health Organization, *WHO Report on the Tuberculosis Epidemic 1997* (Geneva: World Health Organization, 1997) (emphasis added).
Around this time, a great many public health experts claimed that MDRTB
was untreatable, in part because of high costs; for a discussion, see Michael D.
Iseman, David L. Cohn, and John A. Sbabaro, "Directly Observed Treatment of Tuberculosis—We Can't Afford Not to Try It," *New England Journal
of Medicine* 328, no. 8 (1993): 576–578; and Veronica L.C. White and John
Moore-Gillon, "Resource Implications of Patients with Multidrug Resistant
Tuberculosis," *Thorax* 55, no. 11 (2000): 962–963.

96. For an extended discussion of the DOTS-Plus model, see Julie Talbot,
Joseph Rhatigan, and Jim Yong Kim, "The Peruvian National Tuberculosis
Control Program," HBS no. GHD-002 (Boston: Harvard Business School
Publishing, 2011), Global Health Delivery Online, www.ghdonline.org/cases/
(accessed October 16, 2012).

97. Carole Mitnick, Jaime Bayona, Eda Palacios, Sonya Shin, Jennifer
Furin, Felix Alcántara, Epifanio Sánchez, Madeleny Sarria, Mercedes Becerra,
Mary C. Smith Fawzi, Saidi Kapiga, Donna Neuberg, James H. Maguire,
Jim Yong Kim, and Paul Farmer, "Community-Based Therapy for Multidrug-
Resistant Tuberculosis in Lima, Peru," *New England Journal of Medicine* 348,
no. 2 (2003): 119, 122.

98. Paul E. Farmer, Jim Yong Kim, Carole D. Mitnick, and Ralph Timperi,
"Responding to Outbreaks of Multidrug-Resistant Tuberculosis: Introducing

DOTS-Plus," in *Tuberculosis: A Comprehensive International Approach*, ed. Lee B. Reichman and Earl S. Hershfield (New York: Decker, 2000), 447–469.

99. Mitnick, Bayona, et al. "Community-Based Therapy for Multidrug-Resistant Tuberculosis in Lima, Peru," 119, 122.

100. Goble, Iseman, et al., "Treatment of 171 Patients with Pulmonary Tuberculosis Resistant to Isoniazid and Rifampin."

101. Farmer, Kim, et al., "Responding to Outbreaks of Multidrug-Resistant Tuberculosis: Introducing DOTS-Plus."

102. Sonya S. Shin, Martin Yagui, Luis Ascencios, Gloria Yale, Carmen Suarez, Neyda Quispet, Cesar Bonilla, Joaquin Blaya, Allison Tayloe, Carmen Contreras, and Peter Cegielski, "Scale-Up of Multidrug-Resistant Tuberculosis Laboratory Services, Peru," *Emerging Infectious Diseases* 14, no. 5 (2008): 701–708.

103. See Michael D. Iseman, "MDR-TB and the Developing World—A Problem No Longer to Be Ignored: The WHO Announces 'DOTS Plus' Strategy," *International Journal of Tuberculosis and Lung Disease* 2, no. 11 (1998): 867; Stop TB Partnership, *The Global Plan to Stop TB, 2006–2015: Actions for Life, Towards a World Free of Tuberculosis* (Geneva: World Health Organization, 2006), http://whqlibdoc.who.int/publications/2006/9241593997_eng .pdf (accessed October 15, 2012); Paul E. Farmer and Jim Y. Kim, "Community-Based Approaches to the Control of Multidrug-Resistant Tuberculosis: Introducing 'DOTS-Plus,'" *British Medical Journal* 317, no. 7159 (1998): 671–674.

104. Rajesh Gupta, Jim Yong Kim, Marcos A. Espinal, Jean-Michel Caudron, Bernard Pecoul, Paul E. Farmer, and Mario C. Raviglione, "Responding to Market Failures in Tuberculosis Control," *Science* 293, no. 5532 (August 10, 2001): 1051.

105. Salmaan Keshavjee, "Role of the Green Light Committee Initiative in MDR-TB Treatment Scale-Up," presentation at the World Health Organization ministerial meeting, Beijing, April 3, 2009, www.who.int/tb_beijingmeet ing/media/press_pack/presentations/day3_presentation4.pdf (accessed October 15, 2012).

106. Salmaan Keshavjee and Paul E. Farmer, "Time to Put Boots on the Ground: Making Universal Access to MDR-TB Treatment a Reality," *International Journal of Tuberculosis and Lung Disease* 14, no. 10 (2010): 1222.

107. Médecins Sans Frontières, *DR-TB Drugs under the Microscope: The Sources and Prices of Medicines for Drug-Resistant Tuberculosis*, 2011, www .doctorswithoutborders.org/publications/reports/2011/Report_Summary_DR -TB_Drugs_Under_the_Microscope.pdf (accessed October 15, 2012).

108. Keshavjee and Farmer, "Time to Put Boots on the Ground."

109. World Bank, *World Development Report 1993*, 116.

110. World Health Organization, *Treatment of Tuberculosis*.

111. See, for example, World Health Organization, "WHO Global Tuberculosis Program" (1997).

112. Mario C. Raviglione and Mukund W. Uplekar, "WHO's New Stop TB Strategy," *Lancet* 367, no. 9514 (2006): 952–955.

Suicide in China, pages 220–221

1. World Health Organization, *World Health Report 2001—Mental Health: New Understanding, New Hope* (Geneva: World Health Organization, 2001), x, www.who.int/whr/2001/en/whr01_en.pdf (accessed October 15, 2012).

2. Vikram Patel and Arthur Kleinman, "Poverty and Common Mental Disorders in Developing Countries," *Bulletin of the World Health Organization* 81, no. 8 (2003): 611–612. See also Arthur M. Kleinman, "Global Mental Health: A Failure of Humanity," *Lancet* 374, no. 9690 (2009): 603–604.

3. World Health Organization, *World Health Report 2001—Mental Health*, 37.

4. Michael R. Phillips, Huaqing Liu, and Yanping Zhang, "Suicide and Social Change in China," *Culture, Medicine, and Psychiatry* 23, no. 1 (1999): 25, 30.

5. "Women and Suicide in Rural China," *Bulletin of the World Health Organization* 87, no. 12 (December 2009): 885, www.who.int/bulletin/volumes/87/12/09-011209/en/index.html (accessed October 15, 2012).

6. World Health Organization, *World Health Report 2001—Mental Health*, 37.

7. Since 1978, the government has instituted economic reforms such as liberalizing trade, encouraging private businesses, and opening the country to direct foreign investment. Along with a large increase in economic growth and an improvement in livelihood for many, there has been a sharp rise in income inequality and underinvestment in public services. See chapter 4 for more information on the association between neoliberalism and support for social services such as health care.

8. After the tumultuous political and economic transformations of the 1990s, post-Soviet states exhibit some of the highest suicide rates in the world. Latvia and Lithuania both have rates higher than 40 per 100,000 (the highest in the world), and nine of the fifteen countries with the highest suicide rates were part of the former USSR (all with rates above 15 per 100,000). See José Manoel Bertolote and Alexandra Fleischmann, "A Global Perspective in the Epidemiology of Suicide," *Suicidology* 7, no. 2 (2002): 6–8.

9. Phillips, Liu, and Zhang, "Suicide and Social Change in China," 40.

10. Poisoning from insecticide ingestion and medication overdose account for 32.3 percent to 66.6 percent of completed suicides in China. See Jianlin Ji, Arthur Kleinman, and Anne Becker, "Suicide in Contemporary China: A Review of China's Distinctive Suicide Demographics in Their Sociocultural Context," *Harvard Review of Psychiatry* 9, no. 1 (2001): 4.

11. Although this statistic could be an artifact of help-seeking patterns for highly stigmatized illness and a health system with limited capacity for identifying and treating mental disorders, the percentage of suicides associated with neuropsychiatric conditions in China is likely lower than the 90 percent estimated globally; see ibid., 1.

12. See, for example, M. Giovanna Merli and Adrian E. Raftery, "Are Births Underreported in Rural China? Manipulation of Statistical Records in Response to China's Population Policies," *Demography* 37, no. 1 (2000): 109–

126; Penny Kane and Ching Y. Choi, "China's One-Child Family Policy," *British Medical Journal* 319, no. 7215 (1999): 992–994.

13. Amartya Sen, "Missing Women: Social Inequality Outweighs Women's Survival Advantage in Asia and North Africa," *British Medical Journal* 304, no. 6827 (1992): 587–588. Sen explains that one could expect women to live longer than men because of biological factors (male fetuses have a higher rate of miscarriage, for example) and social factors (more men die from violent causes). In Europe and North America, the female-to-male ratio hovers around 1.05 to 1.

CHAPTER 9

Jonathan Weigel and Arjun Suri contributed equally to this chapter.

1. Arthur Kleinman and Bridget Hanna, "Religious Values and Global Health," in *Ecologies of Human Flourishing,* ed. Donald K. Swearer and Susan Lloyd McGarry, Center for the Study of World Religions (Cambridge, Mass.: Harvard University Press, 2011), 76.

2. Ibid., 83. See also Kearsley A. Stewart, Gerald T. Keusch, and Arthur Kleinman, "Values and Moral Experience in Global Health: Bridging the Local and the Global," *Global Public Health* 5, no. 2 (2010): 115–121.

3. Arthur Kleinman, "The Art of Medicine: The Divided Self, Hidden Values, and Moral Sensibility in Medicine," *Lancet* 377, no. 9768 (2011): 805.

4. Because it confers moral value based on the outcomes or consequences of actions (not on the motives behind them), utilitarianism is known as a *consequentialist* moral theory.

5. Conversely, in the twentieth century, conservatives have invoked utilitarianism to argue that laissez-faire capitalism acts to benefit the good of the many. See, for example, Friedrich Hayek, *Law, Legislation, and Liberty,* vol. 2, *The Mirage of Social Justice* (Chicago: University of Chicago Press, 1973), 17–23; and Friedrich Hayek, *Studies in Philosophy, Politics, and Economics* (New York: Touchstone Books, 1969), 173.

6. Will Kymlicka, *Contemporary Political Philosophy* (Oxford: Oxford University Press, 1990), 11.

7. This is Robert Nozick's critique of what he terms "welfare hedonism." Even if a machine could generate the most pleasurable sensations possible, including a "feeling of accomplishment," he asked, would we choose to use it? See "The Experience Machine" in Robert Nozick, *Anarchy, State, and Utopia* (New York: Basic Books, 1977), 42–45.

8. Robert E. Black, Saul S. Morris, and Jennifer Bryce, "Where and Why Are 10 Million Children Dying Each Year?" *Lancet* 361, no. 9376 (2003): 2226–2234. See also Jim Yong Kim, "Bridging the Delivery Gap in Global Health," MIT lecture, November 19, 2007, http://video.mit.edu/watch/bridging-the-delivery-gap-to-global-health-9317/ (accessed October 22, 2012).

9. "Antiretroviral (ARV) Ceiling Price List," Clinton Health Access Initiative (CHAI), last modified May 2012, http://d2pd3b5abq75bb.cloudfront.net/2012/07/12/15/03/07/163/CHAI_ARV_Ceiling_Price_List_May_2012.pdf (accessed October 22, 2012). This figure is calculated based on the 2010 price

of a first-line regimen of d4T (30 mg), 3TC (150 mg), and NVP (200 mg), which costs $79 per person per year.

10. These questions were developed by Peter Singer in his book *The Life You Can Save: Acting Now to End World Poverty* (New York: Random House, 2009), 10–11.

11. Ibid., 15–16.

12. Peter Singer, "Famine, Affluence, and Morality," in *International Ethics,* ed. Charles R. Beitz, Marshall Cohen, Thomas Scanlon, and A. John Simmons (Princeton, N.J.: Princeton University Press, 1985), 249–252.

13. Singer, *The Life You Can Save,* 18.

14. See Jeffrey A. Schaler, ed., *Peter Singer under Fire: The Moral Iconoclast Faces His Critics* (Chicago: Open Court, 2009).

15. See Linda Polman, *The Crisis Caravan: What's Wrong with Humanitarian Aid?* (New York: Metropolitan Books, 2010); Dambisa Moyo, *Dead Aid: Why Aid Is Not Working and How There Is a Better Way for Africa* (New York: Farrar, Straus and Giroux, 2009); and William Easterly, *The Elusive Quest for Growth: Economists' Adventures and Misadventures in the Tropics* (Cambridge, Mass.: MIT Press, 2001).

16. Singer, *The Life You Can Save,* 7.

17. This is Derek Parfit's principal critique of utilitarianism in his book *Reason and Persons* (New York: Oxford University Press, 1984). According to utilitarianism, he argues, if a state could double its population while reducing the well-being of each citizen by half, it should do so.

18. Singer points out that the American health insurance system already rations care by assigning prices to interventions—prices only some Americans can afford—and by privileging individuals who have insurance over the uninsured (one study found that the death rate after car accidents was 37 percent higher among the uninsured). In other words, the U.S. health care system rations care according to ability to pay instead of other—arguably more equitable—randomized methods. See Peter Singer, "Why We Must Ration Health Care," *New York Times,* July 15, 2009, www.nytimes.com/2009/07/19/magazine/19healthcare-t.html?pagewanted=all (accessed October 22, 2012).

19. "The Few: A Special Report on Global Leaders," *Economist,* January 20, 2011, www.economist.com/node/17929075 (accessed October 25, 2012).

20. Thomas Pogge, *World Poverty and Human Rights,* 2nd ed. (Cambridge: Polity Press, 2008), 10.

21. Pauline Kleingeld and Eric Brown, "Cosmopolitanism," in *Stanford Encyclopedia of Philosophy* (Spring 2011), ed. Edward N. Zalta, http://plato.stanford.edu/archives/spr2011/entries/cosmopolitanism (accessed October 25, 2012).

22. Pogge, *World Poverty and Human Rights,* 20–24.

23. John Rawls, *A Theory of Justice* (Cambridge, Mass.: Harvard University Press, 1971), 54. Social goods (wealth, power, opportunity) and natural goods (health, intelligence, talents) are divided among individuals, Rawls argues, by a natural lottery. Possessing such goods is thus a matter of brute luck and therefore morally arbitrary. A boy born with a severe disability should not be punished for his bad luck by getting no compensation; a girl born into

great fortune should not be rewarded for her good luck by getting to hoard her resources at the expense of those born into indigence. Justice can be realized only if redistribution of wealth and opportunity counterbalance the random allotment of social and natural goods at birth. By starting from this original position, Rawls thought it possible to outline a social contract that most of us would agree to if we, too, faced the natural lottery from behind a "veil of ignorance." The result, Rawls argued, would be liberal egalitarianism: "all social values—liberty and opportunity, income and wealth, and the social bases of self-respect—are to be distributed equally unless an unequal distribution of any, or all, of these values is to everyone's advantage."

24. Ibid., 401; Pogge, *World Poverty and Human Rights*, 111–114. Although his later work speaks to questions of justice between states, Rawls never extends the implications of the difference principle beyond a given nation, which he takes as a "self-contained" system. See John Rawls, *The Law of Peoples; With "The Idea of Public Reason Revisited"* (Cambridge, Mass.: Harvard University Press, 2001).

25. Pogge asks how the world can be carved up, however crudely, into great regions of wealth (the "global North") and poverty (the "global South") if it is in fact up to individual nations to grow or stagnate. This simple evidence points us toward global forces and structures such as trade, foreign policy, and international law.

26. Pogge, *World Poverty and Human Rights*, 15–16 (emphasis added).

27. Ibid., 118.

28. Ibid., 102.

29. "The White Man's Shame," *Economist*, September 25, 1999, 89; quoted in ibid., 20.

30. Joseph E. Stiglitz and Andrew Charlton, *Fair Trade for All: How Trade Can Promote Development* (New York: Oxford University Press, 2005), 120.

31. "Hearing: Building on Success: New Directions in Global Health," U.S. Senate Committee on Foreign Relations, 111th Cong., 2nd sess., March 10, 2010, www.foreign.senate.gov/hearings/building-on-success-new-directions -in-global-health (accessed October 25, 2012).

32. See, for example, Carolyn Nordstrom's work tracing landmine provenance (*Shadows of War: Violence, Power, and International Profiteering in the Twenty-First Century* [Berkeley: University of California Press, 2004]). She writes, "Should any quaint notions exist that mercenaries and human rights violators only get weapons from 'sources in non-democratic locations,' anyone who has walked in warzones, myself included, can easily attest to the wide range of supplies available from all the major sellers in the world. In one square kilometer of land in central Angola I visited with Halo Trust (the British de-mining NGO), they removed land mines manufactured in thirty-one countries" (95).

33. Peter Lurie and Sidney Wolfe, "Unethical Trials of Interventions to Reduce Perinatal Transmission of the Human Immunodeficiency Virus in Developing Countries," *New England Journal of Medicine* 337, no. 12 (1997): 853–856; Brenda Waning, Ellen Diedrichsen, and Suerie Moon, "A Lifeline to Treatment: The Role of Indian Generic Manufacturers in Supplying Antiretro-

viral Medicines to Developing Countries," *Journal of the International AIDS Society* 13 (2010): 35; Pogge, *World Poverty and Human Rights*, 21. This topic is further examined, as are Pogge's critiques of Rawls, in Paul Farmer, "Rich World, Poor World," *Partner to the Poor*, ed. by Haun Saussy (Berkeley: University of California Press, 2010).

34. Pogge, *World Poverty and Human Rights*, 22.

35. See Jeffrey D. Sachs and Andrew M. Warner, "Sources of Slow Growth in African Economies," *Journal of African Economies* 6, no. 3 (1997): 335–376; and Paul Collier and Benedikt Goderis, *Commodity Prices, Growth, and the Natural Resource Curse: Reconciling a Conundrum*, 2007, Centre for the Study of African Economies Working Paper CSAE WSP/2007-15, http://economics.ouls.ox.ac.uk/13218/1/2007-15text.pdf (accessed October 26, 2012).

36. There are many Cold War examples of military regimes receiving substantial foreign assistance from the United States and its allies to prevent left-leaning groups from taking power. Foreign aid to the governments of dictators François and Jean-Claude Duvalier in Haiti, for example, was justified by labeling the island as a bulwark against communism, citing the perceived security threat of Cuba, only a few miles off Haiti's northwest coast.

37. Pogge, *World Poverty and Human Rights*, 119.

38. Ibid., 120.

39. See, for example, Seema Jayachandran and Michael Kremer, "Odious Debt," *American Economic Review* 96, no. 1 (2006): 82–85.

40. President Yoweri Museveni of Uganda has even argued that global warming can be understood as an act of aggression by the rich world against the poor world. He has repeatedly demanded compensation for damage caused by climate change—for example, declining crop yields in the semi-arid Sahel (home to many Ugandan farmers). See also "Drying Up and Flooding Out," *Economist*, May 10, 2007, www.economist.com/node/9163426 (accessed October 25, 2012).

41. For more on how demand for cocaine and other drugs fuels organized crime and political instability in Central America, see "The Tormented Isthmus," *Economist*, April 14, 2011, www.economist.com/node/18558254 (accessed October 25, 2012).

42. Singer, *The Life You Can Save*, 30. On overfishing, see Sharon Lafraniere, "Europe Takes Africa's Fish, and Boatloads of Migrants Follow," *New York Times*, January 14, 2008, www.nytimes.com/2008/01/14/world/africa/14fishing.html?pagewanted=all&_r=0 (accessed October 25, 2012); and Elisabeth Rosenthal, "Europe's Appetite for Seafood Propels Illegal Trade," *New York Times*, January 15, 2008, www.nytimes.com/2008/01/15/world/europe/15fish.html?pagewanted=all (accessed October 25, 2012). On human responsibilities, see, for example, Pogge, *World Poverty and Human Rights*, 31–32.

43. Pogge, *World Poverty and Human Rights*, 121.

44. Solomon Benatar, "Moral Imagination: The Missing Component in Global Health," *PLoS Medicine* 2, no. 12 (2005): e400.

45. Amartya Sen, *Development as Freedom* (New York: Anchor Books, 2000), 36.

46. This excerpt is drawn from Martha Nussbaum, "Capabilities as Fundamental Entitlements: Sen and Social Justice," *Feminist Economics* 9, nos. 2–3 (2003): 41–42.

47. Sen, *Development as Freedom,* 74. In philosophical jargon, the approach of seeking the moral value of an action by looking to its end is known as *teleological* reasoning and is traditionally associated with Aristotle.

48. Although he does not develop the normative position at length, as does Nussbaum, Sen does make it clear that the capabilities approach should be used to evaluate social progress and development policy: "The success of a society is to be evaluated, in this view, primarily by the substantive freedoms that members of that society enjoy" (*Development as Freedom,* 18).

49. Martha Nussbaum, "Human Functioning and Social Justice: In Defense of Aristotelian Essentialism," *Political Theory* 20, no. 2 (1992): 205.

50. Nussbaum, "Capabilities as Fundamental Entitlements," 36.

51. Nussbaum, "Human Functioning and Social Justice," 229.

52. This is a common critique of Nussbaum's approach, and it is one that has plagued teleological thinkers since Aristotle himself proposed that the best flute go to the best flute player. See, for example, "Honor and Resentment," Michael Sandel's critique of a disability rights case among high school cheerleaders in West Texas, in Sandel's book *Public Philosophy: Essays on Morality in Politics* (Cambridge, Mass.: Harvard University Press, 2005), 97–100.

53. Nussbaum, "Capabilities as Fundamental Entitlements," 40.

54. Sen, *Development as Freedom,* 21–23. Although it is often assumed that the shorter life expectancy of African Americans relates to the incidence of violent crime, in fact, recent studies have shown that lack of social services, especially health care, is of primary importance.

55. Ibid., 21.

56. Aristotle, *The Nicomachean Ethics,* trans. William David Ross, rev. ed. (Oxford: Oxford University Press, 1980), bk. 1, sec. 6, p. 7; quoted in Sen, *Development as Freedom,* 14, 289.

57. Nussbaum, "Capabilities as Fundamental Entitlements," 38.

58. See, for example, Paul E. Farmer, Simon Robin, St. Luc Ramilus, and Jim Yong Kim, "Tuberculosis, Poverty, and 'Compliance': Lessons from Rural Haiti," *Seminars in Respiratory Infections* 6, no. 4 (1991): 254–260; and Paul Farmer, *Infections and Inequalities: The Modern Plagues* (Berkeley: University of California Press, 1999).

59. Nussbaum, "Human Functioning and Social Justice," 225.

60. Ibid., 233.

61. John Gray, "Contractarian Method, Private Property, and the Market Economy," in *Liberalisms: Essays in Political Philosophy,* by John Gray (London: Routledge, 1989), 161–198.

62. Amartya Sen, *Inequality Reexamined* (Cambridge, Mass.: Harvard University Press, 1992), 127. Also see Martha C. Nussbaum, *Sex and Social Justice* (New York: Oxford University Press, 1999).

63. See, for example, S. Charusheela, "Social Analysis and the Capabilities

Approach: A Limit to Martha Nussbaum's Universalist Ethics," *Cambridge Journal of Economics* 33, no. 6 (2009): 1135–1152.

64. Ingrid Robeyns, "In Defence of Amartya Sen," *Post-Autistic Economic Review,* no. 17 (December 2002), article 5, www.paecon.net/PAEReview /issue17/Robeyns17.htm (accessed October 30, 2012).

65. Sen, *Development as Freedom,* 33.

66. Ibid., 36.

67. Ibid., 50.

68. Amartya Sen, "Health: Perception versus Observation," *British Medical Journal* 324, no. 7342 (2002): 860–861.

69. Sen, *Development as Freedom,* 47.

70. Ibid., 46.

71. See, for example, Michael Marmot, "Health in an Unequal World," *Lancet* 368, no. 9552 (2006): 2081–2094.

72. Sen, *Development as Freedom,* 92.

73. A landmark document that makes this point is World Bank, *World Development Report 1993: Investing in Health* (Oxford: Oxford University Press, 1993).

74. Sudhir Anand and Martin Ravallion, "Human Development in Poor Countries: On the Role of Private Incomes and Public Services," *Journal of Economic Perspectives* 7, no. 1 (1993): 133–150.

75. Martha Alter Chen, *A Quiet Revolution: Women in Transition in Rural Bangladesh* (Cambridge, Mass.: Schenkman Books, 1983).

76. Nussbaum, *Sex and Social Justice,* chap. 3.

77. Chen, *A Quiet Revolution,* 35.

78. Ibid., 8; Nussbaum, *Sex and Social Justice,* 92–93.

79. Nussbaum, *Sex and Social Justice,* 121–126.

80. Sue Pedersen, "National Bodies, Unspeakable Acts: The Sexual Politics of Colonial Policy-Making," *Journal of Modern History* 63, no. 4 (1991): 657–678. See also Kirsten Bell, "Genital Cutting and Western Discourses on Sexuality," *Medical Anthropology Quarterly* 19, no. 2 (2005): 125–148; and Lucrezia Catania, Omar Abdulcadir, Vincenzo Puppo, Jole Baldaro Verde, Jasmine Abdulcadir, and Dalmar Abdulcadir, "Pleasure and Orgasm in Women with Female Genital Mutilation/Cutting (FGM/C)," *Journal of Sexual Medicine* 4, no. 6 (2007): 1666–1678.

81. Steve Feierman, Arthur Kleinman, Kearsley Stewart, Paul Farmer, and Veena Das, "Anthropology, Knowledge-Flows, and Global Health," *Global Public Health* 5, no. 2 (2010): 122–128.

82. Micheline R. Ishay, *The History of Human Rights: From Ancient Times to the Globalization Era* (Berkeley: University of California Press, 2004), chap. 2.

83. Ibid., 221.

84. Peter Uvin, *Human Rights and Development* (West Hartford, Conn.: Kumarian Press, 2004), 10.

85. Some extend the breadth of social and economic rights to include "the right not to starve to death or die in childbirth; the right to treatment, even for chronic and difficult-to-treat afflictions such as AIDS or multidrug-resis-

tant tuberculosis; the right to primary schooling; and the right to clean water" (Paul Farmer, keynote address, 134th annual meeting of the American Public Health Association, Boston, November 5, 2006).

86. See Isaiah Berlin, *Four Essays on Liberty* (New York: Oxford University Press, 1969).

87. Adam Smith wrote: "The education of the common people requires, perhaps, in a civilized and commercial society, the attention of the public" (*An Inquiry into the Nature and Causes of the Wealth of Nations* [New York: J. M. Dent, 1921], 265; originally published 1776).

88. Thomas Paine, *Rights of Man,* ed. Claire Grogan (Peterborough, Ontario: Broadview Press, 2011), 179–303.

89. Indeed, Mill's *On Liberty* (1859) is a passionate defense of individual liberty and the dangers of paternalism to the cultivation of "individuality," which Mill saw as the root of human achievement (see Mill, *"On Liberty" and Other Writings,* ed. Stefan Collini [Cambridge: Cambridge University Press, 1989]). David Brink argues that Mill saw the state as a guarantor of certain minimum requirements that would allow the individual to have an opportunity to self-develop:

> Mill's perfectionist liberalism is part of classical liberal tradition that grounds liberal essentials in a conception of the good that prizes the exercise of a person's rational capacities. In Mill's version, the good consists in forms of self-government that exercise the very deliberative capacities that make one a moral agent. He concludes that the state cannot foster this kind of good by regular use of paternalistic or moralistic intervention. Liberties of thought and action are central to the exercise of these deliberative powers. *But equally essential are certain positive conditions, such as health, education, a decent minimum standard of living, and fair opportunities for self-realization.* Even paternalistic intervention can sometimes be justified when, without it, people's deliberative powers will be severely compromised (emphasis added) (David Brink, "Mill's Moral and Political Philosophy," *Stanford Encyclopedia of Philosophy* [Fall 2008], ed. Edward N. Zalta, http://plato.stanford.edu/archives/fall2008/entries/mill-moral -political/ [accessed October 25, 2012]).

90. Asbjørn Eide, "Economic, Social, and Cultural Rights as Human Rights," in *Economic, Social, and Cultural Rights: A Textbook,* ed. Asbjørn Eide, Catarina Krause, and Allan Rosas (Dordrecht: Martinus Nijhoff, 2001), 13.

91. Hannah Arendt, *The Origins of Totalitarianism* (New York: Harcourt, 1973), 299.

92. Hannah Arendt, "'The Rights of Man': What Are They?" *Modern Review* 3, no. 1 (1949): 25–37.

93. For a concise overview of Arendt's theory of action, see Maurizio Passerin d'Entreves, "Hannah Arendt," *Stanford Encyclopedia of Philosophy* (Fall 2008), ed. Edward N. Zalta, http://plato.stanford.edu/archives/fall2008/ entries/arendt/ (accessed October 25, 2012).

94. Whether such foundations have normative force has been a topic of great debate. See, for example, Peg Birmingham, *Hannah Arendt and Human Rights: The Predicament of Common Responsibility* (Bloomington: Indiana University Press, 2006); and Serena Parekh, *Hannah Arendt and the Chal-*

lenge of Modernity: A Phenomenology of Human Rights (New York: Routledge, 2008).

95. United Nations, "The Universal Declaration of Human Rights," Article 25 and Preamble, www.un.org/en/documents/udhr/ (accessed October 25, 2012).

96. Johannes Morsink, *The Universal Declaration of Human Rights: Origins, Drafting, and Intent* (Philadelphia: University of Pennsylvania Press, 1999), 21–24. Six nations did abstain from the vote, all of them Soviet-bloc countries. This abstention was significantly different than voting against it, however: in fact, these nations argued that the document should go further in condemning fascism and Nazism.

97. Uvin, *Human Rights and Development*, 11.

98. Philip Alston, "Economic and Social Rights," in *Human Rights: An Agenda for the Next Century*, ed. Louis Henkin and John Lawrence Hargrove (Washington, D.C.: American Society of International Law, 1994), 137, 152. ICESCR was adopted by the UN General Assembly in 1966 and went into effect in 1976. The United States, enmeshed in Cold War politics, was not a signatory.

99. Morsink, *Universal Declaration of Human Rights*, 15.

100. Philip Alston, "U.S. Ratification of the Covenant on Economic, Social, and Cultural Rights: The Need for an Entirely New Strategy," *American Journal of International Law* 84, no. 2 (1990), 365–393.

101. Amnesty International, *Voices for Freedom: An Amnesty International Anthology* (London: Amnesty International Publications, 1986), 106.

102. "Human Rights: Righting Wrongs," *Economist*, August 16, 2001, www.economist.com/node/739385 (accessed October 25, 2012).

103. Michael Ignatieff, *Human Rights as Politics and Idolatry* (Princeton, N.J.: Princeton University Press, 2001), 56. Indeed, though Ignatieff's argument is often used to remove social and economic claims from human rights frameworks, his standard—that rights must specify only the minimum conditions of life—should in fact work in favor of including health care (and even nutrition and housing).

104. See, for example, Henry Shue, *Basic Rights: Subsistence, Affluence, and U.S. Foreign Policy* (Princeton, N.J.: Princeton University Press, 1980).

105. United Nations Development Programme (UNDP), *Human Development Report 2003: Millennium Development Goals: A Compact among Nations to End Poverty* (New York: Oxford University Press, 2003), 85.

106. Matt Bonds, "A Note from the Millennium Villages Project, Rwanda: Breaking the Disease-Driven Poverty Trap," *Consilience: The Journal of Sustainable Development*, no. 1 (2008): 98–111.

107. Kenneth Roth, "Defending Economic, Social, and Cultural Rights: Practical Issues Faced by an International Human Rights Organization," *Human Rights Quarterly* 26, no. 1 (2004): 63–73.

108. Maurice Cranston, "Human Rights: Real and Supposed," in *Political Theory and the Rights of Man*, ed. David Daiches Raphael (Bloomington: Indiana University Press, 1967), 43–51.

109. The Constitutional Right to Housing in South Africa: *The Government of the Republic of South Africa vs. Irene Grootboom*, CCT11/00 (Con-

stitutional Court of South Africa, October 4, 2000), www.case.hks.harvard
.edu/casetitle.asp?caseNo=1627.0 (accessed October 31, 2012).

110. Amartya Sen, for example, explores the links between rights, which
he defines as ethical pronouncements of "what should be done," and laws.
The social contract requires that citizens uphold certain obligations (laws) to
the state in exchange for enjoying certain freedoms (rights). Justiciable rights
(those enforceable in court) generally stem from laws, while laws, in turn, can
formalize the moral claims embodied in rights. See Amartya Sen, *The Idea of
Justice* (London: Allen Lane, 2009), 357–358.

111. Jeremy Bentham, *The Works of Jeremy Bentham,* vol. 8 (Edinburgh:
William Tait, 1839), 523.

112. This distinction was made by Tom Paine and supported, two centuries later, by Oxford philosopher of jurisprudence Herbert Hart. See Amartya
Sen, "Agency, Inequality, and Human Rights," *The Daily Star,* December 29,
2006, www.thedailystar.net/2006/12/29/d61229090198.htm (accessed October 25, 2012).

113. Paul Farmer, *Pathologies of Power: Health, Human Rights, and the
New War on the Poor* (Berkeley: University of California Press, 2003), xiii.

114. Ibid., i-51.

115. United Nations Economic and Social Council, Committee on Economic, Social, and Cultural Rights, "General Comment no. 14, The Right to
the Highest Attainable Standard of Health," August 11, 2000, www.unhchr
.ch/tbs/doc.nsf/o/40d009901358b0e2c1256915005090be?Opendocument (accessed October 25, 2012).

116. Rachel Hammonds and Gorik Ooms, "World Bank Policies and
the Obligation of Its Members to Respect, Protect, and Fulfill the Right to
Health," *Health and Human Rights* 8, no. 1 (2004): 23.

117. Jonathan M. Mann, "AIDS and Human Rights: Where Do We Go
from Here?" *Health and Human Rights* 3, no. 1 (1998): 146.

118. The zealous belief in allowing the market to allocate health care in
poor countries is perhaps best expressed in John S. Akin, Nancy Birdsall, and
David M. De Ferranti, *Financing Health Services in Developing Countries:
An Agenda for Reform,* 1987 World Bank Policy Study (Washington, D.C.:
World Bank, 1987)—a report that crystallizes neoliberal approaches to global
health.

119. The World Bank Poverty Reduction Strategy Papers are available at
http://apps.who.int/hdp/database/PRSPwhat.aspx? (accessed October 25, 2012).

120. World Bank, "The World Bank Holds Its Regional Annual Stakeholders
Consultation on HIV/AIDS in Antananarivo," press release, March 31, 2008,
http://web.worldbank.org/WBSITE/EXTERNAL/COUNTRIES/AFRICA
EXT/MADAGASCAREXTN/0,,contentMDK:21712111~pagePK:1497618~piP
K:217854~theSitePK:356352,00.html?cid=3001 (accessed October 25, 2012).

121. For example, Leslie London argues that "none of the Bretton Woods
institutions' policy advice to recipient countries makes more than token
acknowledgment of human rights obligations, and certainly not in relation to
socio-economic rights" ("What Can Ten Years of Democracy in South Africa
Tell Us?" *Health and Human Rights* 8, no. 1 [2004]: 13).

122. World Bank, "Human Rights Day: Interview with Alfredo Sfeir-Younis," December 10, 2003, http://web.worldbank.org/WBSITE/EXTER NAL/NEWS/0,,contentMDK:20143686~menuPK:34457~pagePK:34370~p iPK:34424~theSitePK:4607,00.html (accessed October 25, 2012).

123. See Jim Yong Kim, Joyce V. Millen, Alec Irwin, and John Gershman, eds., *Dying for Growth: Global Inequality and the Health of the Poor* (Monroe, Maine: Common Courage Press, 2000).

124. It is important to note that this defense of "gradualism" cannot be taken to reflect World Bank policy present or past, although it tends to cohere with the de facto health-sector strategy of structural adjustment. However, in the 1993 *World Development Report* (discussed in chapter 4), the bank explicitly called for investing in health for economic development, a reversal of the gradualist logic that Alfredo Sfeir-Younis outlined. Although the World Bank avoids human rights language, a great many of its initiatives support the goal of human development and the realization of certain basic conditions that others would call rights.

125. Guy Carrin, *Strategies for Health Care Finance in Developing Countries—With a Focus on Community Financing in Sub-Saharan Africa*, ed. Marc C. Vereecke (London: Macmillan, 1992), 68.

126. Clinton Health Access Initiative, "Antiretroviral (ARV) Ceiling Price List."

127. Matthew H. Bonds, Donald C. Keenan, Pejman Rohani, and Jeffrey D. Sachs, "Poverty Trap Formed by the Ecology of Infectious Diseases," *Proceedings of the Royal Society,* Series B, 277 (2010): 1185–1192; Bonds, "A Note from the Millennium Villages Project, Rwanda." See also Jeffrey D. Sachs, *The End of Poverty: Economic Possibilities for Our Time* (New York: Penguin, 2005), 64–65.

128. Pundy Pillay, "Human Resource Development and Growth: Improving Access to and Equity in the Provision of Education and Health Services in South Africa," *Development Southern Africa* 23, no. 1 (2006): 63; Sen, *Inequality Reexamined.*

129. Sachs, *The End of Poverty,* 56.

130. Bonds, "A Note from the Millennium Villages Project, Rwanda."

131. John Rawls, *Justice as Fairness: A Restatement* (Cambridge, Mass.: Harvard University Press, 2003), 58.

132. Paul Farmer, Margaret Connors, and Janie Simmons, eds., *Women, Poverty, and AIDS: Sex, Drugs, and Structural Violence* (Monroe, Maine: Common Courage Press, 1996), 316–322. In many countries, an important risk factor for HIV among women is poverty; economic and political empowerment is thus a highly effective treatment.

133. Wendell Berry, *What Are People For?* (Toronto: HarperCollins, 1990), 135. Many, including several authors of this chapter, would not write off the market as a powerful tool to distribute medical care to the sick and even the destitute, as Berry might. His point is nonetheless important: we should begin analysis of global health (or any great social challenge) with justice and then figure out implementation, not the other way around, as is so often the case.

134. Harri Englund, *Prisoners of Freedom: Human Rights and the African Poor* (Berkeley: University of California Press, 2006), 47–70.

135. Development workers, according to Ferguson, often conceive of Lesotho as an agrarian society, when in fact it is primarily a labor reserve; poverty there is more affected by South African labor policy than by agricultural techniques. See James Ferguson, *The Anti-Politics Machine: "Development," Depoliticization, and Bureaucratic Power in Lesotho* (Minneapolis: University of Minnesota Press, 1994), 112–117.

136. "When applied in historical circumstances arising out of different cultural histories," write John L. Comaroff and Jean Comaroff, the concept of civil society "is liable to have [little] purchase on local realities" (*Civil Society and the Political Imagination in Africa: Critical Perspectives* [Chicago: University of Chicago Press, 1999], 17).

137. Some may recall here the category of *cultural rights,* which includes such provisions as the right to maintain a language or participate in cultural life and begins to address this understanding of human nature as essentially social and communal. To some extent, this may be true, but given that the language of "rights" still uses as its metric the individual rather than the community, there may still be tension among the views of Marx, Sandel, Taylor and others as well as within the human rights discourse in general.

138. Michael J. Sandel, *Liberalism and the Limits of Justice* (Cambridge: Cambridge University Press, 1982), 55. Such critiques of individualism go back to Hegel and indeed to Aristotle.

139. Karl Marx, "On the Jewish Question," in *The Marx-Engels Reader,* ed. Robert C. Tucker, 2nd ed. (New York: Norton, 1978), 35.

140. Some human rights frameworks seek to alleviate the symptoms of oppression—to manage inequality—instead of changing the oppressive system itself. In Marx's terms, rights address inequality in the distribution of goods but not the deeper, more insidious inequalities in our (global) society, which for him meant the inequalities in the mode of production. Put simply, because a human rights approach outlines a basic minimum standard, it may distract from more far-reaching calls for true equality. To some extent, this concern is addressed in the "capabilities approach" outlined earlier in this chapter; however, even this framework, with its more comprehensive list of what humans should enjoy, still speaks to the language of "minimum standard" rather than "maximum equality." See, for example, Alain Badiou, *The Communist Hypothesis* (London: Verso, 2010), 2.

141. Fareed Zakaria, "Culture Is Destiny: A Conversation with Lee Kuan Yew," *Foreign Affairs* 73, no. 2 (March–April 1994): 111.

142. Makau Mutua has similar concerns but also observes that the concept of responsibilities (in relation to rights) resonates in many African societies. In fact, he argues that African conceptions of responsibility to others, to the community, might enhance the global human rights discourse. See Makau Mutua, *Human Rights: A Political and Cultural Critique* (Philadelphia: University of Pennsylvania Press, 2002), 71–94. Others also seek reconciliation between human rights and alternate discourses. Charles Taylor, for example, accepts that there may be two "mutually incompatible justifications" for a certain set

of norms, but he argues that "Asian values" and human rights have many areas of substantive overlap. See Charles Taylor, "Conditions of an Unforced Consensus on Human Rights" (paper presented at the Carnegie Council on Ethics and International Affairs workshop entitled "The Growth of East Asia and Its Impact on Human Rights," Bangkok, March 24–27, 1996), 2.

143. Amartya Sen, "Human Rights and Asian Values: What Lee Kuan Yew and Le Peng Don't Understand about Asia," *New Republic* 217, no. 2/3 (1997): 33–38.

144. See, for example, Kymlicka, *Contemporary Political Philosophy,* chap. 6.

145. Feierman, Kleinman, et al., "Anthropology, Knowledge-Flows, and Global Health," 122–128.

146. Paul Farmer, "Never Again? Reflections on Human Values and Human Rights," in *Partner to the Poor: A Paul Farmer Reader,* ed. Haun Saussy (Berkeley: University of California Press, 2010), p. 494.

147. Chidi Anselm Odinkalu, "Why More Africans Don't Use Human Rights Language," *Human Rights Dialogue* 2, no. 1 (1999), www.carnegie council.org/publications/archive/dialogue/2_01/articles/602.html/:pf_printable (accessed October 25, 2012).

148. Nelson Mandela, "Address by President Nelson Mandela at the 53rd United Nations General Assembly," September 21, 1998, New York, http://db.nelsonmandela.org/speeches/pub_view.asp?pg=item&ItemID=NMS631& txtstr (accessed October 9, 2012).

149. Although our focus is principally on rights-based efforts of a smaller scale, what would the realization of health as a human right look like on a national level? A number of countries have health systems that offer universal coverage, which is, in some sense, a vindication of the right to health. In Sweden, for example, the government pays for and provides comprehensive health care for all its citizens. Individuals can top up the public package by seeking private health care, though the great majority do not. By making health services available to all citizens, universal health care systems rest on an understanding, sometimes implicit, of health as a condition of human experience that is too fundamental to leave up to individuals' and employers' ability to pay. In other words, such systems rest on the notion of health as a human right. In fact, the Swedish government uses rights language in reference to its health system. (See, for example, *The Constitution of Sweden* [Stockholm: Ministry of Justice, 2007].) The Cuban and Keralan health systems, considered in chapter 7, offer further examples of efforts to promote the right to health on a national scale. In contrast, the U.S. health system, discussed in both chapters 7 and 11, takes primarily a market-based approach. A vast and complex network of public and private payers shares the burden of health care expenditures in the United States (though unsustainably rising costs demand significant reform).

150. United Nations Children's Fund (UNICEF), "South Africa Country Profile: November 2009," www.unicef.org/southafrica/SAF_children_profile 1109.pdf (accessed October 20, 2012).

151. A rights-based approach to development "integrates norms, standards,

and principles of the international human rights framework into the plans, policies, and processes of development" whereby states and other parties—including donors—are "accountable and transparent in different institutional and policy fora" (A. Frankovits, introduction to *Human Rights in Development Yearbook 2002: Empowerment, Participation, Accountability, and Non-Discrimination: Operationalising a Human Rights–Based Approach to Development,* ed. Martin Scheinin and Markku Suksi [Leiden: Martinus Nijhoff, 2002]: 3–14). See also Peris Sean Jones, "On a Never-Ending Waiting List: Toward Equitable Access to Anti-Retroviral Treatment? Experiences from Zambia," *Health and Human Rights* 8, no. 2 (2005): 96.

152. Farmer, "Never Again?" 494; Farmer, *Pathologies of Power,* 22.

153. Indeed, philosopher Brian Barry argues that the universal moral force of human rights demands that wealthier nations help poorer ones protect the human rights of their citizens (*Why Social Justice Matters* [London: Polity Press, 2005], 28).

154. This section of the chapter has been adapted, with extensive quotation, from Kleinman and Hanna, "Religious Values and Global Health," 73–87, with permission from the Center for the Study of World Religions and Harvard University Press. For a more extended discussion of the religious roots of global health, please refer to the original essay.

155. William James, *The Varieties of Religious Experience* (Cambridge, Mass.: Harvard University Press, 1985; originally published 1902).

156. Albert Schweitzer, "The Call to Mission" (sermon preached on Sunday, January 6, 1905, at St. Nicolas Church, Strasbourg, Alsace), in Schweitzer, *Essential Writings,* ed. James Brabazon (Maryknoll, N.Y.: Orbis Books, 2005), 79–80.

157. The rise in democratic religious and evangelical movements in the United States during the nineteenth century is referred to as the Second Great Awakening. (Jonathan Edwards, among others, is often credited as the leader of the First Great Awakening in the 1740s.) See Nathan O. Hatch, *The Democratization of American Christianity* (New Haven, Conn.: Yale University Press, 1989) for more information about these movements and the idea of the Second Great Awakening (see esp. 220–226). Also see Jon Butler, *Awash in a Sea of Faith: Christianizing the American People* (Cambridge, Mass.: Harvard University Press, 1990) for a somewhat different view.

158. See International Committee of the Red Cross (ICRC), "The History of the Emblems," April 1, 2007, www.icrc.org/web/eng/siteeng0.nsf/html/emblem-history (accessed October 19, 2012).

159. For a brief biography of Dunant, see the website of the Nobel Prizes (he was awarded the Nobel Peace Prize in 1901): http://nobelprize.org/nobel_prizes/peace/laureates/1901/dunant-bio.html (accessed October 30, 2012).

160. Mary Brown Bullock, *An American Transplant: The Rockefeller Foundation and Peking Union Medical College* (Berkeley: University of California Press, 1980), 2. Also see Carsten Flohr, "The Plague Fighter: Wu Lien-teh and the Beginning of the Chinese Public Health System," *Annals of Science* 53 (1996): 361–380.

161. For more information about the relationship between the Rockefeller

Foundation and Peking Union Medical College, along with Yale-in-China, see Bullock, *An American Transplant*. For more on Hume and Yale-in-China, see Lian Xi, *The Conversion of Missionaries: Liberalism in American Protestant Missions in China, 1907–1932* (University Park: Penn State University Press, 1997).

162. See Kleinman and Hanna, "Religious Values and Global Health."

163. See Marcos Cueto, "The Origins of Primary Health Care and Selective Primary Health Care," *American Journal of Public Health* 94, no. 11 (2004): 1864–1874.

164. See, for example, Peter Adamson, "The Mad American," in *Jim Grant: UNICEF Visionary,* ed. Richard Jolly (Florence, Italy: UNICEF, 2001).

165. David Bornstein, *How to Change the World: Social Entrepreneurs and the Power of New Ideas* (New York: Oxford University Press, 2007), 250.

166. Leonardo Boff, *Faith on the Edge: Religion and Marginalized Existence,* trans. Robert R. Barr (San Francisco: Harper and Row, 1989), 23.

167. See, for example, Gustavo Gutiérrez, *A Theology of Liberation: History, Politics, and Salvation* (Maryknoll, N.Y.: Orbis Books, 1973). Gutiérrez and Paul Farmer have just completed a book, *In the Company of the Poor,* which is coming out this year from Orbis Books.

168. Farmer, *Pathologies of Power,* chap. 5.

169. See Kaiser Family Foundation, "Bush Discusses PEPFAR during Visits to Rwanda, Ghana," February 20, 2008, http://dailyreports.kff.org/Daily -Reports/2008/February/20/dr00050492.aspx (accessed October 19, 2012).

170. George W. Bush, *Decision Points* (New York: Crown, 2010), 31–33.

171. See, for example, Alex Hindman and Jean Reith Schroedel, *U.S. Response to HIV/AIDS in Africa: Bush as a Human Rights Leader?* Claremont Graduate University Working Paper, 2009, www.cgu.edu/PDFFiles/SPE/ workingpapers/politics/humanrightspaper_hindman_schroedel.pdf (accessed October 19, 2012).

172. See, for example, James D. Wolfensohn, *A Global Life: My Journey among Rich and Poor, from Sydney to Wall Street to the World Bank* (New York: PublicAffairs, 2010).

173. See, for example, Paula Goldman, "From Margin to Mainstream: Jubilee 2000 and the Rising Profile of Global Poverty Issues in the United States and the United Kingdom" (PhD diss., Department of Anthropology, Harvard University, 2010).

174. See, for example, Gudran Dahl, *Responsibility and Partnership in Swedish Aid Discourse* (Uppsala: Nordic Africa Institute, 2001).

175. See, for example, Eugene P. Heideman, *From Mission to Church: The Reformed Church in America Mission to India* (Grand Rapids, Mich.: Eerdmans, 2001), 664.

176. World Health Organization, "Faith-Based Organizations Play a Major Role in HIV/AIDS Care and Treatment in Sub-Saharan Africa," press release, February 8, 2007, www.who.int/mediacentre/news/notes/2007/np05/ en/index.html (accessed October 25, 2012).

177. See, for example, Simon Montlake, "Taiwan Charity Has Global

Reach," *Wall Street Journal,* March 11, 2010, http://online.wsj.com/article/ SB10001424052748704353404575114661869717700.html (accessed October 19, 2012).

178. See, for example, Warren Frederick Ilchman, Stanley Nider Katz, and Edward L. Queen II, eds., *Philanthropy in the World's Traditions* (Bloomington: Indiana University Press, 1998).

179. Waraporn Kongsuwan and Teris Touhy, "Promoting Peaceful Death for Thai Buddhists: Implications for Holistic End-of-Life Care," *Holistic Nursing Practice* 23, no. 5 (2009): 289–296; Yaowarat Matchim and Myra Aud, "Hospice Care: A Cross-Cultural Comparison between the United States and Thailand," *Journal of Hospice and Palliative Nursing* 11, no. 5 (2009): 262–268.

180. See the introduction to Arthur Kleinman, Yunxiang Yan, Jing Jun, Sing Lee, Everett Zhang, Pan Tianshu, Wu Fei, and Guo Jinhua, *Deep China: The Moral Life of the Person, What Anthropology and Psychiatry Tell Us about China Today* (Berkeley: University of California Press, 2011).

181. Arthur Kleinman, *What Really Matters: Living a Moral Life amidst Uncertainty and Danger* (New York: Oxford University Press, 2006).

182. Eugene Wang's article about Huang Yu's pen-and-ink piece contains a reproduction of the drawing; see Eugene Y. Wang, "The Winking Owl: Visual Effect and Its Art Historical Thick Description," *Critical Inquiry* 26, no. 3 (2000): 435–473. The painting *Head of the Medical Student (Study for Les Demoiselles d'Avignon),* by Pablo Picasso, is owned by the Museum of Modern Art (MOMA) in New York and can be seen on MOMA's website as well as in the museum.

183. See, for example, John W. Dietrich, "The Politics of PEPFAR: The President's Emergency Plan for AIDS Relief," *Ethics and International Affairs* 21, no. 3 (Fall 2007): 277–292.

Clara Barton and the American Red Cross, page 278

1. For a biographical note on Clara Barton, see "Our Founder," on the website of the American Red Cross, www.redcross.org/about-us/history/clara -barton (accessed October 20, 2012).

2. Clara Barton to Hosea Starr Ballou, April 19, 1899, Clara Barton Papers, 1862–1911, Andover-Harvard Theological Library, Harvard Divinity School, Cambridge, Mass. Hosea Starr Ballou was the son of the grandnephew of Hosea Ballou.

3. Clara Barton to Mrs. Jennie S. M. Nintur, October 6, 1904, Clara Barton Papers. Barton often addressed her female correspondents as "sister"; Nintur was not actually her relative.

CHAPTER 10

1. Nirmala Ravishankar, Paul Gubbins, Rebecca J. Cooley, Katherine Leach-Kemon, Catherine M. Michaud, Dean T. Jamison, and Christopher J. L. Murray, "Financing of Global Health: Tracking Development Assistance

for Health from 1990 to 2007," *Lancet* 373, no. 9681 (2009): 2115. See also Susan Okie, "Global Health: The Gates–Buffett Effect," *New England Journal of Medicine* 355, no. 11 (2006): 1084–1088.

2. Ravishankar, Gubbins, et al., "Financing of Global Health," 2118.

3. Jeffrey D. Sachs, *The End of Poverty: Economic Possibilities for Our Time* (New York: Penguin, 2005), 299.

4. Ibid., 56. See also Matthew H. Bonds, Donald C. Keenan, Pejman Rohani, and Jeffrey D. Sachs, "Poverty Trap Formed by the Ecology of Infectious Diseases," *Proceedings of the Royal Society,* Series B, 277 (2010): 1185–1192; Matt Bonds, "A Note from the Millennium Villages Project, Rwanda: Breaking the Disease-Driven Poverty Trap," *Consilience: The Journal of Sustainable Development,* no. 1 (2008): 98–111.

5. Sachs, *The End of Poverty,* 19–20.

6. Joseph Hanlon, Armando Barrientos, and David Hulme, *Just Give Money to the Poor: The Development Revolution from the Global South* (Sterling, Va.: Kumarian Press, 2010), 4.

7. Sachs, *The End of Poverty,* 57–58.

8. Ibid., 312. Despite the Western media's emphasis on corruption in Africa, Sachs points out that, according to the Freedom House index, the level of corruption in African states is no different on average than that for other low-income countries globally.

9. Ibid., 320, 269.

10. William Easterly, *The White Man's Burden: Why the West's Efforts to Aid the Rest Have Done So Much Ill and So Little Good* (New York: Penguin, 2006), 157.

11. William Easterly and Tobias Pfutze, *Where Does the Money Go? Best and Worst Practices in Foreign Aid,* Brookings Global Economy and Development Working Paper no. 21, June 2008, 19. For more on inefficiencies in the administration of development aid, see Giles Bolton, *Africa Doesn't Matter: How the West Has Failed the Poorest Continent and What We Can Do about It* (New York: Arcade, 2008).

12. Easterly, *The White Man's Burden,* 108.

13. Ibid., 370.

14. Amartya Sen, "The Man without a Plan," *Foreign Affairs,* March/April 2006, www.foreignaffairs.com/articles/61525/amartya-sen/the-man-without-a-plan?page=show (accessed November 15, 2012).

15. See Dambisa Moyo, *Dead Aid: Why Aid Is Not Working and How There Is a Better Way for Africa* (New York: Farrar, Straus and Giroux, 2009). Moyo, a Zambian economist, joins the ranks of the aid skeptics and argues that aid reduces investment and savings, causes inflation, stifles exports, and breeds cultures of dependency and corruption. She calls for an end to all aid to Africa in five years and instead offers a number of market-based reforms that could stimulate growth: freer and fairer trade agreements, participation in capital markets, and foreign direct investment as well as microlending and venture finance models to unlock illiquid assets of the poor, such as land lacking legal title. For Moyo, market-based reform is the key to reducing global poverty. Some would suggest that a similar logic drove the structural adjust-

ment reforms of the International Monetary Fund and the World Bank in the 1980s, an approach that was counterproductive for many of its adopters, as chapter 4 demonstrates.

16. Paul Collier, a former World Bank economist and current professor at Oxford, addresses this question in *The Bottom Billion: Why the Poorest Countries Are Failing and What Can Be Done about It* (Oxford: Oxford University Press, 2007). Most of Collier's research seeks to identify specific aid programs that work in specific settings. For example, when a country experiences a turnaround (such as ending a civil war), Collier argues that foreign aid, like a natural resources windfall (say, the discovery of oil), can distract from the hard work of building a new government and reforming institutions. Aid functions as a prize, and officials may spend more time seeking to get a piece of that prize than rebuilding their country (ibid., 114). He acknowledges that technical assistance (consultants, managers, engineers, legal advisors, and so on) can be useful in post-conflict or turnaround settings, as government officials and civil society seek to build transparent and accountable institutions. Thus he recommends such technical assistance for the first four years after a turnaround. Then, once a stable institutional infrastructure is in place, development aid should kick in. It should be given in regular amounts and over a long period so that the government and other beneficiaries can use it on substantial investments.

Collier identifies other aid modalities that work in specific circumstances. For example, landlocked countries are at an added disadvantage because they face higher transport costs, which discourage trade. They can, however, benefit from spill-over growth among their neighbors: on average, 1 percent growth in one country triggers 0.4 percent growth in its neighbors (ibid., 56). However, spill-overs depend on transportation links between countries: if Niger has poor transportation infrastructure, it will benefit less if neighboring Nigeria experiences good growth. Improving transport links between landlocked countries and their neighbors, therefore, is a fertile area for aid projects. In sum, Collier believes that aid is often flawed but remains one of the key instruments for generating growth in poor countries; greater scrutiny is required to identify specific programs that work in specific circumstances.

17. Abhijit V. Banerjee and Esther Duflo, *Poor Economics: A Radical Rethinking of the Way to Fight Global Poverty* (New York: PublicAffairs, 2011).

18. Edward Miguel and Michael Kremer, "Worms: Identifying Impacts on Education and Health in the Presence of Treatment Externalities," *Econometrica* 72, no. 1 (2004): 159–217. For an update on long-run health gains, see also Sarah Baird, Joan Hamory Hicks, Edward Miguel, and Michael Kremer, *Worms at Work: Long-Run Impacts of Child Health Gains,* working paper, Abdul Latif Jameel Poverty Action Lab, October 2011, www.poverty actionlab.org/publication/worms-work-long-run-impacts-child-health-gains (accessed November 20, 2012).

19. See, for example, Nick Black, "Why We Need Observational Studies to Evaluate the Effectiveness of Health Care," *British Medical Journal* 312, no. 7040 (1996): 1215–1218; Robert William Sanson-Fisher, Billie Bonevski, Law-

rence W. Green, and Cate D'Este, "Limitations of the Randomized Controlled Trial in Evaluating Population-Based Health Interventions," *American Journal of Preventive Medicine* 33, no. 2 (2007): 155–161.

20. Paul Farmer, "Partners in Help: Assisting the Poor over the Long Term," *Foreign Affairs,* July 29, 2011, www.foreignaffairs.com/articles/68002/paul-farmer/partners-in-help?page=show (accessed November 19, 2012).

21. For information on the accompaniment approach, with particular reference to Haiti, see United Nations Office of the Special Envoy for Haiti, "Has Aid Changed? Channeling Assistance to Haiti before and after the Earthquake," June 2011, video presentation, by Katherine Gilbert, www.lessonsfromhaiti .org/press-and-media/videos/presentation-accompany-haiti/; published report, www.lessonsfromhaiti.org/download/Report_Center/has_aid_changed_en .pdf (both accessed March 7, 2013).

22. Collier, *The Bottom Billion,* 99–123.

23. United Nations Office of the Special Envoy for Haiti, "Has Aid Changed?" 15, www.lessonsfromhaiti.org/download/Report_Center/has_aid_changed_en.pdf (accessed March 7, 2013).

24. Center for Economic and Policy Research, "Haitian Companies Still Sidelined from Reconstruction Contracts," April 19, 2011, www.cepr.net/ index.php/blogs/relief-and-reconstruction-watch/haitian-companies-still-sidelined-from-reconstruction-contracts (accessed November 14, 2012).

25. ActionAid International, *Real Aid: An Agenda for Making Aid Work,* 2005, 22, www.actionaid.org/sites/files/actionaid/real_aid.pdf (accessed November 14, 2012).

26. Hanlon, Barrientos, and Hulme, *Just Give Money to the Poor,* 38–39.

27. Juan A. Rivera, Daniela Sotres-Alvarez, Jean-Pierre Habicht, Teresa Shamah, and Salvador Villalpando, "Impact of the Mexican Program for Education, Health, and Nutrition (Progresa) on Rates of Growth and Anemia in Infants and Young Children: A Randomized Effectiveness Study," *Journal of the American Medical Association* 291, no. 21 (2004): 2563–2570; Paul Gertler, "Do Conditional Cash Transfers Improve Child Health? Evidence from PROGRESA's Control Randomized Experiment," *American Economic Review* 94, no. 2 (2004): 336–341. See also Julio Frenk, "Bridging the Divide: Global Lessons from Evidence-Based Health Policy in Mexico," *Lancet* 368, no. 9539 (2006): 954–961.

28. Farmer, "Partners in Help."

29. For more on this example, see Paul Farmer, *Haiti after the Earthquake* (New York: PublicAffairs, 2011), 211.

30. Betsy McKay, "Global Fund to Resume New Health Grants," *Wall Street Journal,* May 9, 2012, http://online.wsj.com/article/SB1000142405270 23042036045773937326178865576.html (accessed November 15, 2012).

31. The Digicel Foundation's education aid in Haiti offers one compelling example of accompaniment. Digicel launched its foundation arm in Haiti less than a year after it set up its first mobile phone networks in 2006. The largest mobile phone provider in the country today, Digicel has also emerged as a substantial funder of education efforts in rural Haiti, building or rebuilding more than twenty schools across the country. The foundation also supports partner-

ships with school lunch programs and vaccination initiatives. This model of private sector engagement and philanthropy has yielded durable partnerships and effective aid delivery. For more information, see http://fondationdigicel haiti.org/about/ (accessed November 15, 2012).

32. See, for example, Jim Yong Kim, Joseph Rhatigan, Sachin H. Jain, Rebecca Weintraub, and Michael E. Porter, "From a Declaration of Values to the Creation of Value in Global Health: A Report from Harvard University's Global Health Delivery Project," *Global Public Health* 5, no. 2 (2010): 181–188. For a full list of GHD cases, see www.ghdonline.org/cases/ (accessed November 15, 2012).

33. For more information, see "Access to Life-Saving Health Information: Not a Luxury, a Necessity," *Health and Human Rights,* January 5, 2010, http://hhrjournal.org/index.php/hhr/article/view/339/551 (accessed November 15, 2012).

34. Farmer, *Haiti after the Earthquake,* 165.

35. Sachs, *The End of Poverty,* 269.

36. For more on these conditions, which have included the "global gag rule" and the prostitution pledge, see Nils Daulaire, "Global Health for a Globally Minded President," *Health Affairs* 28, no. 2 (2009): w199–w204, http://content.healthaffairs.org/content/28/2/w199.full.html (accessed November 15, 2012).

37. Prabhat Jha, Anne Mills, Kara Hanson, Lilani Kumaranayake, Lesong Conteh, Christoph Kurowski, Son Nam Nguyen, Valeria Oliveira Cruz, Kent Ranson, Lara M.E. Vaz, Shengchao Yu, Oliver Morton, and Jeffrey D. Sachs, "Improving the Health of the Global Poor," *Science* 295, no. 5562 (March 15, 2002): 2036.

38. Jeffrey Sachs, "Development Aid in Five Easy Steps," *Project Syndicate,* May 26, 2010, www.project-syndicate.org/commentary/sachs166/English (accessed November 15, 2012).

39. Kaiser Family Foundation, "Americans Say Maintain or Increase Funding for Global Health and Development, But Take Care of Problems at Home First in the Recession," press release, May 7, 2009, www.kff.org/kaiserpolls/posr050709nr.cfm?RenderForPrint=1 (accessed November 15, 2012).

40. WorldPublicOpinion.org, "American Public Vastly Overestimates Amount of U.S. Foreign Aid," November 29, 2010, www.worldpublicopinion.org/pipa/articles/brunitedstatescanadara/670.php (accessed November 15, 2012).

41. Clay Ramsay, Stephen Weber, Steven Kull, and Evan Lewis, "American Public Opinion and Global Health," WorldPublicOpinion.org, May 20, 2009, www.worldpublicopinion.org/pipa/pdf/may09/WPO_IOM_May09_rpt.pdf (accessed November 15, 2012).

42. On aid as a percentage of the U.S. budget, see U.S. Global Leadership Coalition, "Myths and Facts about the International Affairs Budget," www.usglc.org/wp-content/uploads/2011/01/Myths-and-Facts-About-the-International-Affairs-Budget.pdf (accessed November 15, 2012).

43. Sachs, "Development Aid in Five Easy Steps."

44. World Health Organization, "The Abuja Declaration: Ten Years On,"

2011, 2, www.who.int/healthsystems/publications/Abuja10.pdf (accessed November 15, 2012).

45. Ibid.

46. See Partners In Health, "Tackling Acute and Chronic Disasters," Partners In Health 2010 Annual Report, http://parthealth.3cdn.net/fdb20a0a7ef6b 71153_06m6icn3q.pdf (accessed March 7, 2013); Public Radio International (PRI), "Haiti: A Year and a Half after the Earthquake," *The World,* July 15, 2011, www.pri.org/stories/business/nonprofits/haiti-a-year-and-a-half-after -the-earthquake4907.html (accessed March 7, 2013); and United Nations Office of the Secretary-General's Special Adviser on Community-Based Medicine and Lessons from Haiti, "Assistance Tracker," www.lessonsfromhaiti.org/assis tance-tracker/ (accessed March 7, 2013). For more on the modalities for foreign aid in Haiti after the earthquake, see Farmer, *Haiti after the Earthquake.*

CHAPTER 11

1. See, for example, Jon Cohen, "Global Health: The New World of Global Health," *Science* 311, no. 5758 (January 13, 2006): 162–167. Also see chapter 5 for a detailed discussion of the worldwide response to the AIDS epidemic and the development of a vision based in global health equity.

2. David M. Morens, Gregory K. Folkers, and Anthony S. Fauci, "The Challenge of Emerging and Re-Emerging Infectious Diseases," *Nature* 430, no. 6996 (July 8, 2004): 242–249.

3. See, for example, Elliot Marseille, Paul B. Hofmann, and James G. Kahn, "HIV Prevention before HAART in Sub-Saharan Africa," *Lancet* 359, no. 9320 (2002): 1851; Andrew Creese, Katherine Floyd, Anita Alban, and Lorna Guinness, "Cost-Effectiveness of HIV/AIDS Interventions in Africa: A Systematic Review of the Evidence," *Lancet* 359, no. 9318 (2002): 1635–1642.

4. See World Health Organization, *Global Tuberculosis Report 2012,* http:// apps.who.int/iris/bitstream/10665/75938/1/9789241564502_eng.pdf (accessed November 15, 2012); and World Health Organization, *World Malaria Report 2011,* www.who.int/malaria/world_malaria_report_2011/9789241564403_ eng.pdf (accessed November 15, 2012). Globally, the TB death rate fell by 41 percent between 1990 and 2012, and the world is on track to achieve the global target of a 50 percent reduction by 2015 (WHO, *Global Tuberculosis Report 2012,* 1). Between 2000 and 2011, the estimated incidence of malaria globally decreased by 17 percent, and malaria-specific mortality rates fell by 26 percent. The percentage of households owning at least one insecticide-treated bed net has risen from 3 percent in 2000 to 50 percent in 2011 (WHO, *World Malaria Report 2011,* ix).

5. See, for example, Badara Samb, Tim Evans, Mark Dybul, Rifat Atun, Jean-Paul Moatti, Sania Nishtar, Anna Wright, Francesca Celletti, Justine Hsu, Jim Yong Kim, Ruairi Brugha, Asia Russell, and Carissa Etienne (World Health Organization Maximizing Positive Synergies Collaborative Group), "An Assessment of Interactions between Global Health Initiatives and Country Health Systems," *Lancet* 373, no. 9681 (2009): 2137–2169; Institute of Medicine, *The U.S. Commitment to Global Health: Recommendations for*

the Public and Private Sectors (Washington, D.C.: National Academies Press, 2009), 512–513; Julio Frenk, "Bridging the Divide: Global Lessons from Evidence-Based Health Policy in Mexico," *Lancet* 368, no. 9539 (2006): 954–961; Paul E. Farmer, Fernet Léandre, Joia S. Mukherjee, Marie Sidonise Claude, Patrice Nevil, Mary C. Smith-Fawzi, Serena P. Koenig, Arachu Castro, Mercedes C. Becerra, Jeffrey Sachs, Amir Attaran, and Jim Yong Kim, "Community-Based Approaches to HIV Treatment in Resource-Poor Settings," *Lancet* 358, no. 9279 (2001): 404–409; David A. Walton, Paul E. Farmer, Wesler Lambert, Fernet Léandre, Serena P. Koenig, and Joia S. Mukherjee, "Integrated HIV Prevention and Care Strengthens Primary Health Care: Lessons from Rural Haiti," *Journal of Public Health Policy* 25, no. 2 (2004): 137–158; Jaime Sepúlveda, Flavia Bustreo, Roberto Tapia, Juan Rivera, Rafael Lozano, Gustavo Oláiz, Virgilio Partida, Lourdes García-García, and José Luis Valdespino, "Improvement of Child Survival in Mexico: The Diagonal Approach," *Lancet* 368, no. 9551 (2006): 2017–2027.

6. Thomas Pogge, *World Poverty and Human Rights,* 2nd ed. (Cambridge: Polity Press, 2008), 24. Pogge also notes that the income shortfall of the 2.5 billion people living (or dying) in severe poverty is estimated at $300 billion, or 1 percent of the combined gross national product of OECD countries.

7. World Health Organization, *World Health Report 2006: Working Together for Health* (Geneva: World Health Organization, 2006). See also Pooja Kumar, "Providing the Providers: Remedying Africa's Shortage of Health Care Workers," *New England Journal of Medicine* 356, no. 25 (2007): 2564–2567.

8. Julio Frenk, José L. Bobadilla, Jaime Sepulveda, and Malaquais López Cervantes, "Health Transition in Middle-Income Countries: New Challenges for Health Care," *Health Policy and Planning* 4, no. 1 (1989): 29–39.

9. See United Nations, *The Millennium Development Goals Report,* 2012, http://mdgs.un.org/unsd/mdg/Resources/Static/Products/Progress2012/English2012.pdf (accessed November 15, 2012).

10. United Nations, "Millennium Development Goals: Goal 4—Reduce Child Mortality," Fact Sheet, UN Department of Public Information, September 2010, www.un.org/millenniumgoals/pdf/MDG_FS_4_EN.pdf (accessed November 15, 2012).

11. World Health Organization and World Bank, "High-Level Forum on the Health Millennium Development Goals," December 2003, www.who.int/hdp/en/IP1-overview.pdf (accessed November 15, 2012).

12. World Health Organization, "Children: Reducing Mortality," Fact Sheet no. 178, September 2012, www.who.int/mediacentre/factsheets/fs178/en/ (accessed November 15, 2012).

13. Amy L. Rice, Lisa Sacco, Adnan Hyder, and Robert E. Black, "Malnutrition as an Underlying Cause of Childhood Deaths Associated with Infectious Diseases in Developing Countries," *Bulletin of the World Health Organization* 78, no. 10 (2000): 1207–1221.

14. Richard Horton, "A New Global Commitment to Child Survival," *Lancet* 368, no. 9541 (2006): 1041–1042.

15. GAVI Alliance, "2000–2010: A Decade of Saving Lives," December

8, 2010, www.gavialliance.org/library/publications/gavi-fact-sheets/current/true/page/2/ (accessed February 6, 2013).

16. For data on weight gain, see Harold Alderman, Joseph Konde-Lule, Isaac Sebuliba, Donald Bundy, and Andrew Hall, "Effect on Weight Gain of Routinely Giving Albendazole to Preschool Children during Child Health Days in Uganda: Cluster Randomised Controlled Trial," *British Medical Journal* 333, no. 7559 (2006): 122.

Concerning reduced school absenteeism, see Edward Miguel and Michael Kremer, "Worms: Identifying Impacts on Education and Health in the Presence of Treatment Externalities," *Econometrica* 72, no. 1 (2004): 159–217.

For evidence of higher cognitive exam scores, see Catherine Nokes, Sally M. Grantham-McGregor, Anthony W. Sawyer, Edward S. Cooper, and Donald A. P. Bundy, "Parasitic Helminth Infection and Cognitive Function in School Children," *Proceedings: Biological Sciences* 247, no. 1319 (1992): 77–81.

For data on higher wages earned in adulthood, see Sarah Baird, Joan Hamory Hicks, Edward Miguel, and Michael Kremer, *Worms at Work: Long-Run Impacts of Child Health Gains,* working paper, Abdul Latif Jameel Poverty Action Lab, October 2011, www.povertyactionlab.org/publication/worms -work-long-run-impacts-child-health-gains (accessed November 20, 2012).

17. Michael Kremer, "School-Based Deworming: Big Impact for Small Change," Harvard Kennedy School lecture, May 15, 2010, www.hks.harvard .edu/var/ezp_site/storage/fckeditor/file/pdfs/degree-programs/mpaid/mpaid -10th-michael-kremer-slideshow.pdf (accessed November 15, 2012).

18. World Health Organization, "Community-Based Management of Severe Acute Malnutrition: A Joint Statement by the World Health Organization, the World Food Programme, the United Nations System Standing Committee on Nutrition, and the United Nations Children's Fund," May 2007, www.who.int/nutrition/topics/statement_commbased_malnutrition/en/index .html (accessed November 15, 2012).

19. Isabelle Defourny, Gwenola Seroux, Issaley Abdelkader, and Géza Harczi, "Management of Moderate Acute Malnutrition with RUTF in Niger," *MSF Report,* 2007, www.msf.org.au/uploads/media/mod_acc_mal_Niger.pdf (accessed November 15, 2012); Steve Collins and Kate Sadler, "Outpatient Care for Severely Malnourished Children in Emergency Relief Programmes: A Retrospective Cohort Study," *Lancet* 360, no. 9348 (2002): 1824–1830; Michael A. Ciliberto, Heidi Sandige, MacDonald J. Ndekha, Per Ashorn, André Briend, Heather M. Ciliberto, and Mark J. Manary, "Comparison of Home-Based Therapy with Ready-to-Use Therapeutic Food with Standard Therapy in the Treatment of Malnourished Malawian Children: A Controlled, Clinical Effectiveness Trial," *American Journal of Clinical Nutrition* 81, no. 4 (2005): 864–870.

20. Eleanor Oakley, Jason Reinking, Heidi Sandige, Indi Trehan, Gregg Kennedy, Kenneth Maleta, and Mark Manary, "A Ready-to-Use Therapeutic Food Containing 10% Milk Is Less Effective than One with 25% Milk in the Treatment of Severely Malnourished Children," *Journal of Nutrition* 140, no. 12 (2010): 2248–2252; Collins and Sadler, "Outpatient Care for Severely Malnourished Children in Emergency Relief Programmes"; El Hadji Issakha Diop,

Nicole Idohou Dossou, Marie Madeleine Ndour, André Briend, and Salimata Wade, "Comparison of the Efficacy of a Solid Ready-to-Use Food and a Liquid, Milk-Based Diet for the Rehabilitation of Severely Malnourished Children: A Randomized Trial," *American Journal of Clinical Nutrition* 78, no. 2 (2003): 302–307.

21. See Martin Enserink, "The Peanut Butter Debate," *Science* 322, no. 5898 (October 2, 2008): 36–38; Paul Farmer, "Partners in Help: Assisting the Poor over the Long Term," *Foreign Affairs,* July 29, 2011, www.foreign affairs.com/articles/68002/paul-farmer/partners-in-help?page=show (accessed November 19, 2012); and Andrew Rice, "The Peanut Solution," *New York Times,* September 2, 2010, www.nytimes.com/2010/09/05/magazine/05 Plumpy-t.html (accessed November 15, 2012).

22. United Nations, "Millennium Development Goals—Goal 5: Improve Maternal Health," Fact Sheet, UN Department of Public Information, September 2010, www.un.org/millenniumgoals/pdf/MDG_FS_5_EN_new.pdf (accessed November 15, 2012).

23. The eleven countries were Afghanistan, Bangladesh, the Democratic Republic of the Congo, Ethiopia, India, Indonesia, Kenya, Nigeria, Pakistan, Sudan, and the United Republic of Tanzania. See World Health Organization, United Nations Children's Fund, United Nations Population Fund, and the World Bank, *Trends in Maternal Mortality: 1990 to 2008* (Geneva: World Health Organization, 2010), 1, 17.

24. United Nations, "Millennium Development Goals—Goal 5: Improve Maternal Health."

25. Institute for Health Metrics and Evaluation, "Building Momentum: Global Progress toward Reducing Maternal and Child Mortality" (report presented at the Women Deliver Conference, Washington, D.C., June 7, 2010), 7.

26. Isabella Danel and Ada Rivera, "Honduras, 1990–1997," in *Reducing Maternal Mortality: Learning from Bolivia, China, Egypt, Honduras, Indonesia, Jamaica, and Zimbabwe,* ed. Marjorie A. Koblinsky (Washington, D.C.: World Bank, 2003), 51–62.

27. Joia S. Mukherjee, Donna J. Barry, Hind Satti, Maxi Raymonville, Sarah Marsh, and Mary Kay Smith-Fawzi, "Structural Violence: A Barrier to Achieving the Millennium Development Goals for Women," *Journal of Women's Health* 20, no. 4 (2011): 593–597; Louise Ivers and Kimberly Cullen, "Food Insecurity: Special Considerations for Women," *American Journal of Clinical Nutrition* 94, no. 6 (2011): 1740S-1744S.

28. See Kate Kerber, Joseph de Graft-Johnson, Zulfiqar Bhutta, Pius Okong, Ann Starrs, and Joy Lawn, "Continuum of Care for Maternal, Newborn, and Child Health: From Slogan to Service Delivery," *Lancet* 370, no. 9595 (2007): 1358–1369; and Allan Rosenfield, Caroline J. Min, and Lynn P. Freedman, "Making Motherhood Safe in Developing Countries," *New England Journal of Medicine* 356, no. 14 (2007): 1395–1397.

29. Santoso S. Hamijoyo and Donald S. Chauls, "Community Participation in the Indonesian Family Planning Program: The Village Perspective and Management Strategies," Management Sciences for Health, 1992; Siswanto Agus Wilopo and W. Henry Mosley, "The Relationship of Child Survival

Intervention Programs to the Practice of Contraception: A Case Study in Indonesia," Johns Hopkins Population Center, 1993; Tasnim Partapuri, Robert Steinglass, and Jenny Sequeira, "Integrated Delivery of Health Services during Outreach Visits: A Literature Review of Program Experience through a Routine Immunization Lens," *Journal of Infectious Diseases* 205, suppl. 1 (2012): S23.

30. Mukherjee, Barry, et al., "Structural Violence," 596.

31. John Cleland, Stan Bernstein, Alex Ezeh, Anibal Faundes, Anna Glasier, and Jolene Innis, "Family Planning: The Unfinished Agenda," *Lancet* 368, no. 9549 (2006): 1810–1827; Sue J. Goldie, Lynne Gaffikin, Jeremy D. Goldhaber-Fiebert, Amparo Gordillo-Tobar, Carol Levin, Cédric Mahé, and Thomas C. Wright, "Cost-Effectiveness of Cervical-Cancer Screening in Five Developing Countries," *New England Journal of Medicine* 353, no. 20 (2005): 2158–2168; Sue J. Goldie, Meredith O'Shea, Nicole Gastineau Campos, Mireia Diaz, Steven Sweet, and Sun-Young Kim, "Health and Economic Outcomes of HPV 16,18 Vaccination in 72 GAVI-Eligible Countries," *Vaccine* 26, no. 32 (2008): 4080–4093.

32. UNAIDS, *World AIDS Day Report 2012: Results,* www.unaids.org/en/resources/publications/2012/name,76120,en.asp (accessed January 29, 2013).

33. World Health Organization, *World Malaria Report 2011,* 72–73.

34. World Health Organization, "The Top 10 Causes of Death," Fact Sheet no. 310, June 2011, www.who.int/mediacentre/factsheets/fs310/en/index.html (accessed November 15, 2012); United Nations, "Millennium Development Goals—Goal 6: Combat HIV/AIDS, Malaria and Other Diseases," Fact Sheet, UN Department of Public Information, September 2010, www.un.org/millenniumgoals/pdf/MDG_FS_6_EN.pdf (accessed January 31, 2013).

35. The RTS,S Clinical Trials Partnership, "First Results of Phase 3 Trial of RTS,S/AS01 Malaria Vaccine in African Children," *New England Journal of Medicine* 365, no. 20 (2011): 1863–1875; Stu Hutson, "Half-Century-Old TB drugs Get a Facelift in New Cocktails," *Nature Medicine* 16, no. 20 (2010): 1346. These developments are being accelerated by the PATH Malaria Vaccine Initiative and the TB Alliance.

36. Myron S. Cohen, Ying Q. Chen, et al., "Prevention of HIV-1 Infection with Early Antiretroviral Therapy," *New England Journal of Medicine* 365, no. 6 (2011): 493–505.

37. For more information on HIV vaccine progress, see HIV Vaccine Trials Network, www.hvtn.org/ (accessed January 31, 2013).

38. Anthony S. Fauci, "25 Years of HIV," *Nature* 453, no. 7193 (May 15, 2008): 289–290.

39. UNAIDS, *World AIDS Day Report 2012: Results,* 6.

40. Ibid., 8, 16.

41. Jennifer Kates, Adam Wexler, Eric Lief, Carlos Avila, and Benjamin Gobet, "Financing the Response to AIDS in Low- and Middle-Income Countries: International Assistance from Donor Governments in 2011," UNAIDS and Kaiser Family Foundation, July 2012, www.kff.org/hivaids/upload/7347-08.pdf (accessed November 25, 2012); Kaiser Family Foundation, Kaiser Daily Global Health Policy Report, "Global Fund Cancels Round 11 Grants,

Approves New Strategy and Organization Plan," November 29, 2011, http://globalhealth.kff.org/Daily-Reports/2011/November/29/GH-112911-Global -Fund-Round-11.aspx (accessed January 8, 2013).

42. United Nations General Assembly, "Political Declaration on HIV/AIDS: Intensifying Our Efforts to Eliminate HIV/AIDS," June 8, 2011, www .un.org/ga/search/view_doc.asp?symbol=A/65/L.77 (accessed November 25, 2012); Office of the White House Press Secretary, "The Obama Administration to Participate in the 19th International AIDS Conference," press release, July 16, 2012, www.whitehouse.gov/the-press-office/2012/07/16/obama-admin istration-participate-19th-international-aids-conference (accessed November 20, 2012).

43. Kates, Wexler, et al., "Financing the Response to AIDS in Low- and Middle-Income Countries."

44. For more information, see World Health Organization, *Global Plan to Combat Neglected Tropic Diseases, 2008–2015,* March 2007, esp. 28–34, www.who.int/neglected_diseases/NTD%20Global%20plan_%20January %202007.pdf (accessed November 20, 2012).

45. Peter J. Hotez, David H. Molyneux, Alan Fenwick, Jacob Kumaresan, Sonia Ehrlich Sachs, Jeffrey D. Sachs, and Lorenzo Savioli, "Control of Neglected Tropical Diseases," *New England Journal of Medicine* 357, no. 10 (2007): 1018.

46. Hoyt Bleakley, "Disease and Development: Evidence from Hookworm Eradication in the American South," *Quarterly Journal of Economics* 122, no. 1 (2007): 73–117; Kapa D. Ramaiah, Pradeep K. Das, Edwin Michael, and Helen L. Guyatt, "The Economic Burden of Lymphatic Filariasis in India," *Parasitology Today* 16, no. 6 (2000): 251–253.

47. Pierre Chirac and Els Torreele, "Global Framework on Essential Health R&D," *Lancet* 367, no. 9522 (2006): 1560–1561.

48. Bernard Pécoul, "New Drugs for Neglected Diseases: From Pipelines to Patients," *PLoS Medicine* 1, no. 1 (2004): e6.

49. This dynamic was described in precisely these terms concerning drugs to treat multidrug-resistant TB (see chapter 8). See, for example, Salmaan Keshavjee, Kwonjune Seung, et al., "Stemming the Tide of Multidrug-Resistant Tuberculosis: Major Barriers to Addressing the Growing Epidemic," in Institute of Medicine, *Addressing the Threat of Drug-Resistant Tuberculosis: A Realistic Assessment of the Challenge. Workshop Summary* (Washington, D.C.: National Academies Press, 2009), 67, www.iom.edu/~/media/Files/Activity%20Files/Research/DrugForum/IOM_MDRTB_whitepaper_2009 _01_14_FINAL_Edited.pdf (accessed October 15, 2012), with data drawn from World Health Organization/International Union against Tuberculosis and Lung Disease, Global Project on Anti-Tuberculosis Drug Resistance Surveillance, *Anti-Tuberculosis Drug Resistance in the World: Report no. 4* (Geneva: World Health Organization, 2008), www.who.int/tb/publications/2008/drs_report4_26feb08.pdf (accessed November 15, 2012); and Médecins Sans Frontières, *DR-TB Drugs under the Microscope: The Sources and Prices of Medicines for Drug-Resistant Tuberculosis,* 2011, www.doctorswithout

borders.org/publications/reports/2011/Report_Summary_DR-TB_Drugs_ Under_the_Microscope.pdf (accessed November 15, 2012).

50. Sylvie Bisser, François-Xavier N'Siesi, Veerle Lejon, Pierre-Marie Preux, Simon Van Nieuwenhove, Constantin Miaka Mia Bilenge, and Philippe Büscher, "Equivalence Trial of Melarsoprol and Nifurtimox Monotherapy and Combination Therapy for the Treatment of Second-Stage *Trypanosoma brucei gambiense* Sleeping Sickness," *Journal of Infectious Diseases* 195, no. 3 (2007): 322–329.

51. Manica Balasegaram, Steve Harris, Francesco Checchi, Sara Ghorashian, Catherine Hamel, and Unni Karunakara, "Melarsoprol versus Eflornithine for Treating Late-Stage Gambian Trypanosomiasis in the Republic of the Congo," *Bulletin of the World Health Organization* 84, no. 10 (2006): 783–789.

52. François Chappuis, Nitya Udayraj, Kai Stietenroth, Ann Meussen, and Patrick A. Bovier, "Eflornithine Is Safer than Melarsoprol for the Treatment of Second-Stage *Trypanosoma brucei gambiense* Human African Trypanosomiasis," *Clinical Infectious Diseases* 41, no. 5 (2005): 748–751; Gerardo Priotto, Loretxu Pinoges, Isaac Badi Fursa, Barbara Burke, Nathalie Nicolay, Guillaume Grillet, Cathy Hewison, and Manica Balasegaram, "Safety and Effectiveness of First Line Eflornithine for *Trypanosoma brucei gambiense* Sleeping Sickness in Sudan: Cohort Study," *British Medical Journal* 336, no. 7646 (2008): 705–708; Simon Van Nieuwenhove, Paul J. Schechter, Johan Declercq, George Boné, Joanne Burke, and Albert Sjoerdsma, "Treatment of Gambiense Sleeping Sickness in the Sudan with Oral DFMO (DL-α-difluoromethylornithine), an Inhibitor of Ornithine Decarboxylase; First Field Trial," *Transactions of the Royal Society of Tropical Medicine and Hygiene* 79, no. 5 (1985): 692–698.

53. Jürg Utzinger, Xiao-Nong Zhou, Maurice G. Chen, and Robert Bergquist, "Conquering Schistosomiasis in China: The Long March," *Acta Tropica* 96 (2005): 69–96.

54. Boakye A. Boatin and Frank O. Richards Jr., "Control of Onchocerciasis," *Advances in Parasitology* 61 (2006): 349–394; Hotez, Molyneux, et al., "Control of Neglected Tropical Diseases."

55. World Health Organization, "Onchocerciasis Control Programme in West Africa (OCP)," www.who.int/apoc/onchocerciasis/ocp/en/ (accessed November 15, 2012).

56. Andy Crump and Satoshi Omura, "Ivermectin, 'Wonder Drug' from Japan: The Human Use Perspective," *Proceedings of the Japan Academy, Series B, Physical and Biological Sciences* 87, no. 2 (2011): 13–28.

57. See, for example, Jeremy A. Greene, "Making Medicines Essential: The Emergent Centrality of Pharmaceuticals in Global Health," *Biosocieties* 6, no. 1 (2011): 10–33.

58. Hotez, Molyneux, et al., "Control of Neglected Tropical Diseases." However, stories of pharmaceutical donations to combat NTDs and other treatable and preventable global scourges are still few and far between. See the box titled "Intellectual Property and Global Health Equity," later in this chapter.

59. David H. Molyneux, "Elimination of Transmission of Lymphatic Filariasis in Egypt," *Lancet* 367, no. 9515 (2006): 966–968; Khalfan A. Mohammed, David H. Molyneux, Marco Albonico, and Francesco Rio, "Progress towards Eliminating Lymphatic Filariasis in Zanzibar: A Model Programme," *Trends in Parasitology* 22, no. 7 (2006): 340–344.

60. David H. Molyneux, Peter J. Hotez, and Alan Fenwick, "'Rapid-Impact Interventions': How a Policy of Integrated Control for Africa's Neglected Tropical Diseases Could Benefit the Poor," *PLoS Medicine* 2, no. 11 (2005): e336.

61. Jeffrey Bethony, Simon Brooker, Marco Albonico, Stefan M. Geiger, Alex Loukas, David Diemert, and Peter J. Hotez, "Soil-Transmitted Helminth Infections: Ascariasis, Trichuriasis, and Hookworm," *Lancet* 367, no. 9521 (2006): 1521–1532; Miguel and Kremer, "Worms: Identifying Impacts on Education and Health."

62. Ruth Levine and the What Works Working Group, "Case 9: Controlling Trachoma in Morocco," in *Millions Saved: Proven Successes in Global Health,* by Ruth Levine and the What Works Working Group (Washington, D.C.: Center for Global Development, 2004), 83–89.

63. "Schistosomiasis Control Initiative," Imperial College London, School of Public Health, 2012, www1.imperial.ac.uk/publichealth/departments/ide/research_groups/thesci/ (accessed November 15, 2012).

64. World Health Organization, "Dracunculiasis Eradication," *Weekly Epidemiological Record* 83, no. 18 (2008): 159–167, www.who.int/wer/2008/wer8318.pdf (accessed November 26, 2012).

65. In the late 1990s, many of us exhorted Lilly to make available two second-line tuberculosis medicines and then to transfer technology to Chinese companies. And Lilly did so. See Jim Yong Kim, Joia S. Mukherjee, Michael L. Rich, Kedar Mate, Jaime Bayona, and Mercedes C. Becerra, "From Multidrug-Resistant Tuberculosis to DOTS Expansion and Beyond: Making the Most of a Paradigm Shift," *Tuberculosis* 83, nos. 1–3 (2003): 59–65; and Rajesh Gupta, J. Peter Cegielski, Marcos A. Espinal, Myriam Henkens, Jim Y. Kim, Catherina S.B. Lambregts-van Weezenbeek, Jong-Wook Lee, Mario C. Raviglione, Pedro G. Suarez, and Francis Varaine, "Increasing Transparency in Partnerships for Health—Introducing the Green Light Committee," *Tropical Medicine and International Health* 7, no. 11 (2002): 970–976.

66. Hotez, Molyneux, et al., "Control of Neglected Tropical Diseases."

67. Ibid.

68. See, for example, François Nosten and Nicholas J. White, "Artemisinin-Based Combination Treatment of Falciparum Malaria," *American Journal of Tropical Medicine and Hygiene* 77, no. 6 suppl. (2007): 181–192.

69. Gerardo Priotto, Serena Kasparian, et al., "Nifurtimox-Eflornithine Combination Therapy for Second-Stage African *Trypanosoma brucei gambiense* Trypanosomiasis: A Multicentre, Randomised, Phase III, Non-Inferiority Trial," *Lancet* 374, no. 9683 (2009): 56–64.

70. Paul Farmer and Louise C. Ivers, "Cholera in Haiti: The Equity Agenda and the Future of Tropical Medicine," *American Journal of Tropical Medicine and Hygiene* 86, no. 1 (2012): 7–8.

71. Abdel R. Omran, "The Epidemiological Transition: A Theory of the

Epidemiology of Population Change," *Milbank Memorial Fund Quarterly* 49, no. 4 (1971): 509–538.

72. Frenk, Bobadilla, et al., "Health Transition in Middle-Income Countries."

73. World Health Organization, *Preventing Chronic Diseases: A Vital Investment*, 2006, www.who.int/chp/chronic_disease_report/en/ (accessed November 25, 2012).

74. Abdallah S. Daar, Peter A. Singer, et al., "Grand Challenges in Chronic Non-Communicable Diseases," *Nature* 450, no. 7169 (November 22, 2007): 494–496; Derek Yach, Corinna Hawkes, C. Linn Gould, and Karen J. Hofman, "The Global Burden of Chronic Diseases: Overcoming Impediments to Prevention and Control," *Journal of the American Medical Association* 291, no. 21 (2004): 2616–2622.

75. World Health Organization Mental Health Gap Action Programme (mhGAP), *Scaling Up Care for Mental, Neurological, and Substance Use Disorders*, 2008, 4, www.who.int/mental_health/mhgap_final_english.pdf (accessed November 26, 2012).

76. David E. Bloom, Elizabeth T. Cafiero, Eva Jané-Llopis, Shafika Abrahams-Gessel, Laksmi R. Bloom, Sana Fathima, Andrea B. Feigl, Tom Gaziano, Mona Mowafi, Ankur Pandya, Klaus Prettner, Larry Rosenberg, Benjamin Seligman, Adam Z. Stein, and Cara Weinstein, *The Global Economic Burden of Non-Communicable Diseases* (Geneva: World Economic Forum, 2011), www3.weforum.org/docs/WEF_Harvard_HE_GlobalEconomicBurdenNon CommunicableDiseases_2011.pdf (accessed November 26, 2012).

77. While cervical cancer is a communicable disease insofar as 99 percent of cases are caused by human papilloma virus (HPV), many believe it should be grouped with noncommunicable diseases because the frameworks for medical intervention are often most concerned with its status as a malignancy. This technical ambiguity is one example of the many definitional problems associated with classifying disease groups and determining priorities.

78. Gene Bukhman and Alice Kidder, "Cardiovascular Disease and Global Health Equity: Lessons from Tuberculosis Control Then and Now," *American Journal of Public Health* 98, no. 1 (2008): 44–54.

79. Gene Bukhman and Alice Kidder, eds., *The Partners In Health Guide to Chronic Care Integration for Endemic Non-Communicable Diseases, Rwanda Edition: Cardiac, Renal, Diabetes, Pulmonary, and Palliative Care* (Boston: Partners In Health, 2011), http://act.pih.org/ncdguide (accessed November 15, 2012).

80. Kirk R. Smith, Sumi Mehta, and Mirjam Maeusezahl-Feuz, "Indoor Air Pollution from Household Use of Solid Fuels," in *Comparative Quantification of Health Risks: Global and Regional Burden of Disease Attributable to Selected Major Risk Factors*, ed. Majid Ezzati, Alan D. Lopez, Anthony Rodgers, and Christopher J.L. Murray (Geneva: World Health Organization, 2004), 1:1435–1493; Gwénaëlle Legros, Ines Havet, Nigel Bruce, and Sophie Bonjour, *The Energy Access Situation in Developing Countries: A Review Focusing on the Least Developed Countries and Sub-Saharan Africa* (New York: United National Development Programme/World Health Orga-

nization, 2009), http://content.undp.org/go/cms-service/stream/asset/?asset_id
=2205620 (accessed November 25, 2012).

81. Peter J. Hotez and Abdallah S. Daar, "The CNCDs and the NTDs:
Blurring the Lines Dividing Noncommunicable and Communicable Chronic
Diseases," *PLoS Neglected Tropical Diseases* 2, no. 10 (2008): e312.

82. World Health Organization, *The Global Burden of Disease: 2004 Update* (Geneva: World Health Organization, 2008), www.who.int/healthinfo/
global_burden_disease/GBD_report_2004update_full.pdf (accessed November 26, 2012).

83. Bukhman and Kidder, *The Partners In Health Guide to Chronic Care
Integration for Endemic Non-Communicable Diseases;* World Health Organization, *Package of Essential Noncommunicable (PEN) Disease Interventions for Primary Health Care in Low-Resource Settings,* 2010, http://whqlib
doc.who.int/publications/2010/9789241598996_eng.pdf (accessed February 1,
2013); World Health Organization, "Prevention and Control of NCDs: Priorities for Investment" (discussion paper, First Global Ministerial Conference on
Healthy Lifestyles and Noncommunicable Disease Control, Moscow, April
28–29, 2011), www.who.int/nmh/publications/who_bestbuys_to_prevent_
ncds.pdf (accessed November 26, 2012). For more on NCD care as a pillar
of health system strengthening, see Rosalind L. Coleman, Geoffrey V. Gill,
and David Wilkinson, "Noncommunicable Disease Management in Resource-
Poor Settings: A Primary Care Model from Rural South Africa," *Bulletin of
the World Health Organization* 76, no. 6 (1998): 633–640.

84. Agnes Binagwaho, "Meeting the Challenge of NCD: We Cannot Wait,"
Global Heart 7, no. 1 (2012): 1–2; Bukhman and Kidder, *The Partners In
Health Guide to Chronic Care Integration for Endemic Non-Communicable
Diseases.* See also Aaron D. A. Shakow, Gene Bukhman, Olumuyiwa Adebona, Jeremy Greene, Jean de Dieu Ngirabega, and Agnes Binagwaho, "Transforming South-South Technical Support to Fight Noncommunicable Diseases," *Global Heart* 7, no. 1 (2012): 35–45.

85. Bukhman and Kidder, *The Partners In Health Guide to Chronic Care
Integration for Endemic Non-Communicable Diseases,* 7.

86. Julio Frenk, keynote address, "Framing the Diagonal Approach," conference on "The Long Tail of Global Health Equity: Tackling the Endemic
Non-Communicable Diseases of the Bottom Billion," Harvard Medical
School, March 2–3, 2011; Amy Roeder, "Conference Calls for Global Focus
on the Burden of Non-Communicable Diseases of the World's Poorest Billion,"
Harvard School of Public Health, *HSPH News,* March 23, 2011, www.hsph
.harvard.edu/news/features/long-tail-bottom-billion-conference/ (accessed
February 20, 2013).

87. Robert Beaglehole, Ruth Bonita, George Alleyne, Richard Horton,
Liming Li, Paul Lincoln, Jean Claude Mbanya, Martin McKee, Rob Moodie,
Sania Nishtar, Peter Piot, K. Srinath Reddy, and David Stuckler, for the *Lancet* NCD Action Group, "UN High-Level Meeting on Non-Communicable
Diseases: Addressing Four Questions," *Lancet* 378, no. 9789 (2011): 449–455.

88. For more on combating the NCDs of the bottom billion, see the "Boston Statement on Non-Communicable Diseases of the Poorest Billion People,"

March 2–3, 2011, http://parthealth.3cdn.net/7612953957373a2e4b_pqm6iv
pfn.pdf (accessed March 26, 2012). As of March 2012, the Boston Statement
had some seventy-two hundred signatories from around the world.

89. Christopher J.L. Murray and Alan D. Lopez, "Alternative Projections
of Mortality and Disability by Cause, 1990–2020: Global Burden of Disease
Study," *Lancet* 349, no. 9064 (1997): 1501–1502.

90. Nancy Beaulieu, David E. Bloom, Lakshmi Reddy Bloom, and Richard
M. Stein, *Breakaway: The Global Burden of Cancer—Challenges and Opportunities. A Report from the Economist Intelligence Unit*, 2009, http://livestrong
blog.org/ (accessed November 25, 2012); CanTreat International, "Scaling Up
Cancer Diagnosis and Treatment in Developing Countries: What Can We Learn
from the HIV/AIDS Epidemic?" *Annals of Oncology* 21, no. 4 (2010): 680–
682; Twalib Ngoma, "World Health Organization Cancer Priorities in Developing Countries," *Annals of Oncology* 17, suppl. 8 (2006): viii9–viii14.

91. Beaulieu, Bloom, et al., *Breakaway*; Panos Kanavos, "The Rising Burden of Cancer in the Developing World," *Annals of Oncology* 17, suppl. 8
(2006): viii15–viii23.

92. Peter Boyle and Bernard Levin, eds., *World Cancer Report 2008* (Lyon:
International Agency for Research on Cancer, 2008); Jacques Ferlay, Hai-
Rim Shin, Freddie Bray, David Forman, Colin Mathers, and Donald Max-
well Parkin, *GLOBOCAN 2008: Estimated Cancer Incidence, Mortality,
Prevalence, and Disability-Adjusted Life Years (DALYs) Worldwide* (Lyon:
International Agency for Research on Cancer, 2010), http://globocan.iarc.fr
(accessed November 25, 2012).

93. I. Magrath and J. Litvak, "Cancer in Developing Countries: Opportunity and Challenge," *Journal of the National Cancer Institute* 85, no. 11
(1993): 863.

94. Ngoma, "World Health Organization Cancer Priorities in Developing
Countries," viii11.

95. For more on palliation and the challenges of cancer care in low-income
countries, see Julie Livingston, *Improvising Medicine: An African Oncology Ward in an Emerging Cancer Epidemic* (Durham, N.C.: Duke University
Press, 2012).

96. See, for example, Joseph W. Carlson, Evan Lyon, David Walton, Wai-
Chin Foo, Amy C. Sievers, Lawrence N. Shulman, Paul Farmer, Vania Nosé,
and Danny A. Milner Jr., "Partners in Pathology: A Collaborative Model to
Bring Pathology to Resource Poor Settings," *American Journal of Surgical
Pathology* 34, no. 1 (2010): 118–123.

97. Peter B. Hesseling, Elizabeth Molyneux, Francine Tchintseme, Jennifer
Welbeck, Peter McCormick, Kathryn Pritchard-Jones, and Hans-Peter Wagner, "Treating Burkitt's Lymphoma in Malawi, Cameroon, and Ghana," *Lancet Oncology* 9, no. 6 (2008): 512–513.

98. Lawrence N. Shulman, Walter Willett, Amy Sievers, and Felicia M.
Knaul, "Breast Cancer in Developing Countries: Opportunities for Improved
Survival," *Journal of Oncology* 2010 (2010): doi:10.1155/2010/595167; Alex
B. Haynes, Thomas G. Weiser, William R. Berry, Stuart R. Lipsitz, Abdel-
Hadi S. Breizat, E. Patchen Dellinger, Teodoro Herbosa, Sudhir Joseph, Pasci-

ence L. Kibatala, Marie Carmela M. Lapitan, Alan F. Merry, Krishna Moorthy, Richard K. Reznick, Bryce Taylor, and Atul A. Gawande, for the Safe Surgery Saves Lives Study Group, "A Surgical Safety Checklist to Reduce Morbidity and Mortality in a Global Population," *New England Journal of Medicine* 360, no. 5 (2009): 491–499; Paul Farmer, Julio Frenk, Felicia M. Knaul, Lawrence N. Shulman, George Alleyne, Lance Armstrong, Rifat Atun, Douglas Blayney, Lincoln Chen, Richard Feachem, Mary Gospodarowicz, Julie Gralow, Sanjay Gupta, Ana Langer, Julian Lob-Levyt, Claire Neal, Anthony Mbewu, Dina Mired, Peter Piot, K. Srinath Reddy, Jeffrey D. Sachs, Mahmoud Sarhan, and John R. Seffrin, "Expansion of Cancer Care and Control in Countries of Low and Middle Income: A Call to Action," *Lancet* 376, no. 9747 (2010): 1186–1193.

99. Farmer, Frenk, et al., "Expansion of Cancer Care and Control."

100. Felicia Marie Knaul, Gustavo Nigenda, Rafael Lozano, Hector Arreola-Ornelas, Ana Langer, and Julio Frenk, "Breast Cancer in Mexico: A Pressing Priority," *Reproductive Health Matters* 16, no. 32 (2008): 113–123; Julio Frenk, Octavio Gómez-Dantés, and Felicia Marie Knaul, "The Democratization of Health in Mexico: Financial Innovations for Universal Coverage," *Bulletin of the World Health Organization* 87, no. 7 (2009): 542–548; Eduardo González-Pier, Cristina Gutiérrez-Delgado, Gretchen Stevens, Mariana Barraza-Lloréns, Raúl Porras-Condey, Natalie Carvalho, Kristen Loncich, Rodrigo H. Dias, Sandeep Kulkarni, Anna Casey, Yuki Murakami, Majid Ezzati, and Joshua A. Salomon, "Priority Setting for Health Interventions in Mexico's System of Social Protection in Health," *Lancet* 368, no. 9547 (2006): 1608–1618.

101. Ministerio de la Protección Social, República de Colombia, *Plan obligatorio de salud,* www.pos.gov.co/Paginas/InicioPOS.aspx (accessed November 26, 2012).

102. Mahmoud M. Sarhan, "Cancer in Jordan: 2020 and Beyond" (presented at the Third Regional Congress of Cancer and Blood Disorders of Childhood, Amman, Jordan, April 14–17, 2010); Salma Jaouni, "Tailoring Strategies to Available Resources. Jordan Breast Cancer Program: A Bottom-Up Model for Early Detection and Screening," http://isites.harvard.edu/fs/docs/icb.topic665673.files/Salma%20Jaouni.pdf (accessed January 31, 2013).

103. Prabhat Jha, M. Kent Ranson, Son N. Nguyen, and Derek Yach, "Estimates of Global and Regional Smoking Prevalence in 1995, by Age and Sex," *American Journal of Public Health* 92, no. 6 (2002): 1002–1006. For more on the global shifts in tobacco use (and associated lung cancers) from rich to poor countries, see Allan M. Brandt, *The Cigarette Century: The Rise, Fall, and Deadly Persistence of the Product that Defined America* (New York: Basic Books, 2007). One telling example: Brandt (ibid., 454) notes that 12 percent of the Chinese central government's budget comes from sales by state-owned tobacco companies.

104. Farmer, Frenk, et al. "Expansion of Cancer Care and Control," 1186.

105. See Agnes Binagwaho, Claire M. Wagner, and Cameron T. Nutt, "HPV Vaccine in Rwanda: Different Disease, Same Double Standard," *Lancet* 378, no. 9807 (2011): 1916; and David Holmes, "Rwanda: An Injection of Hope," *Lancet* 376, no. 9745 (2010): 945–946.

106. See Farmer, Frenk, et al. "Expansion of Cancer Care and Control," 1186.

107. See, for example, Blake C. Alkire, Jeffrey R. Vincent, Christy Turlington Burns, Ian S. Metzler, Paul E. Farmer, and John G. Meara, "Obstructed Labor and Caesarean Delivery: The Cost and Benefit of Surgical Intervention," *PLoS One* 7, no. 4 (2012): e34595; and World Health Organization, *World Health Report 2005: Making Every Mother and Child Count* (Geneva: World Health Organization, 2005), www.who.int/whr/2005/whr2005_en.pdf (accessed November 25, 2012).

108. Massey Beveridge and Andrew Howard, "The Burden of Orthopaedic Disease in Developing Countries," *Journal of Bone and Joint Surgery* (American vol.) 86-A, no. 8 (2004): 1819–1822; World Health Organization, *World Report on Road Traffic Injury Prevention* (Geneva: World Health Organization, 2004), www.who.int/violence_injury_prevention/publications/road_traffic/world_report/summary_en_rev.pdf (accessed November 25, 2012); David Yorston, "High-Volume Surgery in Developing Countries," *Eye* 19, no. 10 (2005): 1083–1089.

109. James L. Cox, "Presidential Address: Changing Boundaries," *Journal of Thoracic and Cardiovascular Surgery* 122, no. 3 (2001): 413–418; Suresh G. Rao, "Pediatric Cardiac Surgery in Developing Countries," *Pediatric Cardiology* 28, no. 2 (2007): 144–148.

110. Haile T. Debas, Richard Gosselin, Colin McCord, and Amardeep Thind, "Surgery," in *Disease Control Priorities in Developing Countries*, 2nd ed., ed. Dean T. Jamison, Joel G. Breman, Anthony R. Measham, George Alleyne, Mariam Claeson, David B. Evans, Prabhat Jha, Anne Mills, and Philip Musgrove (Washington, D.C.: World Bank, 2006), 1245–1259.

111. Farmer and Kim, "Surgery and Global Health."

112. Ambrose E. Wasunna, "Surgical Manpower in Africa," *Bulletin of the American College of Surgeons* 72, no. 6 (1987): 18–19.

113. Louise C. Ivers, Evan S. Garfein, Josué Augustin, Maxi Raymonville, Alice T. Yang, David S. Sugarbaker, and Paul E. Farmer, "Increasing Access to Surgical Services for the Poor in Rural Haiti: Surgery as a Public Good for Public Health," *World Journal of Surgery* 32, no. 4 (2008): 537–542.

114. André B. Lalonde, Pius Okong, Alex Mugasa, and Liette Perron, "The FIGO Save the Mothers Initiative: The Uganda–Canada Collaboration," *International Journal of Gynecology and Obstetrics* 80, no. 2 (2003): 204–212; L. B. Curet, A. Foster-Rosales, R. Hale, E. Kestler, C. Medina, L. Altamirano, C. Reyes, and D. Jarquin, "The FIGO Save the Mothers Initiative: The Central America and USA Collaboration," *International Journal of Gynecology and Obstetrics* 80, no. 2 (2003): 213–221; T. Mekbib, E. Kassaye, A. Getachew, T. Tadesse, and A. Debebe, "The FIGO Save the Mothers Initiative: The Ethiopia-Sweden Collaboration," *International Journal of Gynecology and Obstetrics* 81, no. 1 (2003): 93–102.

115. International Committee of the Red Cross, *Annual Report 2007*, www.icrc.org/eng/resources/documents/annual-report/icrc-annual-report-2007.htm (accessed November 26, 2012).

116. K. A. Kelly McQueen, Joseph A. Hyder, Breena R. Taira, Nadine

Semer, Frederick M. Burkle Jr., and Kathleen M. Casey, "The Provision of Surgical Care by International Organizations in Developing Countries: A Preliminary Report," *World Journal of Surgery* 34, no. 3 (2010): 397–402.

117. Thomas McIntyre, Christopher D. Hughes, Thierry Pauyo, Stephen R. Sullivan, Selwyn O. Rogers Jr., Maxi Raymonville, and John G. Meara, "Emergency Surgical Care Delivery in Post-Earthquake Haiti: Partners In Health and Zanmi Lasante Experience," *World Journal of Surgery* 35, no. 4 (2011): 745–750.

118. K.A. Kelly McQueen, Doruk Ozgediz, Robert Riviello, Renee Y. Hsia, Sudha Jayaraman, Stephen R. Sullivan, and John G. Meara, "Essential Surgery: Integral to the Right to Health," *Health and Human Rights* 12, no. 1 (2010): 137–152; Farmer and Kim, "Surgery and Global Health."

119. Charles Mock, Meena Cherian, Catherine Juillard, Peter Donkor, Stephen Bickler, Dean Jamison, and Kelly McQueen, "Developing Priorities for Addressing Surgical Conditions Globally: Furthering the Link between Surgery and Public Health Policy," *World Journal of Surgery* 34, no. 3 (2010): 381–385.

120. Nadine B. Semer, Stephen R. Sullivan, and John G. Meara, "Plastic Surgery and Global Health: How Plastic Surgery Impacts the Global Burden of Surgical Disease," *Journal of Plastic, Reconstructive, and Aesthetic Surgery* 63, no. 8 (2010): 1244–1248.

121. Sudha Jayaraman, Jacqueline R. Mabweijano, Michael S. Lipnick, Nolan Caldwell, Justin Miyamoto, Robert Wangoda, Cephas Mijumbi, Renee Hsia, Rochelle Dicker, and Doruk Ozgediz, "First Things First: Effectiveness and Scalability of a Basic Prehospital Trauma Care Program for Lay First Responders in Kampala, Uganda," *PLoS One* 4, no. 9 (2009): e6955; Hans Husum, Mads Gilbert, Torben Wisborg, Yang Van Heng, and Mudhafar Murad, "Rural Prehospital Trauma Systems Improve Trauma Outcome in Low-Income Countries: A Prospective Study from North Iraq and Cambodia," *Journal of Trauma* 54, no. 6 (2003): 1188–1196.

122. Debas, Gosselin, et al., "Surgery"; Benjamin C. Warf, Blake C. Alkire, Salman Bhai, Christopher Hughes, Steven J. Schiff, Jeffrey R. Vincent, and John G. Meara, "Costs and Benefits of Neurosurgical Intervention for Infant Hydrocephalus in Sub-Saharan Africa," *Journal of Neurosurgery: Pediatrics* 8, no. 5 (2011): 509–521; Blake Alkire, Christopher D. Hughes, Katherine Nash, Jeffrey R. Vincent, and John G. Meara, "Potential Economic Benefit of Cleft Lip and Palate Repair in Sub-Saharan Africa," *World Journal of Surgery* 35, no. 6 (2011): 1194–1201; Colin McCord and Qumruzzaman Chowdhury, "A Cost Effective Small Hospital in Bangladesh: What It Can Mean for Emergency Obstetric Care," *International Journal of Gynecology and Obstetrics* 81, no. 1 (2003): 83–92; "Conference on Increasing Access to Surgical Services in Resource-Constrained Settings in Sub-Saharan Africa: Final Report," June 4–8, 2007, Bellagio, Italy, www.dcp2.org/file/137/Bellagio%20Report%20-%20Increasing%20Access%20to%20Surgical%20Services.pdf (accessed January 31, 2012).

123. On uninsured Americans, see Catherine G. McLaughlin, ed., *Health Policy and the Uninsured* (Washington, D.C.: Urban Institute Press, 2004). For information on disparities in health outcomes, see Institute of Med-

icine, *Unequal Treatment: Confronting Racial and Ethnic Disparities in Health Care,* ed. Brian D. Smedley, Adrienne Y. Stith, and Alan R. Nelson (Washington, D.C.: National Academies Press, 2002); and Elizabeth A. McGlynn, Steven M. Asch, John Adams, Joan Keesey, Jennifer Hicks, Alison DeCristofaro, and Eve A. Kerr, "The Quality of Health Care Delivered to Adults in the United States," *New England Journal of Medicine* 348, no. 26 (2003): 2635–2645.

On provider incentives and the issue of unnecessary procedures, see Institute of Medicine, *Rewarding Provider Performance: Aligning Incentives in Medicare* (Washington, D.C.: National Academies Press, 2007).

For a discussion of the fragmentation of U.S. health services, see Thomas H. Lee and James J. Mongan, *Chaos and Organization in Health Care* (Cambridge, Mass.: MIT Press, 2009).

On preventable medical errors, see Institute of Medicine, *To Err Is Human: Building a Safer Health System,* ed. Linda T. Kohn, Janet M. Corrigan, and Molla S. Donaldson (Washington, D.C.: National Academies Press, 1999).

On the challenge of treating patients with multiple chronic diseases, see Anand K. Parekh and Mary B. Barton, "The Challenge of Multiple Comorbidity for the U.S. Health Care System," *Journal of the American Medical Association* 303, no. 13 (2010): 1303–1304.

124. Elayne J. Heisler, "The U.S. Infant Mortality Rate: International Comparisons, Underlying Factors, and Federal Programs," Congressional Research Service, April 4, 2012, www.fas.org/sgp/crs/misc/R41378.pdf (accessed February 20, 2013). In 2012, the U.S. infant mortality rate was calculated to be 6.0, roughly comparable to some Eastern European countries but lagging well behind most Western European countries, Canada, and Cuba; see U.S. Central Intelligence Agency, "The World Factbook: Country Comparison: Infant Mortality Rate," 2012 estimates, https://www.cia.gov/library/publications/the-world-factbook/rankorder/2091rank.html (accessed November 25, 2012).

125. Meena Seshamani, "The Costs of Inaction: The Urgent Need for Health Reform," Department of Health and Human Services, March 2009, www.healthreform.gov/reports/inaction/inactionreportprintmarch2009.pdf (accessed November 25, 2012).

126. Paul Starr, *The Social Transformation of American Medicine: The Rise of a Sovereign Profession and the Making of a Vast Industry* (New York: Basic Books, 1982).

127. See, for example, Barbara Starfield, *Primary Care: Balancing Health Needs, Services, and Technology* (New York: Oxford University Press, 1998); Barbara Starfield, Leiyu Shi, and James Macinko, "Contribution of Primary Care to Health Systems and Health," *Milbank Quarterly* 83, no. 3 (2005): 457–502; Katherine Baicker and Amitabh Chandra, "Medicare Spending, the Physician Workforce, and Beneficiaries' Quality of Care," *Health Affairs* 23 (2004): w4-184–w4-197, http://content.healthaffairs.org/content/early/2004/04/07/hlthaff.w4.184/suppl/DC1 (accessed November 25, 2012); Mark W. Friedberg, Peter S. Hussey, and Eric C. Schneider, "Primary Care: A

Critical Review of the Evidence on Quality and Costs of Care," *Health Affairs* 29, no. 5 (2010): 766–772.

128. Andrew Ellner, Christine Pace, Scott Lee, Jonathan L. Weigel, and Paul Farmer, "Embracing Complexity: Towards Platforms for Integrated Health and Social Service Delivery," in *Structural Approaches in Public Health*, ed. Marni Sommer and Richard Parker (New York: Routledge, 2013).

129. Ellner, Pace, et al., "Embracing Complexity"; Rebecca Onie, Paul Farmer, and Heidi Behforouz, "Realigning Health with Care," *Stanford Social Innovation Review* 10, no. 3 (Summer 2012), www.ssireview.org/articles/entry/realigning_health_with_care (accessed November 25, 2012); Diane R. Rittenhouse and Stephen M. Shortell, "The Patient-Centered Medical Home: Will It Stand the Test of Health Reform?" *Journal of the American Medical Association* 301, no. 19 (2009): 2038–2040.

130. Joia S. Mukherjee, Louise Ivers, Fernet Léandre, Paul Farmer, and Heidi Behforouz, "Antiretroviral Therapy in Resource-Poor Settings: Decreasing Barriers to Access and Promoting Adherence," *Journal of Acquired Immune Deficiency Syndromes* 43, suppl. 1 (December 1, 2006): S123–S126; Heidi L. Behforouz, Paul E. Farmer, and Joia S. Mukherjee, "From Directly Observed Therapy to *Accompagnateurs:* Enhancing AIDS Treatment Outcomes in Haiti and in Boston," *Clinical Infectious Diseases* 38, no. 5 suppl. (2004): S429–S436; Heidi L. Behforouz, Audrey Kalmus, China S. Scherz, Jeffrey S. Kahn, Mitul B. Kadakia, and Paul E. Farmer, "Directly Observed Therapy for HIV Antiretroviral Therapy in an Urban U.S. Setting," *Journal of Acquired Immune Deficiency Syndromes* 36, no. 1 (2004): 642–645.

131. Onie, Farmer, and Behforouz, "Realigning Health with Care"; Tammy Yazzie, Alberta Long, Mae-Gilene Begay, Shirley Cisco, Hannah Sehn, Sonya Shin, and Catherine Harry, "Community Outreach and Patient Empowerment: Collaboration with Navajo Nation CHRs," *Journal of Ambulatory Care Management* 34, no. 3 (2011): 288–289.

132. Jeffrey Brenner, "Building an Accountable Care Organization in Camden, N.J.," *Prescriptions for Excellence in Health Care Newsletter Supplement* 1, no. 9 (2010): 1–4.

133. Onie, Farmer, and Behforouz, "Realigning Health with Care."

134. Lisel Blash, Susan Chapman, and Catherine Dower, "The Special Care Center—A Joint Venture to Address Chronic Disease," Center for the Health Professions, University of California at San Francisco, November 2011, www.futurehealth.ucsf.edu/Content/29/2010-11_The_Special_Care_Center_A_Joint_Venture_to_Address_Chronic_Disease.pdf (accessed November 25, 2012).

135. Atul Gawande, "The Hot Spotters: Can We Lower Medical Costs by Giving the Neediest Patients Better Care?" *New Yorker,* January 24, 2011, www.newyorker.com/reporting/2011/01/24/110124fa_fact_gawande#ixzz1UkUOcFbK (accessed November 25, 2012).

136. Rittenhouse and Shortell, "The Patient-Centered Medical Home." See also Andrew Ellner, Amanda Hoey, and Lawrence E. Frisch, "Speak Up! Can Patients Get Better at Working with Their Doctors?" *British Medical Journal* 327, no. 7410 (2003): 303–304.

137. Neal Emery, "Rwanda's Historic Health Recovery: What the U.S.

Might Learn," *Atlantic,* February 2013, http://www.theatlantic.com/health/archive/2013/02/rwandas-historic-health-recovery-what-the-us-might-learn/273226/ (accessed May 19, 2013).

138. See, for example, Michael Marmot, "Health in an Unequal World," *Lancet* 368, no. 9552 (2006): 2081–2094; René Dubos, "Environment and Disease," in *Mirage of Health: Utopias, Progress, and Biological Change,* by René Dubos (New Brunswick, N.J.: Rutgers University Press, 1987; originally published 1959), 95–128; Bruce G. Link and Jo Phelan, "Social Conditions as Fundamental Causes of Disease," *Journal of Health and Social Behavior* 35, special issue (1995): 80–94.

139. Laurie Garrett, "The Challenge of Global Health," *Foreign Affairs* 86, no. 1 (February 2007): 14–38, www.foreignaffairs.com/articles/62268/laurie-garrett/the-challenge-of-global-health (accessed November 25, 2012).

140. Jim Yong Kim, Aaron Shakow, Kedar Mate, Chris Vanderwarker, Rajesh Gupta, and Paul Farmer, "Limited Good and Limited Vision: Multidrug Resistance Tuberculosis and Global Health Policy," *Social Science and Medicine* 61, no. 4 (2005): 847–59.

141. See Nirmala Ravishankar, Paul Gubbins, Rebecca J. Cooley, Katherine Leach-Kemon, Catherine M. Michaud, Dean T. Jamison, and Christopher J.L. Murray, "Financing of Global Health: Tracking Development Assistance for Health from 1990 to 2007," *Lancet* 373, no. 9681 (2009): 2113–2124.

142. Julio Frenk, "Health Reform in an Age of Pandemics," lecture, Commonwealth Club San Francisco, September 30, 2009, http://fora.tv/2009/09/30/Julio_Frenk_Health_Reform_in_an_Era_of_Pandemics#fullprogram (accessed November 25, 2012).

The GAVI Alliance, pages 306–307

1. Tore Godal, "Viewpoint: Immunization against Poverty," *Tropical Medicine and International Health* 5, no. 3 (2000): 160–165; World Health Organization, *The EPI Information System* (Geneva: World Health Organization, 1999).

2. GAVI Alliance, "Origins of GAVI," www.gavialliance.org/about/mission/origins/ (accessed November 15, 2012).

3. GAVI Alliance, "GAVI Takes First Steps to Introduce Vaccines against Cervical Cancer and Rubella," press release, November 17, 2011, www.gavialliance.org/library/news/press-releases/2011/gavi-takes-first-steps-to-introduce-vaccines-against-cervical-cancer-and-rubella/ (accessed November 17, 2012). See also Sue J. Goldie, Lynne Gaffikin, Jeremy D. Goldhaber-Fiebert, Amparo Gordillo-Tobar, Carol Levin, Cédric Mahé, and Thomas C. Wright, "Cost-Effectiveness of Cervical-Cancer Screening in Five Developing Countries," *New England Journal of Medicine* 353, no. 20 (2005): 2158–2168.

4. Chunling Lu, Catherine M. Michaud, Emmanuela Gakidou, Kashif Khan, and Christopher J.L. Murray, "Effect of the Global Alliance for Vaccines and Immunisation on Diphtheria, Tetanus, and Pertussis Vaccine Coverage: An Independent Assessment," *Lancet* 368, no. 9541 (2006): 1088–1095; GAVI

Alliance, "Immunisation Service Support," www.gavialliance.org/support/iss/ (accessed November 17, 2012).

5. GAVI Alliance, "GAVI's Resource Mobilisation Process," www.gavialliance.org/funding/resource-mobilisation/process/ (accessed November 15, 2012).

6. GAVI Alliance and World Bank, "Creating Markets to Save Lives," Advance Market Commitments for Vaccines Factsheet, November 2012, www.gavialliance.org/library/gavi-documents/amc/ (accessed February 6, 2013). See also Tracy A. Lieu, Thomas G. McGuire, and Alan R. Hinman, "Overcoming Economic Barriers to the Optimal Use of Vaccines," *Health Affairs* 24, no. 3 (2005): 666–679.

7. Furthermore, advance market commitments helped decrease the cost of the pentavalent vaccine, a combination vaccine that protects against diphtheria, tetanus, pertussis, hepatitis B, and Hib, from $3.61 per dose to $2.58 per dose—a 29 percent reduction. Similar efforts have reduced the price of monovalent hepatitis B vaccine by 68 percent and that of pneumococcal vaccine by more than 90 percent. See UNICEF Supply Division communications with the GAVI Secretariat, as detailed in GAVI Alliance, "GAVI Impact on Vaccine Market behind Price Drop," www.gavialliance.org/library/news/roi/2010/gavi-impact-on-vaccine-market-behind-price-drop/ (accessed November 15, 2012); Grace Chee, Vivikka Molldrem, Natasha Hsi, and Slavea Chankova, *Evaluation of the GAVI Phase 1 Performance (2000–2005)* (Bethesda, Md.: Abt Associates, 2008).

The Bill and Melinda Gates Foundation, pages 311–312

1. Mary Moran, Javier Guzman, Anne-Laure Ropars, Alina McDonald, Tanja Sturm, Nicole Jameson, Lindsey Wu, Sam Ryan, and Brenda Omune, *Neglected Disease Research and Development: How Much Are We Really Spending?* (Sydney: George Institute for International Health, 2008), 41, www.georgeinstitute.org.au/sites/default/files/pdfs/G-FINDER_2008_Report.pdf (accessed January 31, 2013).

2. Bill and Melinda Gates Foundation, "Global Health Program: What We Do," www.gatesfoundation.org/global-health/Pages/overview.aspx (accessed November 15, 2012).

3. Dipika Sur, Anna Lena Lopez, et al., "Efficacy and Safety of a Modified Killed-Whole-Cell Oral Cholera Vaccine in India: An Interim Analysis of a Cluster-Randomised, Double-Blind, Placebo-Controlled Trial," *Lancet* 374, no. 9702 (2009): 1694–1702.

4. Anne-Emanuelle Birn, "Gates's Grandest Challenge: Transcending Technology as Public Health Ideology," *Lancet* 366, no. 9484 (2005): 517. For a careful look at the challenges of polio eradication, see Svea Closser, *Chasing Polio in Pakistan: Why the World's Largest Public Health Initiative May Fail* (Nashville, Tenn.: Vanderbilt University Press, 2010).

5. Program for Appropriate Technology in Health, "A Model for Malaria Control: MACEPA Aims to Wipe Out Disease Using Tools Available Now," www.path.org/projects/malaria_control_partnership.php (accessed Novem-

ber 15, 2012). MACEPA (the Malaria Control and Evaluation Partnership in Africa) is a research and control initiative aiming to "end malaria in Africa altogether." BMGF hopes that its model will be adopted across the malaria-endemic world.

6. Carole Mitnick, Jaime Bayona, Eda Palacios, Sonya Shin, Jennifer Furin, Felix Alcántara, Epifanio Sánchez, Madeleny Sarria, Mercedes Becerra, Mary C. Smith Fawzi, Saidi Kapiga, Donna Neuberg, James H. Maguire, Jim Yong Kim, and Paul Farmer, "Community-Based Therapy for Multidrug-Resistant Tuberculosis in Lima, Peru," *New England Journal of Medicine* 348, no. 2 (2003): 119, 122; Paul E. Farmer, Jim Yong Kim, Carole D. Mitnick, and Ralph Timperi, "Responding to Outbreaks of Multidrug-Resistant Tuberculosis: Introducing DOTS-Plus," in *Tuberculosis: A Comprehensive International Approach,* ed. Lee B. Reichman and Earl S. Hershfield (New York: Decker, 2000), 447–469; Sonya S. Shin, Martin Yagui, Luis Ascencios, Gloria Yale, Carmen Suarez, Neyda Quispet, Cesar Bonilla, Joaquin Blaya, Allison Tayloe, Carmen Contreras, and Peter Cegielski, "Scale-Up of Multidrug-Resistant Tuberculosis Laboratory Services, Peru," *Emerging Infectious Diseases* 14, no. 5 (2008): 701–708.

The Drug Development Pipeline, pages 313–314

1. Marcia Angell, *The Truth about the Drug Companies: How They Deceive Us and What to Do about It* (New York: Random House, 2004), 41. Angell, former editor-in-chief of the *New England Journal of Medicine,* argues that pharmaceutical companies are less innovative than they claim and exaggerate the cost of development. Pointing to drugs such as Gleevec, Zidovudine, and Epogen, for example, she notes that the cost of discovery and development was closer to $100 million than to the estimated $800 million to $1 billion per drug that the pharmaceutical industry reports.

2. Tufts Center for the Study of Drug Development, "Average Cost to Develop a New Biotechnology Product Is $1.2 Billion, According to the Tufts Center for the Study of Drug Development," *MarketWire,* November 9, 2006, www.marketwire.com/press-release/average-cost-develop-new-biotechnology-product-is-12-billion-according-tufts-center-711827.htm (accessed November 25, 2012).

3. Patrice Trouiller, Piero Olliaro, Els Torreele, James Orbinski, Richard Laing, and Nathan Ford, "Drug Development for Neglected Diseases: A Deficient Market and a Public-Health Policy Failure," *Lancet* 359, no. 9324 (2002): 2188–2189.

4. Robert E. Black, Saul S. Morris, and Jennifer Bryce, "Where and Why Are 10 Million Children Dying Each Year?" *Lancet* 361, no. 9376 (2003): 2226–2234. See also Jim Yong Kim, "Bridging the Delivery Gap in Global Health," MIT lecture, November 19, 2007, http://video.mit.edu/watch/bridging-the-delivery-gap-to-global-health-9317/ (accessed January 31, 2013).

5. Addressing the delivery gap will mean thinking differently about innovation: breakthroughs in *systems* of care, which combine people and informa-

tion technology in novel ways, can be just as important as biomedical innovations that produce new drugs and devices.

6. During the golden age of global health, new public-private partnerships have begun to jumpstart product development for diseases of poverty and innovations in care delivery. By bringing together pharmaceutical and biotech companies, public research institutes, university labs, public and private health care providers, and government and philanthropic donors, such partnerships can bridge the gaps in the pipeline and generate new technology development and delivery initiatives. Examples include the Drugs for Neglected Diseases Initiative, the Medicines for Malaria Venture, the Malaria Vaccine Initiative, and the Global Alliance for TB Drug Development. These and other partnerships have already developed promising new control tools against malaria, cholera, rotavirus, neglected tropical diseases, and other diseases. In recent years, therapeutics against AIDS have leapt across all three gaps better than most.

Intellectual Property and Global Health Equity, pages 326–327

1. Amy Kapczynski, "The Access to Knowledge Mobilization and the New Politics of Intellectual Property," *Yale Law Journal* 117 (2008): 804–885.

2. For example, in 2004, only 5 to 7 percent of brand-name pharmaceutical revenue came from all low- and middle-income countries. This category includes the huge economies of Brazil, China, India, and South Africa—the percentage would be even smaller if we were to look only at low-income countries. See Amy Kapczynski, Samantha Chaifetz, Zachary Katz, and Yochai Benkler, "Addressing Global Health Inequities: An Open Licensing Approach for University Innovations," *Berkeley Technology Law Journal* 20, no. 2 (2005): 1038 n. 33.

3. World Trade Organization, "Declaration on the TRIPS Agreement and Public Health," article 4, adopted November 14, 2001, by the 4th World Trade Organization Ministerial Conference in Doha, Qatar, http://docsonline.wto .org/imrd/directdoc.asp?DDFDocuments/t/WT/Min01/DEC2.doc (accessed November 25, 2012).

4. CPTech, "Compulsory Licensing. Chapter II: Government Use under 28 USC 1498," www.cptech.org/ip/health/cl/us-1498.html (accessed January 7, 2013).

5. Rama Lakshmi, "India-E.U. Trade Pact Could Boost AIDS Treatment Costs, Health Workers Say," *Washington Post,* February 10, 2012.

6. "AIDS Groups Criticise US/EU/Japan for Putting Profits of MNC Drug Makers before Patients," *Economic Times,* June 8, 2011.

7. Kapczynski, Chaifetz, et al., "Addressing Global Health Inequities," 1031, 1069–1072.

8. Padmashree Gehl Sampath, *Economic Aspects of Access to Medicines after 2005: Product Patent Protection and Emerging Firm Strategies in the Indian Pharmaceutical Industry,* United Nations University-INTECH, May 2005, www.who.int/intellectualproperty/studies/PadmashreeGehlSampath Final.pdf (accessed November 25, 2012).

CHAPTER 12

1. For insightful analysis of a different form of activism—the role of federal activism and the United States as an "activist state"—see Paul Pierson and Theda Skocpol, eds., *The Transformation of American Politics: Activist Government and the Rise of Conservatism* (Princeton, N.J.: Princeton University Press, 2007).

2. Adam Hochschild, *Bury the Chains: Prophets and Rebels in the Fight to Free an Empire's Slaves* (New York: Houghton Mifflin, 2005).

3. Irvin Molotsky, "U.S. Approves Drug to Prolong Lives of AIDS Patients," *New York Times*, March 21, 1987, www.nytimes.com/1987/03/21/us/us-approves-drug-to-prolong-lives-of-aids-patients.html (accessed November 25, 2012).

4. ACT UP New York, "Fight Back, Fight AIDS: 15 Years of ACT UP," www.actupny.org/divatv/synopsis75.html (accessed November 25, 2012).

5. Larry Kramer, "The FDA's Callous Response to AIDS," *New York Times*, March 23, 1987, A19.

6. Ibid.

7. See, for example, Walter Sneader, *Drug Discovery: A History* (Hoboken, N.J.: Wiley, 2005). Also see Jeremy A. Greene, *Prescribing by Numbers: Drugs and the Definition of Disease* (Baltimore: Johns Hopkins University Press, 2007).

8. ACT UP New York, "Fight Back, Fight AIDS."

9. Kaiser Family Foundation, "The AIDS Epidemic at 20 Years: Selected Milestones," June 2001, www.pbs.org/newshour/health/aids20_timeline.pdf (accessed November 25, 2012). For more information see PBS, *Frontline* documentary series *The Age of AIDS*, directed by William Cran and Greg Barker, 2006, www.pbs.org/wgbh/pages/frontline/aids/ (accessed November 25, 2012).

10. PBS, *Frontline: The Age of AIDS*; Stephen J. Ceccoli, *Pill Politics: Drugs and the FDA* (Boulder, Colo.: Lynne Rienner, 2003), 107–108.

11. See, for example, a discussion of this grassroots movement in Ellen Chesler, *Woman of Valor: Margaret Sanger and the Birth Control Movement in America* (New York: Simon and Schuster, 1992).

12. Patricia D. Siplon, *AIDS and the Policy Struggle in the United States* (Washington, D.C.: Georgetown University Press, 2002), 5–6.

13. Thomas Morgan, "Mainstream Strategy for AIDS Group," *New York Times*, July 22, 1998, B1, B4, www.nytimes.com/1988/07/22/nyregion/mainstream-strategy-for-aids-group.html (accessed November 25, 2012).

14. Mark Heywood, "South Africa's Treatment Action Campaign: Combining Law and Social Mobilization to Realize the Right to Health," *Journal of Human Rights Practice* 1, no. 1 (2009): 15.

15. Steven Friedman and Shauna Mottiar, "A Rewarding Engagement? The Treatment Action Campaign and the Politics of HIV/AIDS," *Politics and Society* 33, no. 4 (2005): 533.

16. Ibid., 516, 524.

17. Ibid., 515.

18. Heywood, "South Africa's Treatment Action Campaign," 14.

19. For a more detailed discussion of this episode, see Didier Fassin, *When*

Bodies Remember: Experiences and Politics of AIDS in Post-Apartheid South Africa (Berkeley: University of California Press, 2007).

20. Julius B. Richmond and Milton Kotelchuck, "Political Influences: Rethinking National Health Policy," in *Handbook of Health Professions Education*, ed. Christine H. McGuire et al. (San Francisco: Jossey-Bass, 1983), 386–404.

21. George Kembel, "$25 Incubator Shows Good Design Can Save Lives Affordably," *Exponential Times,* lecture, 2009, www.exponentialtimes.net/videos/25-incubator-shows-good-design-can-save-lives-affordably (accessed November 25, 2012).

22. See, for example, Nicholas D. Kristof and Sheryl WuDunn, *Half the Sky: Turning Oppression into Opportunity for Women Worldwide* (New York: Random House, 2009).

23. See, for example, hospitals designed by MASS Design Group in Rwanda and Haiti, www.massdesigngroup.org/our-work/project-index.html (accessed November 25, 2012).

Contributors

MADELEINE BALLARD is a program manager for Tiyatien Health in Konobo, Liberia. A Rhodes Scholar and Harvard College Women's Leadership Award winner, she graduated magna cum laude from Harvard with an AB in social studies. She has been involved with global health initiatives as diverse as Peer Health Exchange, SPINALpedia, and the Harvard Global Health and AIDS Coalition.

MARGUERITE THORP BASILICO is a student at Harvard Medical School and a member of the Harvard Global Health and AIDS Coalition. After graduating from Harvard College with an AB in social studies, she served as national organizer of the Student Global AIDS Campaign. She has worked for Partners In Health in Malawi and was a 2010 Truman Scholar from Colorado.

MATTHEW BASILICO is a joint MD-PhD student in economics at Harvard University. He has worked for Partners In Health, the Clinton Health Access Initiative, and Innovations for Poverty Action in Malawi, where he was also a Fulbright Scholar. He is a graduate of Harvard's social studies program and has been active in political advocacy for global health equity.

ANNE BECKER is the Maude and Lillian Presley Professor of Global Health and Social Medicine, vice chair of the Department of Global Health and Social Medicine, and director of the Social Sciences MD-PhD Program at Harvard Medical School. She is director of the Eating Disorders Clinical and Research Program in the Department of Psychiatry at Massachusetts General Hospital. She is a graduate of Harvard Graduate School of Arts and Sciences, Harvard Medical School, and Harvard School of Public Health.

JACOB BOR is a doctoral candidate studying health economics in the Department of Global Health and Population at the Harvard School of Public Health. He is a graduate student fellow at the Harvard Center for Population and

Development Studies and the Harvard Global Health Institute. He graduated from Harvard College with an AB in social studies.

GENE BUKHMAN is a cardiologist and medical anthropologist. He is director of the Program in Global Non-Communicable Disease and Social Change at Harvard Medical School, where he is an assistant professor of medicine as well as an assistant professor of global health and social medicine. He is also the cardiology director for Partners In Health. His work focuses on policy, planning, and service delivery for non-communicable diseases of poverty.

OPHELIA DAHL co-founded Partners In Health with Paul Farmer, Jim Kim, Todd McCormack, and Tom White in 1987. She has served as executive director of the organization since 2001 and as chair of the board since 2000. She is a graduate of Wellesley College and a recipient of the Union Medal from Union Theological Seminary.

PETER DROBAC is director of Partners In Health in Rwanda, where he works closely with the government of Rwanda to provide high-quality health care and social services in three rural districts. He is an associate physician in the Division of Global Health Equity at Brigham and Women's Hospital, an instructor of medicine at Harvard Medical School, and an internist, pediatrician, and infectious-disease specialist. Dr. Drobac was appointed chair of the board of directors of the Rwanda Biomedical Center.

ANDY ELLNER is codirector of the Center for Primary Care and director of the Program in Global Primary Care and Social Change at Harvard Medical School. He is an associate physician in the Division of Global Health Equity at Brigham and Women's Hospital and practices primary care medicine at the Phyllis Jen Center for Primary Care. He is a graduate of Harvard Medical School, the London School of Hygiene and Tropical Medicine, and the London School of Economics.

PAUL FARMER, the Kolokotrones University Professor at Harvard, is co-founder of Partners In Health and chair of the Department of Global Health and Social Medicine at Harvard Medical School. His most recent books are *To Repair the World* and *Haiti after the Earthquake.* Other titles include *Pathologies of Power: Health, Human Rights, and the New War on the Poor; Infections and Inequalities: The Modern Plagues;* and *AIDS and Accusation: Haiti and the Geography of Blame.* Tracy Kidder's *New York Times* best-seller *Mountains Beyond Mountains: The Quest of Dr. Paul Farmer, A Man Who Would Cure the World,* chronicles the development of Dr. Farmer's work in Haiti and beyond. He is the chief in the Division of Global Health Equity at the Brigham and Women's Hospital.

JEREMY GREENE is the Elizabeth Treide and A. McGehee Harvey Chair in the History of Medicine at the Johns Hopkins School of Medicine. He received his MD and PhD in the history of science from Harvard University in 2005 and completed his residency in internal medicine at the Brigham and Women's Hospital in 2008.

BRIDGET HANNA is a PhD candidate in social anthropology at Harvard University and co-author of *The Bhopal Reader: Remembering Twenty Years of the World's Worst Industrial Disaster.*

CASSIA VAN DER HOOF HOLSTEIN is Chief of Staff to Dr. Paul Farmer, Chief Global Health Delivery Partnership Integration Officer for Partners In Health, and Associate Director of the Global Health Delivery Partnership for the Department of Global Health and Social Medicine at Harvard Medical School. She studied literature at Harvard and got her start in global health in the late Senator Kennedy's Poverty Issues office.

LOUISE C. IVERS is an associate professor of medicine at Harvard Medical School, an associate physician in the Division of Global Health Equity at Brigham and Women's Hospital, and senior health and policy advisor for Partners In Health in Haiti, where she has worked for the past decade. She graduated from the London School of Hygiene and Tropical Medicine and the Harvard School of Public Health and completed both her residency in internal medicine at Massachusetts General Hospital and her fellowship in infectious diseases at Massachusetts General Hospital/Brigham and Women's Hospital.

DAVID JONES is the A. Bernard Ackerman Professor of the Culture of Medicine at Harvard University. In 2001, he received both an MD at Harvard Medical School and a PhD in the history of science at Harvard University. He worked as an intern in pediatrics at Children's Hospital and Boston Medical Center and trained as a psychiatrist at Massachusetts General Hospital and McLean Hospital. His current research focuses on the history of decision-making in cardiac therapeutics.

VANESSA KERRY is an instructor in global health and social medicine at Harvard Medical School and an instructor in medicine at Massachusetts General Hospital. She is director of the Global Public Policy and Social Change Program in the Department of Global Health and Social Medicine and associate director of partnerships and global initiatives at Massachusetts General Hospital's Center for Global Health. She founded and runs Seed Global Health (formerly the Global Health Service Corps), a nonprofit that works to strengthen health systems through teaching and education.

SALMAAN KESHAVJEE is director of the Program in Infectious Disease and Social Change in the Department of Global Health and Social Medicine at Harvard Medical School and senior tuberculosis specialist at Partners In Health. Trained as a physician and social anthropologist, he is an associate professor at Harvard Medical School and in the Division of Global Health Equity at Brigham and Women's Hospital. He served as the chair of the World Health Organization's Green Light Committee Initiative for drug-resistant tuberculosis.

HEIDI KIM is a student at Harvard Business School and a former member of the Harvard Global Health and AIDS Coalition. After graduating from Harvard College with an AB in social studies, she worked as a development assistant at Partners In Health and a consultant at Oliver Wyman. Most recently, she worked at Kiva.org on the launch team for Kiva Zip, an innovative person-to-person lending platform.

JIM YONG KIM is a co-founder of Partners In Health and the current president of the World Bank Group. He served as president of Dartmouth College from 2009 to 2012 and is a former director of the World Health Organization's HIV/AIDS Department.

ARTHUR KLEINMAN is a professor of anthropology at Harvard University and a professor of social medicine at Harvard Medical School. A pioneering figure in medical anthropology, he is the author of numerous influential works including *The Illness Narratives, Patients and Healers in the Context of Culture,* and *What Really Matters.*

JOHN G. MEARA, MD, DMD, MBA, is the director of the Program in Global Surgery and Social Change in the Department of Global Health and Social Medicine at Harvard Medical School. He is also chair of the executive committee of the Harvard Plastic Surgery Training Program. He serves as chief of the Department of Plastic and Oral Surgery at Boston Children's Hospital and is director of the Paul Farmer Global Surgery Fellowship program, in collaboration with Partners In Health.

LUKE MESSAC is an MD-PhD student in the history and sociology of science at the University of Pennsylvania. He has worked in Rwanda for Partners In Health and the Clinton Health Access Initiative. He has been a member of political advocacy organizations committed to global health equity, including the Harvard Global Health and AIDS Coalition, ACT UP Philadelphia, and the American Medical Student Association. He was a 2007 Truman Scholar from New York and a graduate of Harvard College.

ANJALI MOTGI graduated magna cum laude from Harvard College with an AB in social studies. She has worked as an associate at Global Health Strategies, LLC, in New York City. She is currently a JD student at Yale Law School, where she is an editor of the *Yale Law Journal* and the *Yale Journal of Health Policy, Law, and Ethics;* a member of the Supreme Court Clinic; and the scholarship chair of the American Constitution Society.

JOIA MUKHERJEE is an associate professor in the Division of Global Health Equity at the Brigham and Women's Hospital and Harvard Medical School's Department of Global Health and Social Medicine; chief medical officer of Partners In Health; and a consultant to the World Health Organization on health system strengthening as well as on the treatment of HIV and MDRTB in developing countries. She is a graduate of the University of Minnesota in Minneapolis and the Harvard School of Public Health.

MICHAEL E. PORTER is the Bishop William Lawrence University Professor at Harvard Business School. A leading authority on strategy and the competitiveness of nations and regions, his work is widely recognized by governments, corporations, nonprofits, and academic circles across the globe. His work has also redefined thinking about economically distressed urban communities, environmental policy, and the role of corporations in society. He is the author of nineteen books and numerous articles and the co-founder, with Jim Yong Kim and Paul Farmer, of the Global Health Delivery Partnership at Harvard University.

KRISHNA PRABHU is a student at Harvard Medical School and a member of the Harvard Global Health and AIDS Coalition. Krishna graduated with an AB in social studies from Harvard College. He has led numerous global health activism campaigns as a member of the Student Global AIDS Campaign and ACT UP Boston.

GIUSEPPE RAVIOLA is an assistant professor of psychiatry and in global health and social medicine at Harvard Medical School; director of the Psychiatry Quality Program in the Department of Psychiatry at Boston Children's Hospital; director of the Program in Global Mental Health and Social Change in the Department of Global Health and Social Medicine at Harvard Medical School; and director of mental health for Partners In Health. He graduated from Harvard Medical School and the Harvard School of Public Health.

JOSEPH RHATIGAN, MD, is Associate Chief of the Division of Global Health Equity at Brigham and Women's Hospital and the director of the Hiatt Global Health Equity Residency Program. He is an assistant professor at Harvard Medical School and the Harvard School of Public Health.

AMY SIEVERS is a board-certified internist and hematologist/oncologist. She received her MD and MPH from Northwestern University in 2004, completed her residency in internal medicine and global health equity at Brigham and Women's Hospital, and completed her fellowship training in infectious diseases and hematology/medical oncology. She has worked with the Rwandan Ministry of Health to implement screening and care for cervical and breast cancer and has designed programs for cancer care and chemotherapy administration in settings of limited resources.

ARJUN SURI is a student at Harvard Medical School and a member of the Harvard Global Health and AIDS Coalition. A graduate of Harvard College as a social studies major, he was an award-winning teaching fellow in the first iteration of the course on which this textbook is based. He was a 2009 Fulbright Scholar in Peru, where he studied barriers to quality improvement in the public health system.

DAVID WALTON serves as the senior advisor for health and medical infrastructure for Partners In Health as well as the chief operating officer for Hôpital Universitaire de Mirebalais in Haiti. He is also an associate physician at the Brigham and Women's Hospital and an instructor of medicine at Harvard Medical School. He obtained his MD from Harvard Medical School in 2003 and his MPH from the Harvard School of Public Health in 2007.

JONATHAN WEIGEL is a PhD student in political economy and government at Harvard University and a member of the Harvard Global Health and AIDS Coalition. After graduating from Harvard College with a BA in social studies, He studied political theory at Cambridge University on a Harvard-Cambridge Scholarship and then worked as a research assistant to Dr. Paul Farmer.

REBECCA WEINTRAUB is an associate physician at the Brigham and Women's Hospital, an instructor of medicine at Harvard Medical School, and faculty director of the Global Health Delivery Project at Harvard University. She is a graduate of Yale University and Stanford Medical School and completed her residency at Brigham and Women's Hospital. She founded Jumpstart, the largest AmeriCorps program in the country, and currently serves as advisor to several NGOs and technical advisor to Ashoka, a fund for social entrepreneurs.

ALYSSA YAMAMOTO works for Village Health Works, a partner project of Partners In Health. After graduating from Harvard College in 2012 with an AB in the comparative study of religion, she worked as a research assistant to Dr. Paul Farmer. Before joining Partners In Health, she served as a research assistant to Dr. Suerie Moon, co-chair of the Forum on Global Governance for Health at the Harvard Global Health Institute and Harvard School of Public Health.

Acknowledgments

The energy and inspiration for this book have come in great measure from the students and teaching fellows of our undergraduate course. In particular, Marty Alexander, Shom Dasgupta, Bridget Hanna, Emily Harrison, Evan Lyon, April Opoliner, Jessica Perkins, Amy Saltzman, Maria Stalford, Arjun Suri, and Sae Takada have provided invaluable direction to the course over the years. Nancy Dorsinville has been a cherished mentor to both students and course faculty alike. Drawing upon disciplines as diverse as history, social theory, anthropology, and the biological sciences, Societies of the World 25 relies on a passionate, intrepid teaching staff. Year after year, our teaching fellows, guest lecturers, and other supporters have been essential to the course's success. This work is deeply indebted to their insight and direction.

The skills of Mary Renaud and Jan Reiss, who have copyedited each line of this volume, have greatly improved its quality and readability. Jennifer Puccetti's unwavering support and guidance helped the project through many roadblocks (and an earthquake). We also owe a tremendous debt of gratitude to Zoe Agoos and Emily Bahnsen, whose immeasurable contributions ranged from preparing some of the very first lectures in this course to creating a space in the Department of Global Health and Social Medicine in which this project could be completed. Madeleine Ballard, Marguerite Thorp Basilico, Luke Messac, Jonathan Weigel, and Alyssa Yamamoto devoted several months and many sleepless nights to supporting this effort, contributions that were critical to the book. Likewise, Vera Belitsky, Jennie Block, Caitlin Buysse, Nadza Durakovic, Marilyn Goodrich, Mackenzie Hild, Cassia van der Hoof Holstein, Steve Kadish, Victoria Koski-Karell, Sarah Melpignano, Jon Niconchuk, Haun Saussy, Gretchen Williams, and Gina Zanolli provided important creative and managerial support throughout the five years of this project. Keith Joseph, Jenna LeMieux, and Jonas Rigodon, as well as Jessica Goldberg, Niall Keleher, and Dean Yang, supplied space and guidance for this endeavor, even in the middle of rural Malawi, while the HMS "White Heat" Fellowship afforded generous support in Boston (and Mexico). Drs. Sean and Judy Palfrey, with the tutors, students, and dining hall staff of Adams House, enabled a place where this volume could finally be brought to completion. The Maxwell Dworkin crew also provided vital support and minimized welfare losses throughout. As ever, we are deeply grateful to Didi Bertrand Farmer, Jehane Sedky, and Abbey Gardner.

We are grateful to our many mentors and guest lecturers in the course for their intellectual guidance throughout this process. We highlight here some of those who have made consistent and lasting contributions: Arachu Castro, Peter Drobac, Julio Frenk, Jeremy Greene, David Jones, Keith Joseph, Felicia Knaul, Ira Magaziner, Joia Mukherjee, Michael Porter, Joseph Rhatigan, James Robinson, and especially Anne Becker, who taught this course in its new and improved iterations. The responsibility for the content of this volume (including its errors and imperfections), however, lies with us—the authors and contributors.

As this volume is grounded in our experience as practitioners, we are indebted to the many institutions and people with whom we have the privilege of working. Partners In Health and the communities in which it is based have informed our approach and shaped our lives in ways that could never be adequately described. We must settle for acknowledging all those who work at this institution, and in particular Executive Director Ophelia Dahl, for their efforts, which continue to inspire us every day. Likewise, the Department of Global Health and Social Medicine at Harvard Medical School, the Division of Global Health Equity at Brigham and Women's Hospital, the Office of the President at Dartmouth College, and the Harvard Global Health and AIDS Coalition have provided various homes for this project, in one way or another.

Harvard University and Harvard Medical School have over many years offered support, guidance, and encouragement to engage in the challenges of global health equity, whether in a clinic in Rwinkwavu or in a classroom in Cambridge. The preface of this book notes that global health praxis must consist of more than research and teaching alone. These missions of a university also depend on service delivery of the highest quality, as teaching hospitals have demonstrated since their inception. We are deeply indebted to the leadership of President Drew Gilpin Faust and Dean Jeffrey Flier, who have long shared our vision of global health equity and have enabled delivery projects like those described in this text.

Finally, this book is dedicated to our true heroes and teachers, who often share neither language nor nationality nor gender, but their relative social positioning at the bottom of the ladder. Our hope is that this work may one day make a contribution to their ongoing struggle for health equity.

Index

Page numbers in italics indicate references to tables or illustrations.

Aaron Diamond AIDS Research Center (New York), 117
Abdul Latif Jameel Poverty Action Lab (J-PAL), 292–93
Abuja Declaration, 300, *301*
accidents, road traffic, 4, 6
Accra Agenda for Action (2008), 200, *201*, 206
Achmat, Zackie, 276, *276*, 344
acid-fast bacilli (AFB), 152, *153*, 154
Acland, Sarah, 219
ACT UP (AIDS Coalition to Unleash Power), 116, 118, 120, 121, 348; history of, 341–43, *343*; Treatment Action Campaign links with, 344
acupuncture, 77
"acute-on-chronic" events, 180
Adjustment with a Human Face (UNICEF report), 90, 105
Affordable Care Act (2010), 204, 335
Afghanistan, 198, 299
Africa, sub-Saharan, 1, 60, 92, 172, 217; AIDS epidemic in, 3, 44–45, 92; AIDS treatment in, 114, 118, 124, 156; conflict diamonds in, 255; DALYs (disability-adjusted life years) in, 228, 231–32; economic stagnation in, 87; European mortality rates in, 36–37, 40; female genital alteration in, 262; foreign aid and growth in, 290–91, *291*; global disease burden and, 303; health care workers in, 206, 208; hospitals in, 2; liberation theology in, 282; life expectancy in, 5; Millennium Development Goals and, 166; missionary medicine in, 48; neglected tropical diseases (NTDs) in, 318; sleeping sickness in, 49; tuberculosis (TB) in, 194
African Americans, 127, 258
African trypanosomiasis (sleeping sickness), 36, 49, *314*, 316
AIDS, xiii, xvii, 1, 103, 173–75, 248; antiretroviral therapy (ART) and, 116–18, 130–31, 173–74; care delivery for, 189; cost of treatment, 121–26; DALY (disability-adjusted life year) and, 6; deaths from, 4, 117–18, *117*; funding for, 287, 302–3; global income levels and treatment outcomes, 118–121, *121*; golden age of global health and, 111–15; in Haiti, 141, 145–47; health as a human right and, 272, 273; home-based care for, 188; human rights framework and, 271; intellectual property and drugs for, 326; investment in global treatment efforts, 12; McKeown hypothesis and, 64, 66; Millennium Development Goals (MDGs) and, 310–13; poverty and disease risk in

AIDS *(continued)*
  relation to, 17; in Rwanda, 166, 173–76; sorcery attributed as cause of, 146, 187; strange alliances in fight for treatment funding, 126–130, *128*; treatment after golden age of global health, 130–31; tuberculosis and, 156–58; WHO policy against, 25; women in rural Haiti with, 30–31; worldwide visibility of pandemic, 33. *See also* ACT UP; HIV; Treatment Action Campaign
albendazole, *317*, 318, 319
alcohol use, 6, 107, 323
Alma-Ata Declaration, 80, 94, 109, 158; text of, 355–58; thirtieth anniversary of, 103; vision of equity, 303. *See also* International Conference on Primary Health Care
Alzheimer dementia, 4, 6
American Psychiatric Association, 215, 224
Amnesty International, 267
AMPATH, 133, 191, 192
Anand, Sudhir, 232, 261
Annan, Kofi, 119, 126
Anopheles mosquito, 42, 63, 69
anorexia, 17, 223
anthropology, xiv, xxiii, 167, 275; medical, 16, 20, 223; physician-anthropologists, xix; as resocializing discipline, 3; scientific racism and, 28
antibiotics, 11, 63
antidepressants, 213
anti-helminthic drugs, 57
antiretroviral therapy (ART), 113, 114, 115, 157, 160, 276; AIDS stigma and, 173; antiretroviral (ARV) medications, 121, 122; d4t (stavudine, Zerit), 124; food provided to patients of, 178; funding for access to, 350; PEPFAR expansion and, 347; protease inhibitors, 117; strict demands of, 119; triple-combination, 156; universal coverage for AIDS patients, 203
Aravind Eye Hospital (India), 352
Arcade Fire (band), 352
Arendt, Hannah, 264–65
Aristide, Jean-Bertrand, 138–39, 141
Aristide, Mildred, 159
Aristotle, 257, 258
artemisin, 17, 63
ascariasis, *317*
Aspen Pharmacare, 124
asthma, 153, 186, 321
Atlantic Charter, 60

A to Z Textile Mills Ltd., 195, *196*
authority, modes of, 22–24, 58
avian flu, 41
ayurvedic medicine, 76
azithromycin, *317*, 319
AZT (azidothymidine), 116, 156, 341, 342

Baikie, William, 37
Bamako Initiative (1987), 89
Banerjee, Abhijit, 293
Bangladesh, 179, 261, 291; BRAC (Bangladesh Rural Advancement Committee), 193, 246; infant mortality in, 8; smallpox eradication in, 68
"barefoot doctor" movement, 76–77, *76*, 207
Barshefsky, Charlene, 122, 123
Barton, Clara, 281
Becker, Anne, 17
bed nets, 90, 98, 115, 195
Behforouz, Heidi, 333
Behrman, Greg, 116
Belgium, 168
Bellamy, Carol, 103
Benatar, Solly, 255
Bentham, Jeremy, 27, 247
Berger, Peter, xviii–xix, 18, 22; on habitualization, 115; institutionalization concept, 24, 93, 188
Berg Report (1981), 87
Berlin, Isaiah, 264
Berlin Conference (1884), 41, 168
Berry, Wendell, 274
Bhopal (India) gas leak, 29
Biden, Joseph, 347
Bill and Melinda Gates Foundation (BMGF), 101, 113, 198, 306, 311–12
biomedicine, 76, 151, 154, 221–22, 279
biopower, xviii, 25–30, *29*, 33, 224
biosocial analysis, xiv, 2–3, 9; failed policies and, 33; Partners In Health and, 12; social construction of disease categories, 13; sociology of knowledge and, 17–20
Birn, Anne-Emanuelle, 312
birth asphyxia, 5, 6
birth spacing, 94
birth trauma, 5, 6
birth weight, premature and low, 4, 6
Biya, Paul, 291
Black, Maggie, 98
Boff, Leonardo, 282
Bono, 127, 352
Bordes, Ary, 140
Boy Scouts of America, 280

BRAC (Bangladesh Rural Advancement Committee), 193, 198, 246, 350
Brazil, xv, 62, 121–22, 185
breast cancer, 4, 325, 326
breastfeeding, 82, 94, 305
Brenner, Jeffrey, 333
Brigham and Women's Hospital, 185, 325
Bristol-Meyers Squibb (BMS), 124
Britain/British Empire, 36, 341; Colonial Medical Service, 38, 39; end of, 60; National Health Service, 260, 337. *See also* United Kingdom
Broad Street (London) pump, cholera and, 50, *51, 52*
bronchitis, 65
bronchus cancer, 4, 6
Buddhism, 283, 284
Buffett, Warren, 113, 311
bulimia, 17
Bulletin of the World Health Organization, 119–120
bureaucracies, 23–24, 27, 29, 56; health, 50, 58; "iron cage" of, 25, 58, 241–42; neoliberalism and, 74
Burkina Faso, 318
Burroughs Wellcome, 341, 342
Buruli ulcer, 314
Burundi, xv, 178, 318
Bush, George W., 113, 127–28, 282, 345–46
Bush, Laura, *128*
Butaro Hospital (Rwanda), 177, *177*

Caceres, Marco, 349
Cambodia, 296
Camden Coalition of Healthcare Providers, 333–34
Cameroon, *8*, 291, 324
cancer, xvii, 66, 293, 320, 323–25, 328–29
capabilities approach, 255–263
capitalism, 91
cardiologists, xvi
cardiomyopathy, 321
cardiovascular disease, 320
care delivery value chain (CDVC), 189–191, *190, 192, 195*
Carrin, Guy, 272
Carter, Jimmy, 96
"Case Studies in Global Health" (class at Harvard), xiii, 10
Cash, Richard, 95
cash transfer programs, 296
Catholic Church, 47
causality, xiii, xxiii, 292; interrogation of

claims of, 3; malaria and, 18; tuberculosis (TB) and, 155, 156
Caventou, Joseph Beinaimé, 37
CDC (Centers for Disease Control and Prevention), 117, 235, 237, 239
Center for Medicaid and Medicare Innovation, 335
cerebrovascular disease, 4, 6
cervical cancer, 308, 309, 320, 325
CEYLL (cohort expected years of life lost), 231
Chagas disease, 314, 316, 319
Chamberlain, Joseph, 42
Chan, Margaret, 104
charismatic authority, 22–23, 24, 101
chemoprophylaxis, 69
chemotherapy, 151, 234, 241
Chen, Martha, 261
Chernobyl nuclear disaster, 29
child mortality, 96, 103, 166, 259, 304, 305
children: female infanticide in China, 221; formula feeding of, 186; in health care delivery model, 161; malnourished, 140, 155, 174; mental health of, 216; oral rehydration therapy (ORT) for diarrhea, 81, 102, 305; vaccinations of, 27, 97, 98, 99. *See also* UNICEF (United Nations Children's Fund)
Children First (Black), 98
child survival revolution, 83, 98, 100, 102, 109
Chile, 219
China, xv, 11, 62, 96; "barefoot doctor" movement in, 76–77, *76*, 207; life expectancy in, 260; medical schools in, 280, 282; opium trade with British India, 36; suicide in, 216–17, 220–21; Western financial institutions and, 92
chloroquinine, 67
cholera, xxii, 39, 170, 293, 315; in Egypt, 62; global commerce and, 49–50; in Haiti, 181; health disparities and, 3; identification of cholera pathogen, 41–42; in India, 39, 41, 42, 43; London (1854), 50–52, *51, 52*; in the Philippines, 47
Christian Medical College and Hospital (India), 283
Christian missionary medicine, 45–49, *48*, 279
chronic liver disease, 66
chronic respiratory disease, 320
CIDRZ, 133
cinchona tree, bark of, 37

circumcision, male, 310, 331
civil services, 295–96
civil society, 274, 278
Classe, Léon, 168
clinical medicine, 2, 3
Clinton, Bill, administration of, 122–23, 124, 125, 252, 337
Clinton, Hillary, 111, 347
Clinton Health Access Initiative [Clinton HIV/AIDS Initiative] (CHAI), 172, 206
Cold War, 12, 75, 78, 266–67
Collier, Paul, 294
Colombia, 219, 231, 328
colon cancer, 4
colonial medicine, xiii, 35, 36–39, 39, 41; birth of tropical medicine, 41–45, 45; "civilizing process" in colonial discourse, 44, 45; health, development, and legacies of, 60–70; missionary medicine, 45–49, 48; smallpox eradication program and, 69
Columbian Exchange, 35
Columbus, Christopher, 35, 41, 135
community, 23, 156, 160, 207, 357
community health workers (CHWs), 208
condoms, 115, 116, 156, 291
Confucianism, 283, 284
Congo, Democratic Republic of, 20, 21, 99, 170
Conille, Gary, 201
"Consensus Statement on Antiretroviral Treatment for AIDS in Poor Countries," 120, 158
Cooperative Medical System, 76
COPD (chronic obstructive pulmonary disease), 3, 4, 6
Costa Rica, 260
cost-effectiveness analysis, 25, 75, 81, 234, 273; DALY (disability-adjusted life year) and, 228; in debates on child rights and health, 103; MDRTB (multidrug-resistant tuberculosis) and, 212, 234–242; as principal tool of policymaking, 227; prioritized by financial institutions, 94; surgical care and, 330; utilitarianism and, 250–51; *World Development Report* and, 106–8
Crazy Like United States (Watters), 223
Creese, Andrew, 118
Cromwell, William Nelson, 53
Crosby, Alfred, 35
crush injuries, xxi
Cuba, 53–54, 80, 138, 202–3, 246
Cueto, Marcos, 79
cysticercosis/taeniasis, 314

Dallaire, Gen. Romeo, 170
DALYs (disability-adjusted life years), 212, 225–234, 242, 250; burden of disease and, 5, 6, 106; MDRTB (multidrug-resistant tuberculosis) and, 240, 241; mental disorders and, 214; NCDs (noncommunicable diseases) and, 320, 321; neglected tropical diseases (NTDs) and, 316, 317; surgical diseases and, 329
Dana-Farber Cancer Institute, 325, 328
Das, Veena, 11, 30
DATA (Debt, AIDS, Trade, Africa), 127, 129
DDT pesticide, 11–12, 17, 18, 63–64, 66–67, 69
debt crisis, 84, 93, 109
decolonization, 75, 136
deconstructionism, 16
de Ferranti, David, 84
deforestation, 166
dementia, 4, 6
democracy, 56, 60, 247, 273, 291
Democratic Party, 128, 345, 346, 347
demography, xiv
dengue, 314
Denmark, 300
depression, 19, 25, 30, 213, 215; community-based treatment programs for, 219; local context and, 224
Desjarlais, Robert, 216, 218–19
developing countries (developing world), 2, 12, 44, 332, 335; AIDS in, 112, 114, 203; "appropriate technology" and, 250; cost-effectiveness analysis in, 109; cost of generic drugs in, 126; fiscal austerity measures in, 303; foreign aid and, 289; immunization rates in, 83; medical and nursing schools in, 207; mental health in, 217, 218–220; NCDs (noncommunicable diseases) in, 320; neoliberalism and, 86, 87, 92; public-sector health systems in, 202–3, 205; rural majority in, 79
development, 60–62, 66, 210, 293; accompaniment approach and, 294; "big push" schemes, 136–37, 141; freedoms (capabilities) and, 257, 260; human rights and, 273; improvement of health delivery and, 194–96, 196; international development institutions, 21; poverty traps and, 289; sustainable, 295
deworming drugs, 107, 307, 318
diabetes, 25, 178, 215, 323; DALY (disability-adjusted life year) and, 6; deaths from, 4; global epidemic of, 17;

McKeown hypothesis and, 66; type 1, 321; type 2, 320, 321

Diagnostic and Statistical Manual of Mental Disorders (DSM), 19, 215, 222, 223, 224

diagnostics, xiii, 19, 49, 208; "appropriate technology" and, 250; costs of, 130; drug-resistant disease and, 239; as late twentieth-century innovation, 111; malaria eradication program and, 67; McKeown hypothesis and, 64

diarrheal diseases, 3, 107, 131, 194, 307; DALY (disability-adjusted life year) and, 6; deaths from, 4; in Haiti, 140; infant mortality and, 100; oral rehydration therapy (ORT) for, 81, 82, 102; treatment of, 5

diet, Western, 17

diethylcarbamazine, 317, 319

diphtheria-pertussis-tetanus (DPT) vaccination, 81, 101

Discipline and Punish (Foucault), 26

disease burden, 3–9, 4, 6–9, 13, 242; DALY (disability-adjusted life year) and, 226, 229, 230, 232, 233; double burden (communicable and noncommunicable), 320; mental health and, 213, 214–15, 216, 233; "90-10 gap" and, 315; poverty and, 186, 289

"diseased native," 43, 44, 46

doctors (physicians), xvii, 150–51, 332; "brain drain" from developing world, 208–9; health care delivery and, xiv; in missionary medicine, 47, 48; physician-to-population ratio, 140, 203, 206

Doha Declaration (2001), 123, 327

Dominican Republic, xxii, 138

DOTS (directly observed treatment, short course), 235–241

dracunculiasis (guinea-worm disease), 314

drug development pipeline, 313–14, 315, 316

drug-resistant disease, xvii, 239

drug trade, 254

Duarte, José Napoleón, 99

Duflo, Esther, 292, 293

Dunant, Henri, 280

Duvalier, François ("Papa Doc"), 137, 138, 139

Duvalier, Jean-Claude ("Baby Doc"), 137, 138, 138, 139

dysentery, 148

dyspnea (shortness of breath), 153, 155

Earth Institute (Columbia University), 207, 208

Easterly, William, 287–88, 290–92, 296, 298

echinococcosis, 314

ecological imperialism, 35

Ecuador, 219

Egypt, 42, 62, 318

El Salvador, 99

End of Poverty, The (Easterly), 287–88

Englund, Harri, 274

epidemics, xiii, xxii, 38, 119, 234; bio-surveillance and, 33; border crossing by, xvii; "camp," 106; cholera, 39, 41, 43, 49, 106; controlling spread of, xiv; MDRTB, 212, 239, 241, 242; plague, 27, 36; sleeping sickness, 36; trade liberalization and, 105; "virgin-soil epidemics," 35

epilepsy, 178, 219

equity, global health, xiii–xv, xix, 109, 335; activist strategies for, 347–49; advancement of, 349–353; AIDS response and, 111, 112, 130; grassroots activism and, 340–47, 343, 346; health as a human right and, 272, 277; as human rights challenge, 303; intellectual property and, 326–27; liberal cosmopolitanism and, 255; Partners In Health and, 134; UNICEF and, 103

"Erwadi Tragedy," 217

Escobar, Arturo, 60

ethambutol, 150

Ethiopia, 330

ethnography, 187, 188, 275

etiology, 43, 50, 154–55

Europe, 234, 327; AIDS activism in, 118; colonial empires of, 41; Eastern Europe, 92; Haiti and, 136; mental health in, 214, 223

Everybody's Business (WHO report), 197

Falwell, Rev. Jerry, 113

family planning, 94, 104, 107, 114, 309, 357

famine, 140

Fanon, Franz, 44

Fauci, Anthony, 302

FDA (Food and Drug Administration), 116–17, 310, 341, 342

female literacy campaigns, 94

Ferguson, James, 274

Fernandpoulle, Rushika, 334

FFF interventions, 94–104

Financing Health Services in Developing Countries (World Bank report), 89

Finlay, Carlos, 53, 54, 55

"first pass effect," 160–61

floods, 141
fluoxetine (Prozac), 213
food security, 309
foreign aid, 13, *112*, 113, 126, 287–293;
accompaniment approach and aid
reform, 294–301; as double-edged sword,
181; expansion of, 298–301; pitfalls of,
176
Foucault, Michel, xviii, 11, 25, 26–28, 46,
224
France, xv, 27, 35, 130; colonial Haiti and,
135, 139, 148; Declaration of the Rights
of Man and the Citizen (1789), 263
Frenk, Julio, 197–98, 199, 228, 323, 328,
337
Friedman, Milton, 86, *86*, 93
Frist, Sen. William, 127, 283

Garrett, Laurie, 131, 336
Gay Men's Health Crisis, 342
GDP (gross domestic product), 5, 320, 352
gender inequality, 147
General Hospital (Port-au-Prince, Haiti),
148, 165, 180, 297
General International Sanitary Convention
of the American Republics, First, 54
geopolitics, 74
Germany, 130, 167, 168, 264
germ theory, 41–42, 43, 44
Ghana, 61, 206, 208, 324
GHESKIO, 133, 141, 158
Girl Scouts of America, 280
GlaxoSmithKline, 318
Global AIDS Alliance, 127, 129, 345
Global Alliance for Vaccines and Immuni-
zation (GAVI), 101–2, 305–7, 312
Global Alliance to Eliminate Lymphatic
Filariasis, 318
Global Burden of Disease, The (Murray
and Lopez), 227
Global Burden of Disease Study (World
Bank), 106, 226–27
Global Fund to Fight AIDS, Tuberculosis
and Malaria, xviii, 12, 114, 126, 158,
337; accompaniment approach and,
297; Bill and Melinda Gates Foundation (BMGF) and, 311–12; funding for
antiretroviral therapy (ART), 350; Haiti
as first country to receive funding from,
159; in Rwanda, 173
global health, xiii, 42, 71, 245, 332;
as attitude, xv–xvi; as collection of
problems, xv, xvi–xvii, 2, 351; commerce and, 49–60; definition of, 10, 34;
Development Programme (UNDP), 91;

global empire and, 34–49; golden age
of, 111–15, *112*; growth of interest in,
xiv; moral frameworks and, 247–263;
religious values and, 278–285; social science in, 16
global health delivery (GHD), 10, 12–13,
182, 184, 209–10; care delivery value
chain (CDVC), 189–191, *190*, *192*;
critically self-reflective approach to, 20;
definition of, 9; diagonal approach to,
198–99, 210, 331; economic development and, 194–96, *196*; foreign aid
and, 287; human resources for health,
206–9; leveraging of shared delivery
infrastructure, 192–94; local context
and, 185–89, *188*; public sector and,
199–201; strengthening of health systems, 196–206
Global Health Effectiveness Program, xx
globalization, xxii, 223
Global Network for Neglected Tropical
Diseases, 318
GNP (gross national product), 5, 257, 261
GOBI-FFF interventions, 82, 83, 84, 305;
limits of, 101–4; UNICEF and, 94–101,
305
Gore, Al, 122, 123, *123*
Gorgas, Gen. William, 53–54
Gourevitch, Philip, 168, 170
governance, 28, 197
governmentality, 28
governments, 22, 200–201, 295–96, 356,
357
Graham, Franklin, 127, 283
Grameen Bank, 350
Grant, James P., 83, 96–97, *97*, 100–101,
282, 284
Grant, John, 96
Grassi, Giovanni Battista, 53
Great Depression, 87, 337
Green Light Committee (GLC), 239
Griswold, Frank, 283
growth monitoring, 82
Guatemala, 330
Gutiérrez, Father Gustavo, 245

H₁N₁ epidemic, 33
HAART (Highly Active Antiretroviral
Therapy), 117, 118–120, 122, 124, 126
Habyarimana, President, 169–170
Haiti, xv, 133–34, 186, 207, 252; cancer in,
328; Cange squatter settlement, 141–42,
143, *144*, *147*, 330; Central Plateau, 120,
135, 141, *142*, 145, 161, 199; cholera
epidemic in, 41; Cuban medical brigade

in, 203; displaced people in camps, xxii; Duvalier dictatorships, 137, 138, *138*, 139, 142; field experience in, 11; food prices in, 105; health care in, 139–141; history of, 134–39, *138*; HIV/AIDS in, 30–31, 120, 141, 145–47; lack of specialists in, xvii; mental health programs in, 219; NGOs in, xxi, xxii, 150, 181, 201, 205; Péligre Dam, 21, 137, 141, *143*, 150; private-sector health facilities, 200; public-sector health system in, 12, 61, 158, 159, 180; RUTFs in, 308; Rwanda compared with, 165–67, 171–72, 178, 181–82; scaled-up HIV/AIDS treatment in rural areas, 158–165, *162–65*; tuberculosis (TB) in, 148–158; "water refugees" from floods, 141, 142, 144, 145, 147. *See also* Zanmi Lasante (ZL)

Haiti earthquake (2010), xx–xxiii, 134, 161, 179–181, 203, 219; foreign aid and, 295; loss of life and damage in, *179*; surgical services and, 330

Hammonds, Rachel, 270

handwashing, xxii, 115

Hanna, Bridget, 246

Hanson, Kara, 232

Hardiman, David, 47, 48

Harlem Hospital Center, 334

Harvard College, xiii, xvi, xvii, 2; Global Health Delivery Project, 184, 185, 209–10, 297–98; global health equity and, xviii; Student Global AIDS Campaign and, 127

Harvard Medical School, xviii, xx, 2, 325, 328

Hayek, Friedrich von, 85, *86*

Head of the Medical Student (Picasso), 284–85, *284*

health: commodification of, 88–93; definition of, 9

health care delivery, xiv, 16, 175, 294; community participation in, 79–80; improvement of, xvi; model for, 160–61

health disparities, xviii, xix, 3–9, 4, *6–8*

"health for all" agenda, 74, 104, 109; after golden age of global health, 130; rise of neoliberalism and, 84, 93; unraveling of, 271

Health GAP, 345, 348

Health Global Access Project, 127

Health Global Action Project (Health GAP), 121

Health Leads, 334

Health Sector Policy Report, 83

"healthy carrier," 43

heart disease, 17, 66, 215, 320, 323, 331

Helms, Sen. Jesse, 113, 127

hepatitis B, 328

Hepburn, Audrey, 100

herpes, 116

Heywood, Mark, 276, 344

Hinduism, 283

Hispaniola, 35, 135

history, xxiii, 3

HIV, 9, 131, 141, 185–86, 293; AMPATH care, 191, *192*; care delivery for, 189; DALY (disability-adjusted life year) and, 6; deaths from, 4; global health delivery (GHD) and, 185; HAART (Highly Active Antiretroviral Therapy) as pillar of treatment for, 120; health disparities and, 3; McKeown hypothesis and, 66; mother-child transmission of, 127, 156, 277, 336; seroprevalence, 154; sex workers at risk of infection, 285; testing and detection of, *162*; as treatable disease, 112, *118*; tuberculosis and, 148–158; World Bank funding for prevention of, 104, 107. *See also* AIDS

HIV Equity Initiative, 157, 158, 173

Ho, David, 117

Hobsbawm, Eric, 74

Holocaust, the, 265

homosexuality, 19, 113, 127, 224

Honorat, Jacques, 144–45, 146

hookworm, 57, 58, 59, 314, *317*

Hôpital Albert Schweitzer (Haiti), 148, 149

Hôpital Universitaire de Mirebalais (Haiti), xxi–xxii

horizontal health interventions, 71

Horton, Richard, xv, xxi

Horwitz, Allan, 213

hospitals, xvi, 10, 21; in Africa, 2, 208; disciplinary power and, 26–27; in Haiti, xxi, 134, 140, 148, 157, 165, 180; MCRTB spread in, 238; missionary medicine and, 47; resources of urban hospitals, 79; in Rwanda, 173, *174*, *177*; twinning programs and, 331

Hotez, Peter, 318–19, 321

Hougen, Phillip, 129

housing, 140, 185, 209, 268, 269

human rights, 13, 68, 80, 217, 246; capabilities approach and, 258, 262–63; of children, 103; critiques of human rights theory, 274–76; equity and, 303; health as a human right, 259, 270–74; history of, 263–270, *265*, *266*; praxis of, 276–78, *276*, *278*; secular traditions and, 279

Human Rights Watch, 268

Hume, Edward H., 282
Hunter, W. W., 39, 41, 43
Hutus, 28, 167, 168, 169, 170
hyperinflation, 86–87
hypertension, 320, 321, 334

Ignatieff, Michael, 267
IMF (International Monetary Fund), 74,
  85–92, 94, 114, 271
immunization, 80, 98, 107; diphtheria-
  pertussis-tetanus (DPT), 81, 101; fall in
  rates of, 101; GOBI interventions, 82,
  97; in public-sector health systems, 202;
  universal childhood immunization, 94,
  96, 305–6
imperialism, 43, 60–61
income inequality, 249–250
India, 186, 221, 327, 352; Bhopal gas leak,
  29; caste and colonialism in, 28; cholera
  outbreak in, 39, 41, 42, 43; "Erwadi
  Tragedy," 217; generic AIDS drugs
  manufactured in, 121, 125; opium trade
  between British India and China, 36;
  polio in Uttar Pradesh, 187, 188; public-
  sector health system in Kerala, 202, 260;
  rural doctors in, 76, 77; Western financial institutions and, 92
individualism, Western, 275
Indochina, French colony of, 37
Indonesia, 106, 185, 309
infant mortality, 5, 8, 94, 101, 204, 332
infectious-disease practitioners, xvi
inflammatory bowel disease, 321
inflation, 93
influenza, 65
infrastructure, 2, 61, 130; global health
  delivery (GHD) and, 185; in Haiti, 142;
  leveraging of shared delivery infrastructure, 192–94; religious values and, 283;
  shared delivery infrastructure, 201
insecticide-treated bed nets (ITNs), 195
Inshuti Mu Buzima (IMB), 165, 172–78,
  184
institutionalization, 18, 24, 93, 115, 350
intellectual property rights, 121–26,
  326–27
intentions, announcing, 21–22
Interim Haiti Reconstruction Commission,
  181
internally displaced persons (IDP) camps,
  180
International AIDS Conference, 117, 118,
  124, 156
International Bank for Reconstruction and
  Development. See World Bank

International Conference on Primary
  Health Care (Alma Ata, 1978), 78–81,
  79, 355; antecedents of, 12; "health for
  all" agenda and, 74; neoliberalism and,
  86; political will at, 108. See also Alma-
  Ata Declaration
International Covenant on Economic,
  Social, and Cultural Rights (ICESCR),
  267, 270
international health, xiii–xiv, 58, 71, 302;
  definition of, 9, 10, 34; paltry resources
  for, 115
International Sanitary Bureau (ISB), 54,
  55, 56
International Sanitary Conference, 52, 54
International Trachoma Initiative, 318
internship, xvi
"Introduction to Social Medicine" (class at
  Harvard Medical School), xviii
Invisible People, The (Behrman), 116
iodine deficiency, 100
Iran, 185
irrigation reservoirs, 67
ischemic heart disease, 4, 6, 321
Islam, 283
isoniazid, 150, 234
ivermectin, 316, 317, 319

James, William, 43, 279
Japan, 41, 217
Johnson, H.L.E., 54–55
Jolly, Richard, 100
Joseph, Acéphie, 144–47
Jubilee 2000 debt relief movement, 283
justice, social/global, xiv, 16, 246, 257, 275,
  277; foreign aid and, 299; primary health
  care (PHC) and, 356; religious values
  and, 282

Kagame, Paul, 171
Kapczynski, Amy, 124
Kaposi's sarcoma, 328
Kayibanda, President, 169
Kazakhstan, 12
Kenya, 61, 90, 133, 167; AMPATH care in,
  191, 192; deworming program in, 307;
  female genital alteration in, 262; global
  health delivery (GHD) and, 185; health
  care workers in, 208; HIV prevalence
  in, 185–86; randomized controlled trials
  (RCTs) in, 293
Kenyatta Hospital (Nairobi), 79, 106
Keynes, John Maynard, 85
Kleinman, Arthur, 11, 30, 93, 216, 220,
  224; critique of medicalization, 221–22;

on divided self, 284; on health work as moral practice, 246–47; on PTSD, 222–23; on social suffering, 229, 230, 231
knowledge, 58, 155, 350; aysmmetries of, 20; colonial medicine and, 43, 71; economic, 93; local knowledge integrated with clinical medicine, 224; power and, 25–26; social construction of, xviii–xix, 18–19
Koch, Robert, 41–42
Koenig, Serena, 159
Kramer, Larry, 342
Kremer, Michael, 293
Kristof, Nicholas, 352

laboratory technicians, xvii, 206
labor migration patterns, 67
Lambo, Thomas, 219
Lancet, The (journal), xv, 115, 118, 126, 215, 233
Lascahobas Clinic (Haiti), 159, 160–61, 162–64
Latin America, 58, 60, 87, 91, 254, 282
Latvia, 239
Laveran, Charles Alphonse, 53
"Lazarus effect," 157, 174
Leach, Jim, 283
League of Nations Health Committee, 56, 62
Léandier, Fernet, 173
Lebanon, 99
Lee Kuan Yew, 274–75
legitimation, 19
leishmaniasis, 314, 319
leprosy, 314
Lesotho, xv, 178, 274, 309
leukemia, 325
Lévy-Bruhl, Lucien, 44
liberal cosmopolitanism, 251–55
liberation theology, 282
Liberia, 178
life expectancy, 5, 140, 202, 232; gender and, 226; map, 7; public-sector health care and, 260; U.S. ranking in, 204
Livingstone, David, 48
local context, 185–89, 188
Lock, Margaret, 11, 30
Locke, John, 263
Logiest, Col Guy, 169
London School of Tropical Medicine, 42
Lopez, Alan, 227
lower respiratory infections, 4, 6
Luckmann, Thomas, xviii–xix, 18, 22; on habitualization, 115; institutionalization concept, 24, 93, 188
lung cancer, 4, 6

lung disease, 321, 323, 334
Lyautey, Hubert, 37
lymphatic filariasis, 77, 314, 316, 317

Madagascar, 37
Mahler, Halfdan, 76, 78, 79, 80, 83, 93; GOBI criticized by, 102; as medical missionary, 282; religious values of, 284
malaria, xviii, 59, 77, 113, 302; antimalarial drug production, 185; child mortality and, 305; comparison with smallpox eradication program, 68, 69; control of, 95; DALY (disability-adjusted life year) and, 6; DDT spraying and, 17–18; deaths from, 4; febrile malaria treatment, 81; funding for treatment and prevention, 130; in Haiti, 140; health care delivery infrastructure and, 192; health disparities and, 3; Panama Canal construction and, 53; poverty and disease risk in relation to, 17; quinine as treatment for, 37; in Rwanda, 166; as treatable disease, 112; vaccine for, 310
Malaria Control and Evaluation Partnership, 312
Malaria Eradication Programme (MEP), 33, 62–64, 66–67, 71, 75
Malawi (colonial Nyasaland), 1–2, 9, 178, 206, 308; cancer in, 324, 328; field experience in, 11; human rights discourse in, 274; missionary medicine in, 46
Mali, 318
Mallon, Mary ("Typhoid Mary"), 43
malnutrition, 166, 216, 249, 305, 307
Mandela, Nelson, 122, 276, 276
Mann, Jonathan, 9, 271
Manson, Patrick, 42–43, 53
market fundamentalism, 85, 91
Marseille, Elliot, 118
Marx, Karl, 15, 274, 275
Marxism, 15, 274
Mbeki, Thabo, 122, 276, 345
McKeown, Thomas, 64
McKeown hypothesis, 64, 65–66
McNamara, Robert, 83, 84
MDRTB (multidrug-resistant tuberculosis), 13, 25, 207, 212; limits of cost-effectiveness analysis and, 234–242; poverty and disease risk in relation to, 17. See also tuberculosis (TB)
measles, 35, 81, 185
mebendazole, 317, 319
Mectizan, 318
Médecins Sans Frontières (Doctors Without Borders), 120, 124, 307–8, 330

Medicaid, 121, 333, 335, 346
"medical apartheid," 120
medicalization, 19–20, 221–22
medical records, electronic, 161
medical schools, 206–7, 282
medicine, 9, 111, 130
Medicines Act (South Africa, 1997), 122–23, 124, 344–45
MedPharm, 318
melarsoprol, 316
meningitis, 306
Mental Health GAP Action Programme (WHO), 220
mental health/illness, 13, 212, 303, 320; human resources for, 218, *218*; as "odd case," 213–225
Merck, 316, 318
Merton, Robert, xix, 20, 21, 93
Mexico, 58, 84, 87, 199, 228; cash transfer program, 296; Seguro Popular program, 337
miasma, theory of, 50, 51
Middle East, 92, 98
midwives, 140, 357
Miguel, Edward, 293
Mill, John Stuart, 247, 264
Millennium Development Goals (MDGs), 166, 206, 288, 301; eight goals, 304–5, *304*; maternal and child health, *304*, 305–10, 331
Millennium Villages Project, 207
Mirebalais Hospital (Haiti), 165
"Missing Women" (Sen), 221
Mock, Charles, 330
molecular biology, xiv
morbidity, 5, 193, 197, 210; level of medical care and, 259; Millennium Development Goals and, 304; NCDs (noncommunicable diseases) and, 321, 323; psychiatric, 225
Morocco, 37
mortality rates, 5, 193, 197, 210; cancer, 328; for children under five, 8, *166*; DALY (disability-adjusted life year)and, 225, 226; economic development and, 260; of Europeans in colonies, 36–37, 40; infant and child, 8, 94, 100; McKeown hypothesis and, 64, *65*–66; Millennium Development Goals and, 304; NCDs (noncommunicable diseases) and, 321, 323; tuberculosis (TB), 152, *153*
mosquitoes, 53, 61, 63, 64, 67
Mugyenyi, Peter, *128*
Murray, Christopher, 225–28, 230, 231, 232–33

Mycobacterium tuberculosis, 9, 149, 234

Napoleon I, 135
National Institute of Allergy and Infectious Diseases, 302, 310
National Institutes of Health (NIH), 131, 311
national-legal authority, 23, 24
Natsios, Andrew, 119, 120
Navajo Nation, xv, 333
NCDs (noncommunicable diseases), xiii, 320–23
neglected tropical diseases (NTDs), 313–19, 321, 336
Neno District Hospital (Malawi), 2
neoliberalism, 12, 74, 84; antecedents of structural adjustment, 84–87, *85*, *86*; commodification of health, 88–93; food and trade liberalization, 105; selective primary health care (SPHC) and, 103; "Washington consensus," 87–88
neonatal infections, 3, 4, 6
Nepal Community Mental Health Project, 219
Nerette, Blanco, 145–46
Netherlands, 130
Newell, Kenneth, 76
NGOs (nongovernmental organizations), xv, xvi, 10, 182, 203, 328; accompaniment approach and, 294–95; accountability to donors, 200, *201*, 205; AIDS response and, 131; as architects of global health policy, 22; "failing" public health care systems and, xix; in Haiti, xxi, xxii, 150, 181, 201, 205, 296, 301; human rights discourse used by, 275; in Malawi, 1; as partners of universities, xviii; public-sector health systems and, 205–6; Red Cross and, 297; in Rwanda, 172, 301
Nicaragua, 53
nifurtimox-eflornithine combination therapy, 319
Niger, 318
Nigeria, 61, 198, 219
NNRTIs (non-nucleotide reverse transcriptase inhibitors), 117
North, global, 34, 60
North Africa, 92, 98
Norway, 300
Nuremberg War Crimes Trials, 265, *265*
nurses, xvii, 150–51, 206, 357; "brain drain" from developing world, 208–9; health care delivery and, xiv; nurse-midwives, 1
Nussbaum, Martha, 255–262, *256*, 267

Nussle, Rep. Jim, 129
nutrition, 80, 107, 114, 199, 356
Nyasaland. *See* Malawi

Obama, Barack, 312, 346, 347
obesity, 17
obstetric services, 330
Odinkalu, Chidi, 275
OECD (Organisation for Economic Co-
    operation and Development), 250, 252
Office International d'Hygiène Publique
    (OIHP), 49–50, 56, 62
Olyset, 195, *196*
onchocerciasis (river blindness), 314, 316,
    317, 318
oncologists, xvi, xvii
ONE Campaign, 348
Ooms, Gorik, 270
Opportunidades program (Mexico), 199
oral rehydration therapy (ORT), 94, 95, 98,
    100, 101, 305
orthopedists, xvii
Overseas Development Council, 96
Oxfam America, 348

Packard, Randall, 67
PAHO (Pan American Health Organiza-
    tion), 52, 54, 55–56, 58; formation of
    WHO and, 62; on MDRTB treatment,
    237; Pan American Sanitary Conference
    hosted by, 59; on prevalence of tubercu-
    losis in Haiti, 148
Paine, Thomas, 263, 264
Pakistan, 198, 221
Panama Canal, construction of, 52–56, *54*,
    56, 64
Pan American Sanitary Bureau (PASB), 55
pandemic diseases, 33, 245
panopticon prison, 27
Pape, Jean, 158
parasite control, 63, 64, 69, 194
Paris Declaration on Aid Effectiveness
    (2005), 200, *201*, 206
paroxetine (Paxtil), 213
Partnership for Maternal, Newborn, and
    Child Health, 309
Partners In Health, 2, 3, 120, 182, 325;
    biosocial approach of, 12; community
    health worker model and, 207; diagonal
    approach to health care and, 199; global
    health delivery and, 184; in Haiti, 133–
    34, 139, 141, 147, 159–161, 165; health
    as a human right and, 277, 278; local
    context and, 185; MDRTB treatment
    and, 239; in Rwanda, 134, 165, 172–79,

174, *177*; social theory and, 16; surgical
    services and, 330
Pasteur, Louis, 41
Patel, Vikram, 216, 217, 220
pathogens, 63, 319, 329; in Columbian
    Exchange, 35; drug-resistant, 240; iden-
    tification of, 42; international borders
    disregarded by, 10
"Paying for Health Services in Developing
    Counries" (de Ferranti), 84
Peking Union Medical College, 280, 282
Pelletier, Pierre-Joseph, 37
Pérez de Cuéllar, Javier, 99
Peru, 11, 37, 172, 175, 207; Bill and
    Melinda Gates Foundation and, 312;
    National Tuberculosis Program, 235–36,
    236, 238–39, 241
Petryna, Adriana, 29
Pfizer, 318
pharmaceutical companies, 118, 122–23,
    214, 318, 326, 342
pharmacy systems, 192
philanthropists, private, 10, 112
Philippines, 43, 47, 58, 239
Pillay, Navanethem, 268
plague epidemics, 36
Plasmodium falciparum, 17
pneumonia, 65, 113, 116, 131, 305, 320
podoconiosis, 315
Pogge, Thomas, 251–55, 258, 268
policymakers, xviii, 12, 58, 95, 120,
    285, 351; activist strategies and, 348;
    AIDS treatment and, 120, 272; cost-
    effectiveness analysis and, 242; DALYs
    (disability-adjusted life years) and, 227,
    228, 234; global health delivery and,
    184; health care reform in United States
    and, 335; "health for all" agenda and,
    84; MDRTB (multidrug-resistant tuber-
    culosis) and, 212; mental health and,
    212, 214; randomized controlled trials
    (RCTs) and, 293; religious values and,
    282; selective primary health care and,
    94; visionary, 337
polio, xiii, 95, 97, 187, *188*, 198
political economy, xiv, 3, 165, 210, 252,
    258–59
Poor Economics (Bannerjee), 293
post-traumatic stress disorder (PTSD),
    19–20, 215, 222–23
poverty, 59, 89, 127, 133, 245, 298, 304;
    agency constrained by, 147; burden of
    disease and, 186; development projects
    and, 21, 60; disease risk and, 17, 194;
    eradication of extreme poverty, *304*;

poverty *(continued)*
gender inequity and, 309; health care delivery and, 134; liberal cosmopolitanism and, 251–52; mental health and, 215–16; number of people in extreme poverty, 249, 250; perpetuated by social forces, 352; poverty traps, 92–93, 273, 288–89; reduction of, 234, 248, 291, 296; in Rwanda, 172, 175; social suffering and, 30, 144; structural adjustment and, 92; structural violence and, 268; tuberculosis treatment and, 149, 156
power, disciplinary, 25
praziquantel, *317*, 318, 319
premenstrual syndrome, 20
Prescriptions for Hope, 127
President's Emergency Plan for AIDS Relief (PEPFAR), xviii, 12, 111, 113, 285, 323, 337; accompaniment approach and, 297; authorization of, 129, 130, 348; Bush (George W.) and, 345; funding for, 131; funding for antiretroviral therapy (ART), 350; reauthorization of (2008), 347; religious values and, 282–83
Préval, René, 138
preventatives, xiii, 49; costs of, 130; as late twentieth-century innovation, 111; malaria eradication program and, 67; McKeown hypothesis and, 64; unavailability in developing world, 3
Prevention and Access to Care and Treatment (PACT), 333
primary health care (PHC), 69, 75, 83, 104, 356–57; community-based, 207; "horizontal," 131; neoliberalism and, 91; roots of, *75–78, 76, 78*; in Rwanda, 172; shared delivery infrastructure and, 193; strengthened access to, 160
Primary Health Care, Now More Than Ever (WHO report, 2008), 74, 104
Principles of Political Economy (Mill), 264
prisons, 27
privatization, 87, 90, 91, 221
Program for Appropriate Technology in Health (PATH), 312
Progress of Nations report, 100, 103
Protestant churches, 47
Prusoff, William, 124
psychiatrists, xvi
psychosis, 219
psychotropic drugs, 213
public health, xvi, xxiii, 2, 9
public sector, xxiv, 83, 184, 199–201; BRAC and, 193; examples of effective health systems, 202–6; foreign aid and, 138; in Haiti, 12, 158, 159, 161, 180; "market fundamentalism" and, 85; neoliberalism and, 94, 104; as only health provider for the poor, 186; predominantly urban areas served by, 106; resuscitation of, 12; in Rwanda, 172, 173, 174, 175, 178; in sub-Saharan Africa, 1; weakening of, xxi
purposive social action, unintended consequences of, xix, 20–22, 36
pyrazinamide, 150

quarantine regulations, 62
Quiet Revolution, A (Chen), 261
quinine, 37

rabies, 314
race/racial ideology, 30, 35; "Hamitic" myth in Rwanda, 168, 169; scientific racism, 16, 28
Ragon Institute, 310
randomized controlled trials (RCTs), 293
rationalization, 22–25
rational-legal authority, 58
Ravallion, Martin, 261
Ravishankar, Nirmala, 112, 115
Rawls, John, 251–55, 258, 259, 273
ready-to-use therapeutic foods (RUTFs), 307–8
Reagan, Ronald, 84–85, *85*, 87
rectum cancer, 4
Red Crescent, 330
Red Cross, 280, 281, 297, 330
Reed, Walter, 53
refractive errors, 6
rehydration interventions, 5, 62, 94, *95*
religious practices/values, 186–87, 278–285
Republican Party, 113, 128, 346, 347
research, training integrated with, xiv–xv
residency, xvi
respiratory infections, 107
RESULTS, 348
Retrovir, 341, 342
Richmond, Julius, 80, 349–350
rifampin, 234
Rights of Man (Paine), 264
Rockefeller, John D., 280
Rockefeller Foundation, 57, *57*, 58–59; Bellagio conference, 81, 82, *82*, 96; GOBI-FFF interventions funded by, 101
Rockefeller Sanitary Commission, 57
Roll Back Malaria Partnership, 312
Roosevelt, Eleanor, 266, *266*
Roosevelt, Theodore, 54, 55
Ross, Ronald, 42, 53

Rotary Foundation, 198
rotavirus control, 95, 306
Rousseau, Jean-Jacques, 263, 264
Russia, xv, 172, 175, 207; MDRTB treatment in, 239, 312; Russian empire, 41; Stalin regime, 264
Rwanda, xv, 134, 203, 318; cancer in, 328; European colonialism in, 28; field experience in, 11; genocide in, 20, 21, 28, 166, 176; government investment in health sector, 300–301; Haiti compared with, 165–67, 171–72, 178, 181–82; history of, 167–172; lack of specialists in, xvii; *mutuelle* system, 175–76; NCDs (noncommunicable diseases) in, 321–22; Partners In Health (Ishunta Mu Buzima) in, 172–79, *174, 177*; public-sector health system in, 12
Rwinkwavu District Hospital (Rwanda), 173, *174, 177*

Sabin polio vaccine, 95
Sachs, Jeffrey, 126, 287–88, 298, 299, 300
Sachs, Wolfgang, 60
Salmonella typhi, 43
Samaritan's Purse, 127, 283
Sandel, Michael, 274
sanitation, xxii, 15, 62, 80, 102, 357; commodification of health and, 88; Cooperative Medical System and, 76; economic development and, 194; in Haiti, 140; public health infrastructure and, 320
SARS epidemic, 33, 41
Sawyer, Eric, 116, 118
scarcity, socialization for, xxii, 61, 63, 322; global AIDS response and, 115, 130; human rights and, 272; priorities and, 336
schistosomiasis, 77, 314, 316, *317*
schizophrenia, 178, 224
Schweitzer, Albert, 279–280, 284
selective primary health care (SPHC), 12, 81–84, *82*, 92, 108; rise of UNICEF and, 94–104
"Selective Primary Health Care: An Interim Strategy for Disease Control in Developing Countries" (Walsh and Warren), 81
Seligman, Charles Gabriel, 168
Sen, Amartya, 221, 229–230, 255, *256*, 302; on development and freedom, 257, 260; Easterly criticized by, 292; on individual rights, 275
Sergi, Giuseppe, 168
service providers, xv, xvi
sewage/sewer systems, xxii, 50

sexism, 30
sexually transmitted diseases, 107, 221
sex workers, 186, 200, 285, 291
Sfeir-Younis, Alfredo, 271, 272–73
Sierra Leone, 99
Singer, Peter, 248, 249, 255
Siplon, Patricia, 342–43
slavery, 135, 136, 140, 148, 264; abolition of slave trade in British Empire, 341; trans-Atlantic slave trade, 38
sleeping sickness. *See* African trypanosomiasis
smallpox, xvii, 35, 36, 67–70, *70*, 75
Smith, Adam, 264
snakebite, 315
Snow, John, 50–51, 59
Social Construction of Reality, The (Berger and Luckmann), 18
social science, 16
social theory, 15, 31–32, 34
sociology, xiv, 3, 16, 17–20
Socios En Salud, 235, 236, 238
Somalia, 70, 75
sorcery, disease attributed to, 54, 151, *153*, 156, 187
South, global, 34, 60
South Africa, xv, 89, 125, 254, 337; AIDS treatment in, 120, 121, 122, 276–77, *276*; DALYs (disability-adjusted life years) in, 228; poverty reduction in, 296; right to housing in, 268. *See also* Treatment Action Campaign
South Sudan, 254
sovereign power, 26
Soviet Union, 75, 91, 236, 267
Spain, 35, 67, 135
Spanish-American War, 43
Special Care Center (Atlantic City), 334
specialists, xvi
species-being, 274, 275
Spicer, Sean, 129
sputum positivity, 152
Sri Lanka, 260
Stalin, Joseph, 264
Stewart, Frances, 90–91
stomach cancer, 4
STOP AIDS campaigns, 345–47, *346*
stretpmycin, 150
stroke, 215, 320
strongyloidiasis, 315
structural adjustment, xvii, 74, 89, 92, 107; antecedents of, 84–87, *85*, *86*; declining public investment in heatlh programs and, 109; human rights and, 271–72; Washington Consensus and, 87, 88

structural violence, 5, 9, 17, 194, 255; brain drain of medical professionals and, 209; definition of, 30–31; interventions to counter effects of, 147; mental health and, 216; social movements against, 350
Stuckler, David, 89
Student Global AIDS Campaign, 127, 129, 345, 346, 348
substance abuse, 30, 215, 218
Sudan, 99
Suez Canal, 49
suffering, social, xxiii, 17, 30, 144, 229, 230, 231
suicide, 30, 202, 215; gender and, 216, 220–21, 222; McKeown hypothesis and, 66; world rates of, 217
supply chains, 101, 161, 192, 194, 206, 321
surgery, 329–331
surveillance, 27, 29, 56, 67
survival potentials, 231
Sweden, 300
Switzerland, 280, 289

Taíno Indians, 35, 135
Tanzania, 80, 129, 218, 228, 318
Task Force for Global Health (Task Force for Child Survival), 96–97, 307
teaching hospitals, xvi, 165
technologies, xiii, 208, 288; "appropriate technology," 79, 250; communications and transportation, 49; in health care delivery model, 161; of power, 29
Terry, Fiona, 170
tertiary care, 106, 109
tetanus, 101
Thatcher, Margaret, 84–85, 85, 87, 106
Government of the Republic of South Africa vs. Irene Grootboom, 268, 276
Theory of Justice, A (Rawls), 251, 259
therapeutics, 33, 49; for AIDS, 116–17, 342; costs of, 130; drug-resistant disease and, 239; as late twentieth-century innovation, 111; malaria eradication program and, 67; McKeown hypothesis and, 64; unavailability in developing world, 3
tobacco use, 107, 114, 323
totalitarianism, 264
tourism, 17
toxocariasis, 321
trachea cancer, 4, 6
trachoma, 314, 317
traditional authority, 22, 24
training, xiv–xv, xvi, 331
Treatment Action Campaign (South Africa), 121, 121, 276–77, 343–45

trichuriasis, 317, 321
TRIPS (Trade Related Aspects of Intellectual Property Rights), 252
tropical medicine, 41–45
Trouillot, Michel-Rolph, 135
Truman, Harry, 60–61
trypanosomiasis, 192
tsetse fly, 49
tuberculosis (TB), xviii, 1, 49, 113, 302; bacillus associated with, 41; biosocial analysis of, 2; BRAC (Bangladesh Rural Advancement Committee) program and, 193; cure rate, 155–56; DALY (disability-adjusted life year) and, 6; deaths from, 4; falling prevalence of, 310; "first pass effect" in detection of, 160–61; in Haiti, 144, 148–158; health disparities and, 3; HIV patients with, 131, 147; home-based care for, 188; IMF impact on control of, 89; McKeown hypothesis and, 65; mental disorders and, 215; microbe associated with, 9; poverty linked to, 59; in Rwanda, 166, 174; second-line treatment for, 115; sorcery attributed as cause of, 151, 153, 156, 187; as "virgin-soil epidemic," 35. See also MDRTB (multidrug-resistant tuberculosis)
Turkey, 97, 98
Tutsis, 28, 167, 168, 169, 170
Twain, Mark, 43
twinning programs, 331
typhoid fever, 43, 186

Uganda, 89–90, 99, 167, 318, 330
unemployment, 17, 145, 185, 258, 275, 352; as barrier to good health, 133; improvement of economic development and, 194; as structural violence, 166
UNICEF (United Nations Children's Fund), 25, 74, 109, 282, 351; Partners In Health and, 172–73; polio eradication campaign and, 198; primary health care and, 75, 357, 358; reports of, 90; selective primary health care and, 83, 94–104, 95, 97; *State of the World's Children* report, 100, 102
unipolar depressive disorders, 6
United Kingdom, 38, 84, 108, 130, 283. See also Britain/British Empire
United Nations (UN), xv, 22, 62; Development Programme (UNDP), 97; Haiti and, xxii, 138, 148; Joint United Nations Programme on HIV/AIDS (UNAIDS), 114, 115, 129–130, 311; Millennium Project, 288; Rwanda and, 20, 21, 169, 170; UNESCO (UN Educational, Scientific,

and Cultural Organization), 261; Universal Declaration of Human Rights, 200, 265–66, 266, 267, 270. *See also* UNICEF (United Nations Children's Fund); WHO (World Health Organization)

United States, 11, 234; AIDS activism in, 116, 118, 122; Alma-Ata Conference and, 80; Bill of Rights (1791), 263; cancer in, 324; civil rights movement in, 350; foreign-trained doctors and nurses in, 208–9; as global superpower, 62; government spending on global health, 299, 300; Haiti and, 136, 137–39, 252; health care reform debates in, 249; health care workers in, 206; hookworm eliminated in, 57; intellectual property rights and, 327; market-based health care system of, 202, 204; MDRTB (multidrug-resistant tuberculosis) in, 235, 236, 238; mental health in, 214; primary care transformation in, 332–36; suicide rates and gender in, 222; tropical medicine in U.S.-occupied Philippines, 43–44

Universal Declaration of Human Rights, 200

universities, xviii, 127, 259, 350

Universities Allied for Essential Medicines, 327

urbanization, 105

USAID (U.S. Agency for International Development), 25, 44, 96, 119, 157, 319

utilitarianism, 247–251, 259

vaccination, xxii, 19, 62; BCG, 151; diphtheria-pertussis-tetanus (DPT), 81, 307; GAVI Alliance, 305–7; "herd immunity" and, 98; in Lascahobas Clinic, 164; measles, 97, 185; polio, 97, 187, 198; smallpox, 67–68, 97; UNICEF and, 101

Vansina, Jan, 167

Vaughan, Megan, 46–47, 48

vectors, 42, 43, 63, 69, 251

Venediktov, D. D., 78, 80

Venezuela, 138

"vertical" (disease-focused) interventions, 57, 75, 90, 102, 131, 199

Vibrio cholerae, 42

Village Health Works, 350

vitality of praxis, 3

vitamin A distribution, 101

vitamin D deficiency, 95

Wakefield, Jerome, 213

Walsh, Julia, 81, 82, 104

Walton, David, 159

Warren, Kenneth, 81, 82, 83, 104

Washington Consensus, 87–88, 91, 92, 93

water, 102, 131, 185; commodification of health and, 88; economic development and, 194; formula feeding of children and, 186; in Haiti, 140, 150, 180; public health infrastructure and, 320; safety of, 80, 356; waterborne diseases, 186; water-insecurity, xxii

Watters, Ethan, 223

Wealth of Nations (Smith), 264

Weber, Max, 11, 23, 56, 57, 241; on charismatic leadership, 101; on "iron cage" of bureaucracy, 25, 58; on modes of authority, 22–24; on rationalization of the world, 24–25; sociology defined by, 16

White Man's Burden, The (Easterly), 290–91

WHO (World Health Organization), 11, 22, 115, 188, 283, 351; cancer control and, 324; Commission on Macroeconomics and Health, 126; Commission on Social Determinants of Health, 5; cost-effectiveness analysis used by, 25; on disease burden in Africa, 303; Essential Medicines list, 324; formation of, 62; Global Program on AIDS, 271; health defined by, 9; "health for all" agenda and, 105; Mahler and, 77, 78, 83; Malaria Eradication Programme (MEP), 63–64, 66–67, 75; on MDRTB treatment, 237; mental health and, 214, 220, 224; NCDs (noncommunicable diseases) and, 321; neglected tropical diseases (NTDs) and, 314, 315, 316; pre-qualification from, 19; *Primary Health Care* report (2008), 74, 357; smallpox eradication program, 67–70, 70; Stop TB Partnership, 239, 241; five"3 by 5" initiative, 114, 158; *World Health Report*, 204, 215

"Why More Africans Don't Use Human Rights Language" (Odinkalu), 275

Wiese, Jean, 148

William J. Clinton Foundation, 125, 172, 175

Williamson, John, 91

Wolfensohn, James, 203, 283

women: female genital alteration, 262; in health care delivery model, 161; with HIV/AIDS in rural Haiti, 30–31, 144–47; HIV-positive pregnant women, 113; HIV testing for pregnant women, 156; life expectancy, 226; literacy rates, 202, 261; maternal and child health, 336; mental health of, 216; Millennium Development Goals and, 304; suicide rate in China, 216, 220–21; women's rights, 247

Worboys, Michael, 45–49
World Bank, 12, 22, 74, 203, 283, 351; on conditions in Haiti, 140; debt relief offered by, 114; emergence as key player in global health, 75; Global Burden of Disease Study, 106, 226–27; growing role in health, 104–8, 108; human rights and, 271; neoliberalism and, 85–92; reports of, 83, 84, 89, 103; selective primary health care and, 83, 84, 94, 97
World Development Report (World Bank), 83–84, 103, 104, 227; on cost-effectiveness, 106–8, 234; on DOTS, 235, 241; on human rights and development, 273
World Economic Forum, 101
World Health Assembly, 62, 77, 96, 105
World Mental Health (Desjarlais), 216
World Summit for Children, 96, 98, 103
World Trade Organization (WTO), 125, 252, 253, 326, 327
World War I, 60, 168
World War II, 60, 62, 63, 64, 264, 337
Wyman, Walter, 55

Yale University, 124
yaws, 148, 314
yellow fever, 49, 59, 306; carried by slaves from Africa, 148; Panama Canal construction and, 53–55, 54, 55
Young Men's Christian Association, 280
Young Women's Christian Association, 280
Yugoslavia, 99

Zambia, 89, 90, 92, 133, 208, 312, 318
Zanmi Lasante (ZL), 139, 141, 147, 165, 198, 350; diagonal approach to health care and, 199; earthquake relief and, 180; health as a human right and, 277, 278; home-based care and, 188; Ishunta Mu Buzima (IMB) compared with, 172–73; Lascahobas Clinic and, 159–161; local context and, 185, 186; mental health program, 219; Socios En Salud and, 237; surgical services and, 330; tuberculosis-control program, 150–56
Zerit, 124
zidovudine, 336
Zimbabwe, 98, 208

CALIFORNIA SERIES IN PUBLIC ANTHROPOLOGY

The California Series in Public Anthropology emphasizes the anthropologist's role as an engaged intellectual. It continues anthropology's commitment to being an ethnographic witness, to describing, in human terms, how life is lived beyond the borders of many readers' experiences. But it also adds a commitment, through ethnography, to reframing the terms of public debate—transforming received, accepted understandings of social issues with new insights, new framings.

Series Editor: Robert Borofsky (Hawaii Pacific University)

Contributing Editors: Philippe Bourgois (University of Pennsylvania), Paul Farmer (Partners In Health), Alex Hinton (Rutgers University), Carolyn Nordstrom (University of Notre Dame), and Nancy Scheper-Hughes (UC Berkeley)

University of California Press Editor: Naomi Schneider

1. *Twice Dead: Organ Transplants and the Reinvention of Death,* by Margaret Lock

2. *Birthing the Nation: Strategies of Palestinian Women in Israel,* by Rhoda Ann Kanaaneh (with a foreword by Hanan Ashrawi)

3. *Annihilating Difference: The Anthropology of Genocide,* edited by Alexander Laban Hinton (with a foreword by Kenneth Roth)

4. *Pathologies of Power: Health, Human Rights, and the New War on the Poor,* by Paul Farmer (with a foreword by Amartya Sen)

5. *Buddha Is Hiding: Refugees, Citizenship, the New America,* by Aihwa Ong

6. *Chechnya: Life in a War-Torn Society,* by Valery Tishkov (with a foreword by Mikhail S. Gorbachev)

7. *Total Confinement: Madness and Reason in the Maximum Security Prison,* by Lorna A. Rhodes

8. *Paradise in Ashes: A Guatemalan Journey of Courage, Terror, and Hope,* by Beatriz Manz (with a foreword by Aryeh Neier)

9. *Laughter Out of Place: Race, Class, Violence, and Sexuality in a Rio Shantytown,* by Donna M. Goldstein

10. *Shadows of War: Violence, Power, and International Profiteering in the Twenty-First Century,* by Carolyn Nordstrom

11. *Why Did They Kill? Cambodia in the Shadow of Genocide,* by Alexander Laban Hinton (with a foreword by Robert Jay Lifton)

12. *Yanomami: The Fierce Controversy and What We Can Learn from It,* by Robert Borofsky

13. *Why America's Top Pundits Are Wrong: Anthropologists Talk Back,* edited by Catherine Besteman and Hugh Gusterson

14. *Prisoners of Freedom: Human Rights and the African Poor,* by Harri Englund

15. *When Bodies Remember: Experiences and Politics of AIDS in South Africa,* by Didier Fassin

16. *Global Outlaws: Crime, Money, and Power in the Contemporary World,* by Carolyn Nordstrom

17. *Archaeology as Political Action,* by Randall H. McGuire

18. *Counting the Dead: The Culture and Politics of Human Rights Activism in Colombia,* by Winifred Tate

19. *Transforming Cape Town,* by Catherine Besteman

20. *Unimagined Community: Sex, Networks, and AIDS in Uganda and South Africa,* by Robert J. Thornton

21. *Righteous Dopefiend,* by Philippe Bourgois and Jeff Schonberg

22. *Democratic Insecurities: Violence, Trauma, and Intervention in Haiti,* by Erica Caple James

23. *Partner to the Poor: A Paul Farmer Reader,* by Paul Farmer, edited by Haun Saussy (with a foreword by Tracy Kidder)

24. *I Did It to Save My Life: Love and Survival in Sierra Leone,* by Catherine E. Bolten

25. *My Name Is Jody Williams: A Vermont Girl's Winding Path to the Nobel Peace Prize,* by Jody Williams

26. *Reimagining Global Health: An Introduction,* by Paul Farmer, Jim Yong Kim, Arthur Kleinman, and Matthew Basilico

27. *Fresh Fruit, Broken Bodies,* by Seth M. Holmes, MD, PhD